Calcium Antagonists

and the Kidney

Calcium Antagonists
and the
Kidney

Murray Epstein, M.D.
Rodger Loutzenhiser, Ph.D.

HANLEY & BELFUS, INC.
Philadelphia
The C.V. Mosby Company
St. Louis • Toronto • London

Publisher: HANLEY & BELFUS, INC.
                          210 South 13th Street
                          Philadelphia, PA 19107

North American and worldwide sales and distribution:
                          THE C.V. MOSBY COMPANY
                          11830 Westline Industrial Drive
                          St. Louis, MO 63146

In Canada: THE C.V. MOSBY COMPANY
                          5240 Finch Avenue East
                          Unit 1
                          Scarborough, Ontario MlS4P2

Designed by Adrianne Onderdonk Dudden

CALCIUM ANTAGONISTS AND THE KIDNEY   ISBN 0-932883-20-6

Last digit is the print number: 9 8 7 6 5 4 3 2 1

To our wives
Nina Epstein and Kathy Loutzenhiser
and
To our children
David, Susanna and Jonathan Epstein, and Daniel and Jennifer Loutzenhiser

Contents

Contributors

John H. Bauer, M.D.
Professor of Medicine, Division of Nephrology, Department of Medicine, University of Missouri—Columbia School of Medicine, Columbia, Missouri

Phillip Darwin Bell, Ph.D.
Associate Professor of Physiology and Biophysics, Nephrology Research and Training Center, University of Alabama at Birmingham, Birmingham, Alabama

Judith A. Benstein, M.D.
Clinical Instructor of Medicine, Department of Medicine, New York University School of Medicine, New York, New York

Joseph V. Bonventre, M.D., Ph.D.
Associate Professor of Medicine, Department of Medicine, Harvard Medical School; Assistant Physician, Renal Unit, Massachusetts General Hospital, Boston, Massachusetts

Paul Clayton Churchill, Ph.D.
Professor of Physiology, Department of Physiology, Wayne State University School of Medicine, Detroit, Michigan

Ingemar J. A. Dawidson, M.D., Ph.D.
Associate Professor of Surgery, Department of Surgery, University of Texas Southwestern Medical Center, Dallas, Texas

Lance D. Dworkin, M.D.
Assistant Professor of Medicine, Department of Medicine, New York University Medical Center, New York, New York

Murray Epstein, M.D.
Professor of Medicine, Department of Medicine, University of Miami School of Medicine; Attending Physician, Veterans Administration Medical Center, and Jackson Memorial Medical Center, Miami, Florida

Martha Franco, M.D.
Assistant Professor, Institute Nacional de Cardiologia I Chavez, Mexico City, Mexico

William H. Frishman, M.D.
Professor of Medicine, Department of Medicine, Albert Einstein College of Medicine; Director of Medicine, Hospital of the Albert Einstein College of Medicine, Bronx, New York

Norman K. Hollenberg, M.D., Ph.D.
Professor of Medicine and Radiology, Harvard Medical School; Senior Physician, Departments of Medicine and Radiology, Brigham and Women's Hospital, Boston, Massachusetts

Stanley M. Lee, M.D.
Clinical Associate Professor of Pediatrics, Vanderbilt University Medical Center, Nashville, Tennessee

Rodger Loutzenhiser, Ph.D.
Research Associate Professor of Medicine, University of Miami School of Medicine; Nephrology Section, Veterans Administration Medical Center, Miami, Florida

Friedrich C. Luft, M.D.
Professor of Medicine, University of Erlangen-Nürnberg; 4th Medical Clinic, Klinikum Nord, Nürnberg, Federal Republic of Germany

Graham MacGregor, M.A., FRCP
Senior Lecturer, Department of Medicine, Charing Cross Hospital and Westminster Medical School, London, England

Ulrich F. Michael, M.D.
Lecturer in Medicine, Department of Internal Medicine, University of Arizona College of Medicine; Staff, Medical and Research Services, Veterans Administration Medical Center, Tucson, Arizona

B. Miranda, M.D.
Nephrology Service, Hospital 1 de octubre, Madrid, Spain

Jules B. Puschett, M.D.
Professor of Medicine and Director, Renal-Electrolyte Divison, Department of Medicine, University of Pittsburgh School of Medicine, Pittsburgh, Pennsylvania

Garry P. Reams, M.D.
Assistant Professor of Medicine, Division of Nephrology, Department of Medicine, University of Missouri—Columbia School of Medicine, Columbia, Missouri

J. L. Rodicio, M.D.
Nephrology Service, Hospital 1 de octubre, Madrid, Spain

Pål Rooth, Ph.D.
Assistant Professor, Department of Histology and Cell Biology, University of Umeå, Umeå, Sweden

Luis M. Ruilope, M.D.
Nephrology Service, Hospital 1 de octubre, Madrid, Spain

Thomas H. Steele, M.D.
Professor of Medicine, Department of Medicine, University of Wisconsin Medical School, Madison, Wisconsin

Myron H. Weinberger, M.D.
Professor of Medicine, and Director, Hypertension Research Center, Department of Medicine, Indiana University School of Medicine, Indianapolis, Indiana

Gordon H. Williams, M.D.
Professor of Medicine, Department of Medicine, Harvard Medical School; Director, Endocrine-Metabolic Unit and Physician, Brigham and Women's Hospital, Boston, Massachusetts

Preface

Cytosolic calcium is a ubiquitous second messenger. Among the myriad physiological processes regulated by intracellular calcium are cardiac contractility and excitability, vascular smooth muscle contractility, excitation-secretion coupling of endocrine glands, neurotransmitter release, skeletal muscle function, and platelet aggregation. Such considerations might lead one to assume that the pharmacological disruption of transcellular calcium movements by a calcium antagonist would produce indiscriminate uncoupling of numerous vital processes. We have come to learn, however, that calcium antagonists act selectively. Indeeed, it is their selective blockade of calcium movements in discrete target tissues that makes calcium antagonists such successful therapeutic agents and such interesting pharmacological tools.

The introduction of the concept of "calcium antagonism" in 1964 is attributed to Fleckenstein. During the ensuing 25 years, we have witnessed an exponential advance in our knowledge of the pharmacology and clinical application of calcium antagonists. Initially, investigative attention focused on the mechanisms of action of these agents in cardiac and vascular smooth muscle, and the clinical application of calcium antagonists to the management of cardiovascular disorders. More recently, investigations have expanded into the effects of calcium antagonists on other organ systems, exploring a wider range of potential therapeutic applications. These include the central nervous system (migraine prophylaxis), respiratory system (asthma), gastrointestinal system (achalasia), and hematologic system (inhibition of platelet aggregation).

During the past several years, it has become increasingly apparent that calcium antagonists exert profound effects on renal hemodynamics and renal excretory function. It is therefore appropriate to consider the effects of calcium antagonists on the kidney and to ascertain whether their renal effects may eventuate in additional therapeutic applications. A careful reading of this book should provide the reader with the information required to make that judgment.

In this book invited experts were requested to review the current state of our knowledge with regard to the physiologic actions of calcium antagonists modulating renal hemodynamics and excretory function, as well as hormonal alterations. In the first chapter, Dr. Loutzenhiser provides an overview of our current knowledge of the mechanisms of action of calcium antagonists. He considers how calcium antagonists modify excitation-contraction coupling in vascular smooth muscle. He also reviews those smooth muscle activating mechanisms that are not affected by calcium antagonists. An understanding of the renal effects of calcium antagonists requires not only knowledge of the mechanism of action of these agents, but also an appreciation of the diversity of calcium-mobilizing processes and an awareness that not all calcium entry mechanisms are affected by calcium antagonists.

The next contribution by Drs. Hollenberg and Williams provides a framework for the succeeding authors by examining the pivotal role of the kidney in essential hypertension, with a focus on its pathogenesis in this widespread disease. The functional abnormalities involving the renal blood supply in essential hypertension are examined critically, and the role of the kidney as a determinant of the effectiveness of antihypertensive therapy is emphasized.

The next contribution, by Loutzenhiser and Epstein, constitutes a comprehensive review of current concepts of the pharmacology of calcium antagonists on renal hemodynamics. These agents produce vasodilation by modifying the function of calcium channels located on the surface of vascular smooth muscle cells, thereby disrupting excitation-contraction coupling. As emphasized in Chapter 1, the recruitment of calcium-sensitive calcium channels differs with various vasoconstrictors. Thus, renal vasodilation produced by calcium antagonists depends upon the prevailing factors determining basal renal vascular tone. Furthermore, individual sensitivity to calcium antagonists varies due to regional heterogeneity of smooth-muscle–activating mechanisms. The unique architecture of the renal microcirculation and the physiological requirement for differential control of pre- and postglomerular resistances provide a setting in which regional heterogeneity has important renal hemodynamic consequences.

In the next chapter, Dr. Steele extends these observations with the isolated kidney and considers the unique response of the hypertensive kidney both in vivo and in vitro. Dr. Steele proposes that hypertension represents a condition of altered membrane calcium handling that results in exaggerated renal responses to both calcium channel antagonists and agonists.

The next chapter by Dr. Bonventre is devoted to an examination of calcium in the renal mesangial cell. Mesangial cell contraction, and eicosanoid production and proliferation are thought to play a critical role in renal function and dysfunction. Ca^{2+} has been implicated in each of these functions; there is a great deal of interest in defining the role of Ca^{2+} in the mesangial cell. In his chapter, Dr. Bonventre reviews the large body of evidence implicating Ca^{2+} as a critical intracellular mediator of many of the functional responses of the mesangial cell. In contrast, there is a paucity of data regarding calcium antagonists and the mesangium, and additional studies are needed to define this important relationship.

Drs. Bell and Franco next follow with an in-depth review of the critical role that calcium plays in the control and regulation of epithelial cell function. Specifically, they consider the following issues: (1) regulation of cytosolic calcium concentration by renal epithelia; (2) cytosolic calcium regulation of transepithelial transport; and (3) mediation of tubuloglomerular feedback signal transmission by cytosolic calcium. They review evidence supporting the postulate that changes in luminal fluid composition directly alter macula densa cytosolic calcium concentration and further substantiate the hypothesis that macula densa cytosolic calcium serves in the transmission of tubuloglomerular feedback signals.

Dr. Churchill's review focuses on the effects of calcium antagonists on the cellular mechanisms regulating renin release. In contrast to its stimulatory role in most cells, intracellular Ca^{2+} appears to play an inhibitory second messenger role in renin secretion. The available evidence suggests that calcium antagonists and agonists modulate intracellular calcium in renin secreting cells, thereby affecting renin secretion. The stimulatory effects of calcium antagonists on the rate of renin secretion may, therefore, be considered as an extension of the pharmacological action of these agents, namely inhibition of calcium influx.

Drs. Dworkin and Benstein next consider a subject of growing importance, i.e., the concept that alterations in glomerular hemodynamics may contribute importantly to progressive renal injury. They review the large body of experimental evidence demonstrating the salutary effects of pharmacologic interventions with antihypertensive agents that not only reduce systemic blood pressure but also modulate glomerular hemodynamics. As the authors emphasize, widepread application of these therapies to patients with renal disease must await completion of rigorous clinical trials.

In the next two chapters, Dr. Puschett, and Drs. Michael and Lee review the role of calcium antagonists in the prevention or amelioration of experimental acute renal ischemia. They review the available data from studies in diverse animal models and conclude that calcium antagonists afford protection against experimental ischemic acute renal failure in most, but not all, models.

The next three chapters address the increasingly important subject of the effects of calcium antagonists on renal electrolyte handling. Acute studies in isolated perfused kidneys and in experimental animals, as well as in man, consistently demonstrate a diuresis, natriuresis, and generally kaliuresis, even in the face of arterial blood pressure reduction. Clearance methodology suggests that calcium antagonists produce their natriuretic response by exerting hemodynamic effects as well as by acting directly on the tubule. Although studies of the chronic effects of calcium antagonists are not definitive, Ruilope and associates report studies demonstrating that the natriuretic effects of calcium antagonists appear to persist during long-term administration of dihydropyridines, as assessed by the enhanced ability to excrete an intravenous saline load.

The final section of this book is devoted to a discussion of the therapeutic applications of calcium antagonists in the management of hypertension and a consideration of potential applications to a number of clinical renal disorders. Drs. Dawidson and Rooth review the ability of calcium antagonists to ameliorate cyclosporine A nephrotoxicity both in experimental animals and in transplant patients. The next two chapters review the role of calcium antagonists in the current antihypertensive armamentarium. Drs. Reams and Bauer consider the effects of the available calcium antagonists on renal hemodynamics and function. Although additional long-term clinical trials are required, the available data indicate that calcium antagonists do not adversely affect renal function. Dr. Frishman provides a comprehensive review of the effects of the available calcium antagonists on systemic hemodynamics and the utility of these agents in specific hypertensive settings. He also summarizes recent data of a new therapeutic delivery system that may optimize the administration of calcium antagonists, such as nifedipine. This drug delivery system (nifedipine GITS) is an osmotic pump that allows the drug to be released over 18–36 hours without abrupt plasma peaks of drug usually associated with adverse reactions. Dr. Frishman reviews recent data regarding the efficacy of this sustained-release preparation of nifedipine in controlling hypertension.

In the final chapter, Epstein and Loutzenhiser consider the potential applicability of calcium antagonists as renal protective agents in diverse clinical settings. Building on the foundation established by many of the contributions in this book detailing the salutary effects of calcium antagonists on renal hemodynamics, we consider possible future applications of calcium antagonists. As detailed in Chapters 3 and 4, calcium antagonists preferentially attenuate afferent arteriolar vasoconstriction. Thus, it is possible that calcium antagonists might have a role in ameliorating the course of acute renal failure in patients who are at increased risk. We review a number of recent studies indicating that calcium antagonists protect against the development of acute renal failure in the setting of cadaveric renal transplantation. Additional investigation is required to delineate other settings in which calcium antagonists may have a renal protective effect. Potential examples include radiocontrast and aminoglycoside nephrotoxicity. Finally, in light of the increasing attention being focused on the choice of an appropriate antihypertensive agent in the management of the diabetic patient, we consider the available data regarding the use of ACE inhibitors and calcium antagonists for this indication.

In this book, the contributors have examined our current understanding of the actions of calcium antagonists on the kidney. More importantly for clinicians and scientists interested in a wide array of renal functional disorders and hypertension, they have reviewed how calcium antagonists modulate renal function and perhaps alter or reverse renal dysfunction in a number of experimental models of renal dysfunction. We hope that the observations presented herein may suggest future avenues for investigation and clinical application.

Murray Epstein, M.D.
Rodger Loutzenhiser, Ph.D.
University of Miami School of Medicine

Rodger D. Loutzenhiser, Ph.D.

1

Mechanisms of Action of Calcium Antagonists

Over two decades ago, Fleckenstein coined the term calcium antagonist to describe the mechanism mediating the negative inotropic actions of prenylamine and verapamil. He noted that the cardiac actions of these agents on contractility and the cardiac action potential were mimicked by the removal of extracellular calcium, and correctly surmised that these agents interfere with calcium entry.[1,2] Since Fleckenstein's original observation, many diverse compounds have been synthesized and characterized as calcium antagonists. During this time, agents from three classes of calcium antagonists have progressed from the laboratory to clinical application: phenylalkylamines (e.g., verapamil), benzothiazepines (e.g., diltiazem), and dihydropyridines (e.g., nifedipine). These three classes of calcium antagonists can be distinguished by their distinct binding characteristics to proteinic calcium channels. They also exhibit different physical and chemical characteristics. The ability of these compounds to modulate the function of L-type calcium channels, however, is the one common feature that defines these agents as calcium antagonists.

The purpose of this chapter is to present a brief overview summarizing some of the observations that form the basis for our understanding of the mechanism of action of calcium antagonists. This chapter is not intended to be a complete review of the pharmacology of calcium antagonists and calcium channels. The reader is directed to several excellent reviews and texts in which these topics are treated in greater depth.[4-12] Rather examples are presented that illustrate how calcium antagonists modify excitation-contraction coupling in vascular smooth muscle. In addition, those smooth muscle activating mechanisms that are not affected by calcium antagonists are discussed. An understanding of the renal effects of calcium antagonists requires not only knowledge of the mechanism of action of these agents, but also an appreciation of the diversity of calcium-mobilizing processes and awareness that not all calcium entry mechanisms are affected by calcium antagonists.

Calcium Antagonists and Calcium Influx

The unique pharmacology of calcium antagonists is derived not only from the ability of these agents to inhibit calcium entry but also from their striking selectivity of action. Since cytosolic calcium is a ubiquitous modulator of cell function, an indiscriminate blockade of calcium entry would have deleterious consequences. The utility of calcium antagonists derives from their ability to prevent calcium entry into specific target tissues, without altering other calcium-dependent processes. The actions of calcium antagonists have been studied extensively in two tissue types, cardiac and vascular smooth muscle, in which the pharmacologic actions of these agents are most conspicuous.

Electrophysiologic Effects on the Heart

Numerous ionic currents characterize the cardiac action potential. The initial depolarization is mediated predominantly by the activation of the so-called "fast sodium channel." This sodium conductance is affected by local anesthetics and a reduction in this current inhibits myocardial excitability. The prolonged cardiac action potential is associated with a stimulation of calcium entry through the activation of a slow calcium conductance. Fleckenstein and co-workers[1,2] demonstrated that calcium antagonists act on the heart as "slow channel blockers," in that these agents block the slow calcium conductance without appreciably altering the fast sodium channel.

The actions of calcium antagonists on the cardiac action potential and on contractility are perfectly mimicked by a reduction in extracellular calcium.[1-3] Furthermore, an elevation of extracellular calcium to supraphysiologic levels reverses the negative inotropic and electrophysiologic actions of these agents.[1-3] From these initial observations, Fleckenstein and co-workers correctly surmised that these agents interfere with the transmembrane movement of calcium ions. Since these agents appeared to act as functional antagonists of calcium ions, the term "calcium antagonist" was coined to describe their actions.

Vascular Smooth Muscle Contractility and Calcium Influx

Although the ability of calcium antagonists to disrupt excitation-contraction coupling was first noted by their effects on the heart, their pharmacologic utility derives from their ability to selectively attenuate vascular smooth muscle contractility. The vasorelaxant properties of calcium antagonists noted by Fleckenstein and co-workers have been investigated in detail during the past decade (see refs. 7, 11 and 12 for review). Although diverse mechanisms were proposed initially, studies examining the effects of calcium antagonists on ^{45}Ca fluxes revealed that the important mechanism in vascular smooth muscle was similar to that in the heart, an inhibition of calcium influx.[12]

Early observations of the effects of calcium antagonists on smooth muscle contractions suggested that these agents alter calcium entry. The phasic smooth muscle contractions that can be elicited in calcium-free buffers (see below) are relatively unaffected by calcium antagonists, whereas contractions that require extracellular calcium are more sensitive to these agents.[13] Direct evidence of this mechanism of action was adduced from the observation that calcium antagonists prevent deplora-

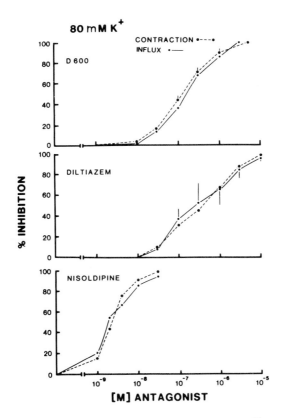

FIGURE 1. Parallel inhibition of tension development (dashed line) and ^{45}Ca uptake (solid line) by D-600 (top), diltiazem (center), and nisoldipine (bottom) in rabbit aorta stimulated with 80 mM KCl. Reproduced with permission from Loutzenhiser and van Breemen, Urban & Schwarzenberg, 1982.[17]

rization-induced ^{45}Ca entry into smooth muscle cells[14–16] although they do not affect the entry of calcium into quiescent tissues.[14] Furthermore, the ability of calcium antagonists to modulate calcium entry correlated precisely with their effects on tension development. Figure 1 illustrates the close concordance between the inhibition of ^{45}Ca uptake and tension development by representative members of each of the three major classes of calcium antagonists. In these studies, calcium uptake and tension were measured in rabbit aortic rings depolarized with 80 mM KCl.[17] As depicted, the dose-response curves describing the inhibition of tension correspond exactly with the curve subtending the inhibition of calcium influx.

The inhibition by calcium antagonists of depolarization-induced calcium entry would explain their vasodilatory effects in settings in which the vasoconstrictor stimulus is coupled to a contractile response via a change in membrane electrical potential (i.e., electromechanical excitation-contraction coupling). For example, receptor-occupation coupled to membrane depolarization would indirectly activate the same calcium entry pathway as that stimulated by KCl (Fig. 2). Some vasoconstrictors stimulate ^{45}Ca uptake in aortic smooth muscle through a pathway that is inhibited by calcium antagonists.[11,12,18] As discussed in greater detail below, however, not

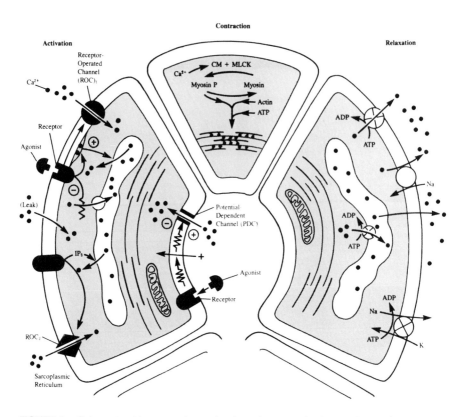

FIGURE 2. Schematic of known and postulated mechanisms of calcium influx, mobilization, and removal in vascular smooth muscle cells. Potential-dependent channels (PDC) may be activated in response to receptor-mediated changes in membrane potential. Receptor-operated calcium channels may be directly or indirectly coupled to receptor activation (ROC1 and ROC2). The passive leak of calcium represents an additional pathway for calcium to enter the cell. Modulation of intracellular calcium release and intracellular calcium sequestration represent additional calcium delivery systems that are coupled to receptor-occupation. Reproduced with permission from Loutzenhiser and Epstein, Hosp Pract, 1987.[21]

all calcium entry pathways are affected by calcium antagonists. For example, in rabbit aorta the ^{45}Ca uptake that is stimulated by norepinephrine (NE) is insensitive to calcium antagonists.[19,20] Partial inhibition of NE-stimulated calcium uptake can be demonstrated with some calcium antagonists.[16,17,19] These effects are seen only at concentrations well above those at which voltage (i.e., KCl) sensitive calcium uptakes are inhibited, and at these high concentrations a concordance between effects on tension and calcium uptake are often lacking (Fig. 3).

Furthermore, although all representatives of each of the three classes of calcium antagonists effectively block KCl-induced calcium entry, not all will affect the stimulation of calcium uptake induced by agonists such as norepinephrine. As an example, Figure 4 illustrates the remarkable selectivity of the dihydropyridine, isradipine, in blocking KCl-, but not NE-induced contractions in rabbit aorta.[20] The effects of this calcium antagonist on ^{45}Ca uptake corresponded to its effects on tension.

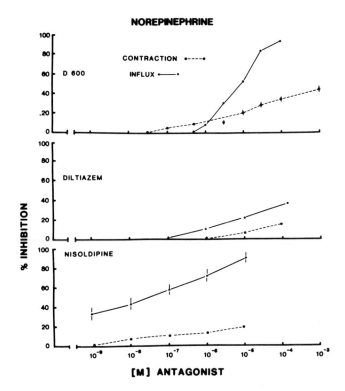

FIGURE 3. Effects of D-600 (top), diltiazem (center), and nisoldipine (bottom) on tension development (dashed line) and ^{45}Ca uptake (solid line) in rabbit aorta treated with norepinephrine (10^{-5} M). Reproduced with permission from Loutzenhiser and van Breemen, Urban & Schwarzenberg, 1982.[17]

Thus, isradipine inhibited KCl-induced ^{45}Ca uptake by 40% at 10^{-9}M, but had no NE-induced ^{45}Ca uptake at 10,000 times this concentration (10^{-5} M).[20]

Effects on Calcium Channels

Electrophysiologic studies using a variety of cell types have revealed a great diversity of calcium channels (for reviews see refs. 9, 10, 22). Most of the calcium channels that have been identified are activated by changes in voltage and can thus be classified as potential-dependent. The putative receptor-operated calcium channel has yet to be identified using electrophysiologic approaches. The potential-dependent calcium channels that have been described can be distinguished from one another by their unit conductances, activating characteristics, and kinetics of inactivation.

At least two types of potential-dependent calcium channels have been discovered in cardiac and vascular smooth muscle: the rapidly inactivating T-type channel and the slowly inactivating L-type calcium channel. The T-type channels are characterized by a rapid inactivation (e.g., within 10 milliseconds), whereas the L-type channels

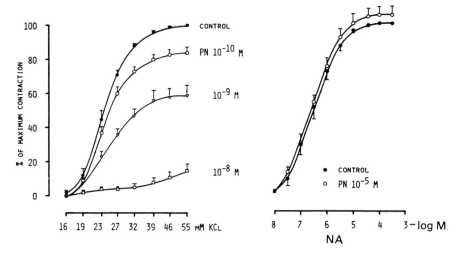

FIGURE 4. Divergent effects of isradipine (PN 200, 110) on the contractile response of rabbit aorta to KCl (left) and norepinephrine (NA, right). Note that isradipine is very effective at inhibiting KCl-induced contractions but is without effect on the contractions elicited by NA. Modified with permission from Hof et al., J Cardiovasc Pharmacol, 1984.[20]

remain activated for several minutes. In addition to their kinetic properties, these channels can also be distinguished by their respective ion selectivities, activation voltages, and their sensitivity to dihydropyridines.[9,10,22−27]

These two channel types exhibit similar properties in cardiac and smooth muscle cells.[22−27] Nevertheless, distinct differences also exist.[23−24] It is thus not certain if cardiac and smooth muscle calcium channels represent unique entities or are homologous proteins exhibiting distinct functional characteristics imparted by their differing environments. It is clear, however, that the L-type calcium channel represents the molecular target site responsible for the pharmacologic actions of calcium antagonists.

The differences in the inactivation characteristics of L- and T-type calcium channels can be utilized to separate the contribution of each channel type to whole-cell calcium currents. The T-type calcium channels are inactivated at membrane potentials of -30 mV and above, whereas inactivation of L-type channels occurs at more positive membrane potentials. Using the recently developed patch-clamp technique, changes in membrane conductance can be studied under conditions in which the membrane potential and intracellular ion composition are experimentally controlled. The amount of current injected to regulate membrane potential is a measure of the ionic flux. The membrane potential can initially be set at a "holding potential" before eliciting depolarization triggering ionic conductance changes.

Figure 5 illustrates how these techniques have been utilized to study the effects of nitrendipine on the currents carried through each type of channel in smooth muscle. In this experiment (taken from a study by Bean et al.[24]), a single cell isolated from the mesenteric artery was voltage-clamped using the patch-clamp technique. A combination of barium and cesium salts was utilized to minimize non-calcium channel currents and to allow measurement of the inward current carried by the passage of barium through calcium channels. The upper tracing illustrates the total

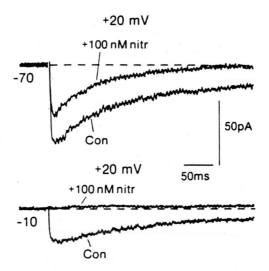

FIGURE 5. Effects of nitrendipine on whole-cell currents carried through T-type and L-type calcium channels in single smooth muscle cells isolated from mesenteric arteries. In upper tracing, nitrendipine blocks the sustained current carried through the L-type channels, but leaves the initial transient current (T-type channels) unaffected when "holding potential: is set to -70 mV. At a more positive holding potential (i.e., -10 mV), the T-type channels are inactivated. Thus in the lower tracing, depolarization to + 20 mV activates only the L-type channels and nitrendipine blocks the entire current. Reproduced with permission from Bean et al., Circ Res, 1986.[24]

calcium current that is stimulated when the membrane potential is suddenly changed from a holding potential of -70 mV to a depolarizing potential of + 20 mV. Note that current is biphasic and that nitrendipine abolishes the "tail" of the current but has little effect on the initial transient current. When the holding potential is set at -10 mV (lower tracing), the initial phasic current is virtually abolished, due to the inactivation of T-type channels. The sustained current that is stimulated by depolarization in this setting is carried by the passage of barium through L-type calcium channels. This current is completely blocked by nitrendipine.

Whole-cell currents such as those depicted in Figure 5 reflect the combined conductance of individual calcium channels. The kinetics and conductance characteristics of individual channels can be directly studied using the excised patch-clamp technique, [27] although such studies are complicated by the relatively small unit conductances of calcium channels. Typically, single calcium channel recordings demonstrate a fluctuating pattern of openings that are best described as a probability function. If the probability of a channel opening is given as "P," whole-cell calcium current would be represented by "P × N × i," where "N" and "i" represent the total number of channels and their unit conductance, respectively.[9] Changes in voltage alter the probability of channel opening (P). At extreme levels of membrane depolarization "P" approaches unity.[9]

Theoretically, agents that alter calcium currents could act by modulating the number of channels (N), channel conductance (i), or the probability of channel opening (P). Analyses of single calcium channel recordings indicate that calcium antagonists inhibit calcium entry by modulating the probability of channel opening.

Kinetic models of calcium channel function suggest that the probability of channel opening is governed by the transition of the channel between an open state, a closed state, and an inactive state, which is both nonconductive and insensitive to voltage.[9,10,28-30] Voltage- and time-dependent inactivation may involve the transition of the channel population into the inactive state. It has been suggested that calcium antagonists bind preferentially to the inactive state of the calcium channel and stabilize this configuration.[28-30]

The hypothesis that calcium antagonists bind to and stabilize the inactive state of the channel is attractive for a number of reasons. This theory would explain the use-dependency of channel inhibition by calcium antagonists (i.e., the enhancement of calcium antagonist sensitivity following a train of action potentials). Theoretically, repetitive depolarizations would increase the population of channels in the inactive state and increase binding affinity of calcium antagonists. It has been suggested that this hypothesis may also explain the fact that vascular smooth muscle exhibits a much greater sensitivity to calcium antagonists than the myocardium.[24] The resting membrane potential of vascular smooth muscle cells is typically more positive than myocardial cells. Furthermore, activation of smooth muscle may involve prolonged depolarization, whereas myocardial cells undergo cycles of depolarization and repolarization. Thus it follows that at any time a greater fraction of smooth muscle calcium channels would be in the inactive state, which is characterized by a higher affinity for dihydropyridines.[31]

The Calcium Antagonist Receptor

The remarkable potency of dihydropyridines and their structure-activity requirements suggest a specific receptor for these agents. It was therefore not surprising that radioligand-binding studies revealed a specific binding for dihydropyridines to high affinity sites in isolated membrane preparations (for review see refs. 7 and 8). The subsequent use of radiolabelled dihydropyridines, which bind with high affinity to their receptors, has been essential in the characterization of the calcium antagonist receptor and in the biochemical characterization of calcium channels. The calcium antagonist receptor has been identified as a subunit of a protein with a molecular weight of approximately 200,000 da that is either identical to or closely associated with the calcium channel (for reviews see refs. 32-35).

Correlation of Pharmacology and Binding

Evidence from both electrophysiological studies and ligand-binding experiments support the concept that the receptor for calcium antagonists is closely associated with or identical to the L-type calcium channel. A comparison of the rank order for ligand binding and inhibition of smooth muscle contraction for a series of dihydropyridines reveals a remarkable correlation between affinity for the ligand receptor and pharmacologic activity (see ref. 7 for review). For example, Figure 6 illustrates the close correlation between binding and mechanical studies of various calcium antagonists on rat aortic tissue. Another functional correlate involves the effects of membrane potential on binding. Electrophysiologic studies indicate differences in the voltage-dependence of calcium channel blockade by dihydropyridines

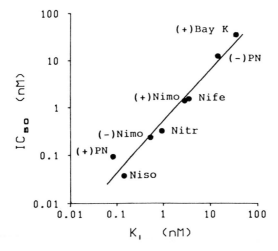

FIGURE 6. Correlation between IC_{50} values for effects of 1,4-dihydropyridines on KCl-induced tension in rat aorta (ordinate) with the K_i value derived from their displacement of ^{3}H-PN 200-110 binding in isolated rat aortic tissue. Individual points represent values obtained with diverse 1,4-dihydropyridines (+ and − denote optical enantiomers): PN, PN 200-110; Niso, nisoldipine; Nimo, nimodipine; Nife, nifedipine; Bay K, Bay K 8644; Nitr, nitrendipine. Reproduced with permission from Wibo and Godfraind, Ann NY Acad Sci, 1988.[36]

and non-dihydropyridines,[36] and ligand-binding studies reflect similar differences in the voltage-dependence of binding.[37]

Although a correlation between pharmacology and binding can be demonstrated in heart and smooth muscle tissues, it should be emphasized that the presence of dihydropyridine receptors cannot be taken as an indication of calcium antagonist sensitivity. Thus, skeletal muscle and brain demonstrate very high levels of dihydropyridine receptors, whereas calcium antagonists exert little pharmacologic activities in these tissues. In skeletal muscle, the dihydropyridine receptor is closely associated with T-tubular membranes and has been postulated to be linked to the voltage sensor.[38] Similarly, although ligand-binding studies indicate the presence of dihydropyridine receptors in brain tissue, it is the dihydropyridine-insensitive "N-type" calcium channels rather than L-channels that modulate neurotransmitter release.[10,39]

Binding Interactions of Calcium Antagonists

Binding studies indicate that all dihydropyridines interact at a common binding site on the receptor. Thus, ^{3}H-nitrendipine is displaced in a competitive fashion by other dihydropyridines. In contrast, an examination of the effects of phenylalkylamines and benzothiazepines on radiolabelled dihydropyridine binding has revealed a complex interaction between the differing classes of calcium antagonists. Verapamil will reduce dihydropyridine binding but is capable of displacing only 50% of the ligand. In contrast, diltiazem actually potentiates dihydropyridine binding.

Such observations suggest that non-dihydropyridines bind at a separate site on the same protein and upon binding exert an allosteric effect on the dihydropyridine binding site. It was originally proposed that verapamil and diltiazem bind to a common site.[40] Recent evidence, however, supports the models proposed by Glossmann et al.[42] and Bolger et al.,[41] in which diltiazem, verapamil, and dihydropyridines occupy distinct binding sites on the calcium channel (for review see ref. 43).

Calcium Agonists

One of the more intriguing developments in the field of calcium antagonists was the discovery several years ago that simple substitutions on the dihydropyridine molecule transform a compound that is a calcium antagonist into a compound with diametrically opposite biologic activity, a calcium agonist.[44] It was subsequently discovered that separate calcium antagonist and agonist activities could even reside in the individual optical enantiomers of a single structure.[45,46] Thus, calcium antagonist and agonist activities may be present in racemic mixtures of such compounds.[45,46]

Calcium agonists exhibit a pharmacologic profile that is opposite to that of calcium antagonists. Thus, calcium agonists are positive inotropic agents and promote vasoconstriction in vascular smooth muscle.[44-47] Their actions on smooth muscle are usually voltage dependent.[44,47] Binding studies suggest that calcium antagonists and agonists compete for the same receptor site[7,8] and their pharmacologic profiles indicate a competitive antagonism.[44-47]

Single-channel recordings from excised membrane patches indicate that calcium agonists increase the probability of calcium channel opening.[29,30] It is suggested that they bind preferentially to the channel in the open state and stabilize this conformation.[29,30] The discovery of these compounds prompted the search for an endogenous calcium channel activator. Although calcium antagonist receptor binding activity has been demonstrated in tissue extracts, the existence of an endogenous calcium channel ligand has not been established.

Calcium-Antagonist Insensitive Mechanisms

Calcium Entry

As described above, not all calcium entry pathways of vascular smooth muscle are sensitive to the actions of calcium antagonists. Norepinephrine stimulates calcium entry into rabbit aortic smooth muscle through a mechanism that is insensitive to blockade by dihydropyridines (Fig. 4). Calcium entry through the norepinephrine-sensitive pathway is additive to that induced by KCl,[19] suggesting an entry mechanism distinct from the potential-dependent calcium channels described above.

Based on such observations, it has been suggested that some smooth muscle agonists may activate receptor-operated calcium channels in vascular smooth muscle.[48,49] These receptor-operated calcium channels (ROCs) are not to be confused with receptor-operated sodium channels (e.g., in analogy to nicotinic receptors), which may be involved in receptor-mediated conductance changes, modulating smooth muscle function by affecting membrane potential.[49,50]

Direct electrophysiologic evidence of receptor-operated calcium channels in vascular smooth muscle is currently lacking. An ATP-activated cation channel that allows both sodium and calcium to enter the cell has been demonstrated.[51] In addition, a thrombin-activated channel with calcium selectivity has been described in platelet membranes.[52] However, a true calcium channel whose gating is directly coupled to adrenergic receptors of vascular smooth muscle has not been found. It is possible that receptor occupation may indirectly activate calcium channels via second messengers. For example, it is suggested that inositol tetrakisphosphate [53] and diacylglycerol [54] are involved in receptor coupling to calcium channels.

Whereas calcium flux studies clearly demonstrate that in large conduit arteries agonists such as norepinephrine activate a calcium entry mechanism that is insensitive to calcium antagonists, such agonists do not necessarily activate the same type of calcium entry process in all blood vessels (see below). It is likely that diverse calcium influx mechanisms are coupled to receptor systems (Fig. 2). For example, the proposed receptor-operated calcium channel is thought to involve a direct activation of a calcium influx pathway. Alternatively, receptor occupation may be indirectly linked to channel function through the actions of second messengers. Receptor occupation may also be linked to L-type calcium channels through changes in membrane conductance and membrane potential. It has been suggested that the calcium antagonist-insensitive calcium influx in some tissues may result from a functional alteration of L-type calcium channels.[24] Thus, a great variety of receptor-coupled calcium influx mechanisms is possible. Furthermore, it is likely that a single agonist may utilize different mechanisms in different types of blood vessels.

Normally, only those calcium entry processes that are activated upon stimulation of the smooth muscle cell are considered to be involved in the contractile process. Nevertheless, it should be noted that even during resting conditions a large amount of calcium enters the cell. This calcium "leak" results from the enormous driving force for calcium entry (ca., 9300 cal/mol) and a resting calcium permeability of $1\text{-}3 \times 10^{-8}$ cm sec^{-1}.[55] This leak pathway is insensitive to calcium antagonists.[12,14] As described in more detail below, the calcium that enters the cell via this leak pathway appears to contribute to vascular tension in some settings. Furthermore, it is possible that the magnitude of the calcium "leak" may be influenced by vasoconstrictor agents. Thus, an increase in lipid fluidity near receptors, or a release of calcium to be bound to extracellular sites on the plasmalemma[56,57] may increase the permeability of the cell to calcium without activating specific calcium channels. To the extent that this pathway contributes to excitation-contraction coupling (see below), the calcium leak represents an additional calcium-antagonist-insensitive calcium entry mechanism.

Calcium Release

Many vasoconstrictor agents release intracellular calcium stores upon activation of their receptors. Thus, in the absence of extracellular calcium these agents elicit a phasic contractile response[58–60] accompanied by a transient elevation in cytosolic calcium.[61] This transient vasoconstriction is due to a receptor-mediated stimulation of phosphatidylinositol hydrolysis, the formation of inositol trisphosphate, and the release of calcium from the sarcoplasmic reticulum.[62,63] Calcium release from the sarcoplasmic reticulum is relatively insensitive to calcium antagonists. Although diltiazem has been reported to inhibit calcium release in rabbit aorta, this effect is seen only at very high concentrations and does not represent a "class action" of calcium antagonists.

It has previously been noted that the contractile responses associated with the release of intracellular calcium tend to be resistant to calcium antagonists.[11,12] The release of intracellular calcium is responsible for the rapid initial phase of the contractile response of conduit arteries to agonists[60,64] and has been implicated in the early biochemical events of contraction. Nevertheless, the sustained phase of the contractile response requires extracellular calcium, as the contractile responses obtained in EGTA and lanthanum are transient. It has been suggested, however, that the release of intracellular calcium is cyclical and supports the sustained component of the contraction. Alternatively, the release of intracellular calcium has been suggested to reflect a mechanism whereby agonists modulate intracellular calcium sequestration.[55,65–69] This mechanism (described in detail below) represents an additional activating mechanism of vascular smooth muscle that is insensitive to calcium antagonists.

The Superficial Calcium Buffer Barrier and Agonist-induced Alterations in Calcium Sequestration

As discussed above, many vasoconstrictor agonists initiate the release of calcium from an intracellularly sequestered calcium pool.[18,55,58–60] This calcium is thought to be released from a portion of the sarcoplasmic reticulum located just beneath the cell surface, where it is positioned to respond to the local generation of inositol trisphosphate.[62,63]

This region of the sarcoplasmic reticulum is also ideally positioned to sequester calcium ions as they enter the cell. Increasing evidence suggests that this region of the sarcoplasmic reticulum acts as an intracellular calcium buffer barrier, modulating the passage of calcium ions from the inner surface of the sarcolemma to the interior regions of the cell.[17,55,65–69] Vasoconstrictor agents not only stimulate calcium influx into the cell but also reduce calcium sequestration by this buffer barrier system. An agonist-induced reduction in calcium sequestration by the superficial sarcoplasmic reticulum represents an additional activating mechanism that is insensitive to calcium antagonists.

Evidence that the superficial sarcoplasmic reticulum functions as a final modulator of calcium delivery to the myofilaments has been adduced from investigations of the refilling of the releasable calcium pool. The administration of norepinephrine to aortic segments placed in calcium-free buffer initiates the release of intracellular calcium, eliciting transient contractile response and depleting the intracellular calcium pool.[58–60] This pool refills rapidly when the tissue is returned to buffer containing calcium.[65,70,71] Furthermore, the rate of refilling of this pool is enhanced when calcium influx is stimulated, for example by KCl-induced depolarization.[65,70,71] Thus, this pool appears to be replenished from calcium that has just entered the cell. In the presence of norepinephrine and other vasoconstrictors that affect this calcium store, the refilling of the pool is inhibited.[17,67,70] Thus, the ability of this pool to sequester calcium after it crosses the cell membrane is reduced by these vasoconstrictors.

Figures 7 and 8 illustrate the effects of calcium sequestration into the releasable store on tension development in response to KCl-induced calcium entry. In Figure 7, aortic rings were first placed in calcium-free buffer. In the top tracing, the releasable store was depleted by the administration of norepinephrine. When the tissues were

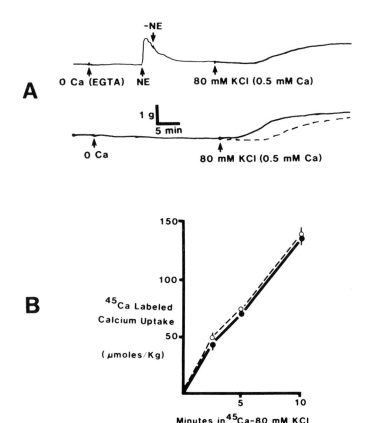

FIGURE 7. *A*, Effects of the intracellular buffer barrier on tension development in isolated rabbit aorta. Prior depletion of the releasable intracellular calcium pool by norepinephrine in calcium-free buffer reduces the rate of tension development when tissues are subsequently placed in 0.5 mM calcium buffer containing 80 mM KCl (dashed line). *B*, ^{45}Ca-uptake in 80 mM KCl (0.5 mM Ca) following exposure to Ca-free buffer alone (solid line) or the depletion of the releasable store in Ca-free buffer (dashed line). Note that the rate of ^{45}Ca uptake was unaffected by depletion of the releasable store.

These results suggest that prior depletion of the releasable intracellular calcium pool modulates tension development without affecting calcium uptake. This indicates an effect on intracellular calcium sequestration into the agonist-sensitive intracellular store. Reproduced with permission from Loutzenhiser and van Breemen, Urban & Schwarzenberg, 1982.[17]

then returned to calcium-replete buffer containing 80 mM KCl, the tissue in which the releasable pool had been depleted exhibited a slower contractile response to KCl (dashed line). Although depletion of the pool reduced the rate of tension development, the rate of ^{45}Ca uptake was not affected (lower panel of Fig. 7). These findings suggest that the releasable store sequesters calcium that has entered the cell. Thus, as this store is refilled, a portion of the calcium entering the cell in response to KCl is diverted into the releasable store and therefore less calcium is available to stimulate contraction.

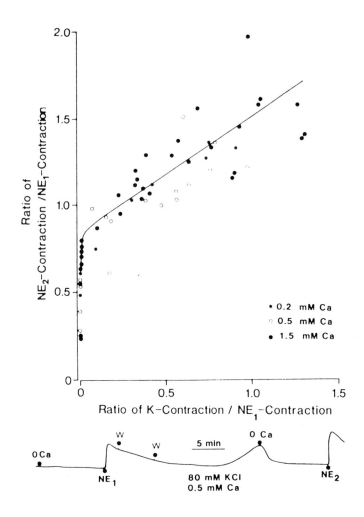

FIGURE 8.   The relationship between the extent of refilling of the releasable intracellular calcium pool and tension development during refilling in 80 mM KCl buffer. The contractile tracing depicted in the lower panel of the figure illustrates the protocol followed. The amount of calcium in the releasable store was assessed by measuring the magnitude of the phasic contraction elicited in Ca-free buffer. The tissue was then placed in Ca-replete buffer containing 80 mM KCl for various periods of time. The maximal amount of tension developed during the "re-filling" of the releasable store was plotted on the abscissa. The absolute tension was factored for each tissue by calculating the ratio of the KCl-induced tension/the initial NE response (NE_1). Thereafter, the tissues were returned to Ca-free buffer and the amount of refilling of the releasable pool was assessed from the size of the second NE-induced response (NE_2). Thus, the degree of refilling of the pool was calculated from the ratio of NE_2/NE_1. A ratio of 1.0 represented complete refilling. Note that KCl-induced tension development was delayed until the releasable pool had refilled to approximately 90% of its resting value. The time course for the delay in tension development increased when extracellular calcium was reduced (data not shown), but the relationship between refilling and KCl-induced tension was not altered. Reproduced with permission from van Breemen, et al., J Cardiovasc Pharmacol, 1987.[67]

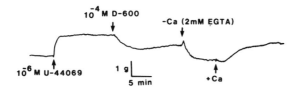

FIGURE 9. Contractile tracing of isolated rabbit aorta illustrating an extracellular calcium-dependent contraction in the presence of complete blockade of stimulated calcium influx. U44069 stimulates a ^{45}Ca influx into rabbit aorta that is completely inhibited by 10^{-5} M D600.[18] Nevertheless, this agonist elicits a sustained contraction that is dependent on extracellular calcium, even in the presence of 10^{-4} M D600. It is postulated that the sustained contraction in this setting is dependent on the "passive" calcium leak pathway and a U44069-induced reduction in calcium sequestration by the releasable store.[17,65] Reproduced with permission from Loutzenhiser and van Breemen, Urban & Schwarzenberg, 1982.[17]

Figure 8 illustrates additional evidence supporting the concept that the site containing the releasable intracellular calcium store functions as a superficial calcium buffering system. In this experiment the relationship between tension development and calcium uptake by the releasable store was assessed more directly. The protocol for these experiments is depicted in the lower panel of the figure. Following a depletion of the releasable pool in calcium-free buffer (i.e., with norepinephrine), tissues were placed in 80 mM KCl buffer containing calcium. The tissues exhibited a slowly developing contraction during refilling in KCl. At various times, tissues were returned to calcium-free buffer, and the extent of refilling of the releasable store was assessed by determining the size of the phasic contractile response to norepinephrine. The concentration of calcium in the KCl buffer was varied (i.e., from 0.2 to 1.5 mM). The duration of exposure to the calcium-containing KCl-buffer was also varied. The degree of refilling of the store was calculated from the ratio of the subsequent phasic response (NE_2) (of lower panel, Fig. 8) divided by the initial size of this response (i.e., NE_1). This parameter was then related to maximal contractile response observed during the exposure to KCl.

The upper panel of Figure 8 illustrates the relationship between the refilling of the releasable store (ordinate) and tension development elicited by KCl during this refilling process (abscissa). Note that the initiation of tension development in response to KCl does not occur until the releasable store refills to approximately 90% of the resting value. The most logical interpretation of these data is that calcium entering the cell was diverted into the releasable store, thereby delaying the onset of tension development. These findings clearly indicate that calcium uptake into the superficial sarcoplasmic reticulum modulates the delivery of calcium to the contractile system in the interior regions of the cell.

Since vasoconstrictors that deplete the releasable calcium store also inhibit its refilling,[17,67,70] it follows that this reduction in calcium sequestration into this superficial buffer barrier would contribute to the delivery of calcium to the myofilaments during vasoconstriction elicited by these agents (Fig. 2). Thus, in the presence of an agent that affects the superficial buffer barrier system, calcium that enters the cell even by passive leak may contribute to tension development. Figure 9 illustrates an example of such a contractile response. The contractile tracing depicted in this figure represents the response of isolated rabbit aorta to the thromboxane agonist U44069. This vasoconstrictor elicits a sustained contractile response following the administration of a concentration of calcium antagonist (10^{-4} M D-600) that completely prevents the U44069-induced ^{45}Ca influx.[18,65] Note that the response to U44069 is dependent on extracellular calcium even though, in this setting, no stimulation of ^{45}Ca influx is apparent.[18] This calcium antagonist-insensitive contractile response is most likely supported by the passive leak of calcium into the cell. Thus, although the calcium that slowly enters the cell through the leak pathway would normally be removed by the superficial buffer barrier, in the presence of U44069 this function of the buffer barrier is suppressed, thereby allowing the passive calcium leak to support a contractile response.[65]

Calcium-Independent Mechanisms

Finally, in addition to altering cell calcium handling, vasoconstrictor agents may also alter the sensitivity of the contractile system to changes in cytosolic calcium. The work of Morgan and co-workers demonstrated that vasoconstrictors such as norepinephrine alter the relationship between cytosolic calcium and tension development.[72,73] They proposed that an activation of protein kinase C, which would occur concomitantly with phosphatidylinositol hydrolysis, may increase the sensitivity of smooth muscle to calcium.[73] Such an increase in the sensitivity of tension development to calcium activity was recently demonstrated in response to norepinephrine in an alpha toxin-permeabilized vascular preparation.[74] Thus, a combination of increased sensitivity to calcium, coupled with a reduction in intracellular calcium sequestration, may represent a heretofore unrecognized vasoconstrictor mechanism that is independent of a stimulation of calcium entry and therefore insensitive to calcium antagonists.

Regional Heterogeneity

Since calcium antagonists do not affect all activating mechanisms of the smooth muscle cell, these agents exhibit an unusual type of specificity. The ability of calcium antagonists to reverse vasoconstriction depends not only on the particular stimulus used to set initial tone but also depends on the vessel type. This follows from the observation that a single agonist may utilize divergent activating mechanisms within different regions of the circulation.

The data depicted in Figure 10 illustrate an example of such regional heterogeneity in the responsiveness to calcium antagonists. In this study, diltiazem was demonstrated to be more effective in reversing norepinephrine-induced vasoconstriction of mesenteric resistance arteries (ca., 200 μm) than those of the superior mesenteric artery or aorta.[75,76] In contrast, diltiazem was equally effective in all three vessels when vasoconstriction was elicited by KCl-induced depolarization. These findings have been interpreted as indicating that the electrical-stimulus elicited by KCl activates an identical type of calcium channel in each vessel type (e.g., L-type calcium channels), whereas receptor activation by the agonists initiates different postreceptor processes exhibiting differing sensitivities to diltiazem. Furthermore, an examination of the effects of diltiazem on ^{45}Ca fluxes revealed that norepinephrine activates a calcium entry mechanism in the mesenteric resistance artery that is more sensitive to inhibition by this calcium antagonist than that elicited by KCl (Fig. 11[77]). The

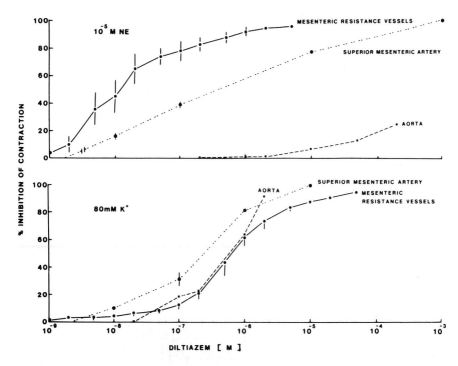

FIGURE 10. An example of regional heterogeneity of sensitivity to calcium antagonists. Upper panel illustrates the divergent effects of diltiazem on norepinephrine-induced tension development in rabbit aortae, superior mesenteric arteries, and mesenteric resistance arteries. In contrast, lower panel illustrates that these same vessels respond similarly to diltiazem when they are pre-constricted by KCl-induced depolarization. Reproduced with permission from Cauvin et al., Blood Vessels, 1984.[77]

remarkable sensitivity to diltiazem of the norepinephrine-induced calcium influx of mesenteric resistance arteries suggests that norepinephrine may activate a calcium channel in this vessel that has a greater sensitivity than the potential-dependent calcium channel. Other interpretations are possible, including an agonist-induced modulation of the sensitivity of the L-type calcium channels in this vessel.[24]

It has been suggested that small resistance vessels are in general more dependent on extracellular sources of activator calcium and thus more sensitive to calcium antagonists.[78] Such a formulation would explain the effectiveness of these agents as antihypertensive agents. Studies in the mesenteric circulation support this concept, but also indicate that differences in calcium influx mechanisms in conduit and resistance vessels play a greater role in the differences between these vessel types.[75–77] As discussed in greater detail elsewhere in this text (see Chapter 3 for review), the segmental resistance vessels of the renal circulation exhibit a unique pattern of sensitivity to calcium antagonists. In a wide variety of settings, the afferent arteriole is sensitive to calcium antagonists, whereas the efferent arteriole is insensitive. Thus in the renal vascular bed, differences in the activating mechanisms of two types of resistance arterioles of similar calibers (ca. 20 μm) is observed. In the kidney,

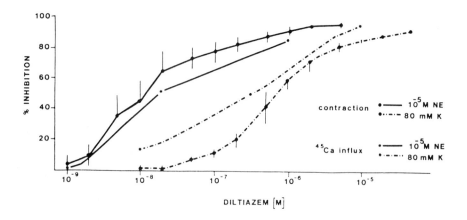

FIGURE 11. Effects of diltiazem on tension development and ^{45}Ca influx in rabbit mesenteric resistance arteries during activation by norepinephrine or KCl. Note that the effects of diltiazem on tension correspond to its effects on calcium entry in both settings. Furthermore, the calcium influx induced by norepinephrine is more sensitive to inhibition by diltiazem than that induced by KCl. Reproduced with permission from Cauvin, et al., Springer-Verlag, 1985.[76]

the efferent arteriole plays a unique role in regulating postglomerular resistance. It remains to be determined if this vessel is singular among resistance arterioles in its insensitivity to calcium antagonists, or if other examples of such regional heterogeneity exist among arterioles in other vascular beds.

Summary

Evidence to date strongly supports the concept that calcium antagonists bind to and modulate the function of a specific proteinic calcium channel, identified as the L-type calcium channel, which is present in the sarcolemma of vascular smooth muscle and myocardial cells. This channel is gated by changes in membrane electrical potential. The binding of calcium antagonists to this channel modulates the gating of the channel by decreasing the "probability" of channel opening.

Modulation of L-type calcium channel activity explains the ability of calcium antagonists to disrupt excitation-contraction coupling in vascular smooth muscle during voltage-mediated activation. However, smooth muscle cells exhibit a great diversity in the mechanisms mobilized to alter cellular calcium handling during vasoconstriction (Fig. 2). Potential-dependent activation of calcium channels represent but one of several possible mechanisms coupled to receptor occupation. It is clear that both calcium-antagonist sensitive calcium channels and insensitive activating mechanisms exist in vascular smooth muscle cells. Furthermore, vascular smooth muscle cells exhibit a unique regional heterogeneity in regard to activating mechanisms, which is reflected by regional variations in responsiveness to calcium antagonists. As discussed in detail in Chapter 3, regional differences in the sensitivity to calcium antagonists are of particular relevance in understanding the effects of these agents on renal hemodynamics.

References

1. Fleckenstein A: Die bedeutung der energiereichen phosphate fur kontraktilitat und tonus des myokards. Verh Dtsch Bes Inn Med 70:81–99, 1964.

2. Fleckenstein A, Kammermeier H, Doring HJ, Freund HJ: Zum wirjungsmechanismus neuartiger koronardilatoren mit gleichzeitig sauerstoff-einsparenden myokard-effeckten, prenylamin und iropveratril. Z Kreislaufforsch 56:716–744, 1967.

3. Fleckenstein A: Calcium antagonists and calcium agonists: Fundamental criteria and classification. In Fleckenstein A, van Breemen C, Gross R, Hoffmeister F (eds): Cardiovascular Effects of Dihydropyridine-type Calcium Antagonists and Agonists. Berlin, Springer-Verlag, 1985, pp 3–31.

4. Fleckenstein A, van Breemen C, Gross R, Hoffmeister F (eds): Cardiovascular Effects of Dihydropyridine-type Calcium Antagonists and Agonists. Berlin, Springer-Verlag, 1985.

5. Morad M, Nayler W, Kazda S, Schramm M: The Calcium Channel: Structure, Function and Implications. Berlin, Springer-Verlag, 1988.

6. Vanhoutte PM, Paoletti R, Govoni S (eds):Calcium Antagonists: Pharmacology and Clinical Research. Ann NY Acad Sci Vol 522, 1988.

7. Janis RA, Silver PJ, Triggle DJ: Drug action and cellular calcium regulation. Adv Drug Res 16:309–591, 1987.

8. Triggle DJ, Janis RA: Calcium channel ligands. Ann Rev Pharmacol Toxicol 27: 347–369, 1987.

9. Tsien RW: Calcium channels in excitable cell membranes. Ann Rev Physiol 45:341–358, 1983.

10. Tsien RW, Hess P, McCleskey EW, Rosenberg RL: Calcium channels: mechanisms of selectivity, permeation, and block. Ann Rev Biophys Biophys Chem 16:265–290, 1987.

11. Godfraind T, Miller R, Wibo M: Calcium antagonism and calcium entry blockade. Pharmacol Rev 38:321–416, 1987.

12. Cauvin C, Loutzenhiser R, van Breemen C: Mechanisms of calcium antagonist-induced vasodilation. Ann Rev Pharmacol 23:373–396, 1983.

13. Godfraind T, Kaba A: Blockade or reversal of the contraction induced by calcium and adrenalin in depolarized arterial smooth muscle. Br J Pharmacol 36:548–560, 1969.

14. Mayer CJ, van Breemen C, Casteels R: The action of lanthanum and D600 on the calcium exchange in smooth muscle cells of the guinea pig taenia coli. Pflugers Arch 337:333–350, 1972.

15. Rosenberger LB, Ticku MK, Triggle DJ: The effects of calcium antagonists on mechanical responses and Ca^{+2} movements in guinea pig ileal longitudinal smooth muscle. Can J Physiol Pharmacol 57:333–347, 1979.

16. van Breemen C, Hwang OK, Meisheri KD: The mechanism of inhibitory action of diltiazem on vascular smooth muscle contractility. J Pharmacol Exp Ther 218:459-463, 1981.

17. Loutzenhiser R, van Breemen C: Mechanisms of stimulated Ca^{+2} influx and consequence of Ca^{+2} influx inhibition. In Merill GF, Weiss HR (eds): Symposium on Calcium Entry Blockers, Adenosine and Neurohumors. Baltimore/Munich, Urban & Schwarzenberg, 1982, pp 73–91.

18. Loutzenhiser R, van Breemen C: Mechanism of activation of isolated rabbit aorta by PGH$_2$ analogue U-44069. Am J Physiol 241:C243–C249, 1981.

19. Meisheri K, Hwang O, van Breemen C: Evidence for two separate Ca^{+2} pathways in smooth muscle plasmalemma. J Membr Biol 59:19–25, 1981.

20. Hof RP, Scholtysik G, Loutzenhiser R, et al: PN 200-110, a new calcium antagonist: Electrophysiological, inotropic, and chronotropic effects on guinea pig myocardial tissue and effects on contraction and calcium uptake of rabbit aorta. J Cardiovasc Pharmacol 6:399–406, 1984.

21. Loutzenhiser R, Epstein M: Calcium antagonists and the kidney. Hosp Pract 22:63–76, 1987.

22. Reuter H: Calcium channel modulation by neurotransmitters, enzymes and drugs. Nature 301:569–574, 1983.

23. Bean BP: Two kinds of Ca channels in canine atrial cells. J Gen Physiol 86:1–30, 1985.

24. Bean BP, Sturek M, Puga A, Hermsmeyer K: Calcium channels in muscle cells isolated from rat mesenteric arteries: modulation by dihydropyridine drugs. Circ Res 59:229–235, 1986.

25. Loirand G, Pacaud P, Mironneau C, Mironneau J: Evidence for two distinct calcium channels in rat vascular smooth muscle cells in short-term primary culture. Pflugers Arch 407:566–568, 1986.

26. Yatani A, Seidel CL, Allen J, Brown AM: Whole-cell and single-channel calcium currents of isolated smooth muscle cells from saphenous vein. Circ Res 60:523–533, 1987.

27. Hammill OP, Marty A, Nehr E, et al: Improved patch-clamp techniques for high-resolution current recording form cells and cell-free membrane patches. Pflugers Arch 391:85–100, 1981.

28. Kokubun S, Reuter H: Dihydropyridine derivatives prolong the open state of Ca channels in cultured cardiac cells. Proc Natl Acad Sci 81:4824–4827, 1984.

29. Hess P, Lansman JB, Tsien RW: Different modes of Ca channel gating behavior favored by dihydropyridine Ca agonists and antagonists. Nature 311:538–544, 1984.

30. Hess P, Lansman JB, Tsien RW: Mechanism of calcium channel modulation by dihydropyridine agonists and antagonists. In Fleckenstein A, van Breemen C, Gross R, Hoffmeister F (eds): Cardiovascular Effects of Dihydropyridine-type Calcium Antagonists and Agonists. Berlin, Springer-Verlag, 1985, pp 34–55.

31. Bean BP: Nitrendipine block of cardiac calcium channels: High-affinity binding to the inactivated state. Proc Natl Acad Sci 81:6388–6392, 1984.

32. Barhanin J, Fosset M, Hoesy M, et al: Biochemistry and molecular pharmacology of Ca^{+2} channels and Ca^{+2} channel proteins. In Morad M, Nayler W, Kazda S, Schramm M: The Calcium Channel: Structure, Function and Implications. Berlin, Springer-Verlag, 1988, pp 159–167.

33. Glossmann H, Striessnig J, Hymel L, et al: The structure of the Ca^{2+} channel: Photoaffinity labeling and tissue distribution. In Morad M, Nayler W, Kazda S, Schramm M: The Calcium Channel: Structure, Function, and Implications. Berlin, Springer-Verlag, 1988, pp 168–192.

34. Seagar MJ, Takahashi M, Catterall WA: Molecular properties of dihydropyridine-sensitive calcium channels from skeletal muscle. In Morad M, Nayler W, Kazda S, Schramm M: The Calcium Channel: Structure, Function and Implications. Berlin, Springer-Verlag, 1988, pp 200–210.

35. Vaghy PL, McKenna E, Schwartz A: Molecular characterization of the 1,4-dihydropyridine receptor in skeletal muscle. In Morad M, Nayler W, Kazda S, Schramm M: The Calcium Channel: Structure, Function, and Implications. Berlin, Springer-Verlag, 1988, pp 211–216.

36. Wibo M, Godfraind T: The mode of action of dihydropyridines in vascular smooth muscle. In Vanhoutte PM, Paoletti R, Govoni S (eds): Calcium Antagonists: Pharmacology and Clinical Research. Ann NY Acad Sci Vol 522, 1988, pp 309–327.

37. Lee KS, Tsien RW: Mechanism of calcium channel blockade by verapamil, D600, diltiazem and nitrendipine in single dialysed heart cells. Nature 302:790–794, 1983.

38. Rios E, Brum G: Involvement of dihydropyridine receptors in excitation-contraction coupling in skeletal muscle. Nature 325:717–720, 1987.

39. Nowycky MC, Fox AP, Tsien RW: Three types of neuronal calcium channel with different calcium agonist sensitivity. Nature 316:440–443, 1985.

40. Murphy KMM, Gould RJ, Largent, Snyder SH: A unitary mechanism of calcium antagonist drug action. Proc Natl Acad Sci 80:860–864, 1983.

41. Bolger GT, Gengo P, Klockowski R, et al: Characterization of binding of the Ca^{2+} channel antagonist, nitrendipine, to guinea pig ileal smooth muscle. J Pharmacol Exp Ther 225:291–309, 1984.

42. Glossmann H, Ferry DR, Goll A, Rombush M: Molecular pharmacology of the calcium channel: Evidence for subtypes, multiple drug receptor sites, channel subunits and the development of a radio iodinated 1,4-dihydropyridine calcium channel label, ^{125}I-iodipine. J Cardiovasc Pharmacol 6:S608-S621, 1984.

43. Glossmann H, Ferry DR, Goll A, Striessnig J, Zernig G: Calcium channels: Introduction into their molecular pharmacology. In Fleckenstein A, van Breemen C, Gross R, Hoffmeister F (eds): Cardiovascular Effects of Dihydropyridine-type Calcium Antagonists and Agonists. Berlin, Springer-Verlag, 1985, pp 113-139.

44. Schramm M, Thomas G, Towart R: Novel dihydropyridines with positive inotropic action through activation of Ca^{2+} channels. Nature 303:535–537, 1983.

45. Hof RP, Ruegg UT, Hof A, Vogel A: Sterioselectivity at the calcium channel: Opposite action of the enantiomers of a 1,4-dihydropyridine. J Cardiovasc Pharmacol 7:689-693, 1985.

46. Franckowiak G, Bechem M, Schramm M, Thomas G: The optical isomers of 1,4-dihydropyridine BAY K 8644 show opposite effects on Ca channels. Eur J Pharmacol 114:223–226, 1985.

47. Loutzenhiser R, Ruegg U, Hof A, Hof RP: Studies on the mechanism of action of the vasoconstrictive dihydropyridine CGP-28392. Eur J Pharmacol 105:229–237, 1984.

48. van Breemen C, Aaronson P, Loutzenhiser R: Na^+, Ca^{2+} interactions in mammalian smooth muscle. Pharmacol Rev 30:167–208, 1979.

49. Bolton T: Mechanisms of action of transmitters and other substances on smooth muscle. Physiol Rev 3:606–718, 1979.

50. Kuriyama H, Ito Y, Suzuki H, Kitamura K, Itoh T: Factors modifying contraction-relaxation cycle in vascular smooth muscle. Am J Physiol 243:H641662, 1982.

51. Benham CD, Tsien RW: A novel receptor-operated Ca^{+2}-permeable channel activated by ATP in smooth muscle. Nature 328:275–278, 1987.

52. Zschauer A, van Breemen C, Buhler FR, Nelson MT: Calcium channels in thrombin-activated human platelet membrane. Nature 334:703–705, 1988.

53. Irvine R, Moor R: Micro-injection of inositol 1,3,4,5-tetrakiphosphate activates sea urchin eggs by a mechanism dependent on external Ca^{+2}. Biochem J 240:917–920, 1986.

54. Vivaudou M, Clapp L, Walsh J, Singer J: Regulation of one type of Ca^{+2} current in smooth muscle cells by diacylglycerol and acetylcholine. FASEB J 2:2497–2504, 1988.

55. Loutzenhiser R, Leyton P, Saida K, van Breemen C: Calcium compartments and calcium mobilization during contraction of smooth muscle. In Grover AK, Daniel EE (eds): Calcium and Smooth Muscle Contractility. Clifton, NJ, Humana Press, 1985, pp 61–92.

56. Tan N, Tashjian A: Receptor-mediated release of plasma membrane-associated calcium and stimulation of calcium uptake by thyrotropin-releasing hormone in pituitary cells in culture. J Biol Chem 256:8994–9002, 1981.

57. Loutzenhiser R, van Breemen C: The involvement of extracellularly bound calcium in the activation of arterial smooth muscle. Blood Vessels 20:295–305, 1983.

58. Deth D, van Breemen C: Agonist induced $^{45}Ca^{+2}$ release from smooth muscle cells of the rabbit aorta. J Memb Biol 30:363–380, 1977.

59. van Breemen C, Deth R: La^{+3} and excitation-contraction coupling in vascular smooth muscle. In Betz E (ed): Symposium on the Role of Ions in Transmission of Signals from Tissue and Blood to the Vascular Smooth Muscle Cells. Basel, Karger, 1976, pp 26–31.

60. Deth R, Casteels R: A study of releasable Ca fractions in smooth muscle cells of the rabbit aorta. J Gen Physiol 69:401–416, 1977.

61. Morgan JP, Morgan KG: Vascular smooth muscle: the first recorded Ca^{2+} transients. Pflugers Arch 395:75–77, 1982.

62. Hashimoto T, Hirata M, Itoh T, Kanamura Y, Kuriyama H: Inositol 1,4,5-trisphosphate activates pharmacomechanical coupling in smooth muscle of the rabbit mesenteric artery. J Physiol 370:605–618, 1986.

63. Somlyo AV, Bond M, Somlyo AP, Scarpa A: Inositol trisphosphate-induced calcium release and contraction in vascular smooth muscle. Proc Nat Acad Sci 82:5231–5235, 1985.

64. Bohr DF: Vascular smooth muscle: Dual effect of calcium. Science 139:597–599, 1963.

65. Loutzenhiser R, van Breemen C: The influence of receptor occupation on Ca^{2+} influx mediated vascular smooth muscle contraction. Circ Res 52:97–103, 1983.

66. van Breemen C, Lukeman S, Loutzenhiser R, Saida S, Cauvin C: Ca^{2+} antagonists in arterial smooth muscle. In Hoffman B (ed): Calcium Antagonists: The State of the Art and Role in Cardiovascular Disease. 1984, pp 13–26.

67. van Breemen C, Lukeman S, Leijten P, Yamamoto H, Loutzenhiser R: The role of the superficial SR in modulating force development induced by Ca^{+2} entry into arterial smooth muscle. J Cardiovasc Pharmacol 8(Suppl 8):S111–S116, 1987.

68. van Breemen C, Hwang K, Loutzenhiser R, Lukeman S, Yamamoto H: Ca entry into vascular smooth muscle. In Fleckenstein A, van Breemen C, Gross R, Hoffmeister F (eds): Cardiovascular Effects of Dihydropyridine-type Calcium Antagonists and Agonists. Berlin, Springer-Verlag, 1985, pp 58–75.

69. Lodge N, van Breemen C: Ca^{+2} pathways mediating agonist-activated contraction of vascular smooth muscle and EDRF release from endothelium. In Morad M, Nayler W, Kazda S, Schramm M: The Calcium Channel: Structure, Function and Implications. Berlin, Springer-Verlag, 1988, pp 283–292.

70. Karaki H, Kuboto H, Urakawa N: Mobilization of stored calcium for phasic contractions induced by norepinephrine in rabbit aorta. Eur J Pharmacol 56:237–245, 1979.

71. Casteels R, Droogmans G: Exchange characteristics of the noradrenaline-sensitive calcium store in vascular smooth muscle cells of rabbit ear artery. J Physiol 317:263–279, 1981.

72. Morgan JP, Morgan KG: Stimulus-specific patterns of intracellular calcium levels in smooth muscle of ferrit portal vein. J Physiol 351:155–157, 1984.

73. Jiang MJ, Morgan KG: Intracellular calcium levels in phorbol ester-induced contractions of vascular smooth muscle. Am J Physiol 253:H1365-H1371, 1987.

74. Nishimura J, Kolber M, van Breemen C: Norephinephrine and GTP-gama-S increase myofilament Ca sensitivity in alpha-toxin permeabilized arterial smooth muscle. Biochem Biophys Res Comm 157:677–683, 1988.

75. Cauvin C, Lukeman S, Cameron J, et al: Differences in norepinephrine activation and diltiazem inhibition of Ca^{+2} channels in isolated rabbit aorta and mesenteric resistance vessels. Circ Res 56:822–828, 1985.

76. Cauvin C, van Breemen C: Effects of Ca^{+2} antagonists on isolated rabbit mesenteric resistance vessels as compared to rabbit aorta. In Fleckenstein A, van Breemen C, Gross R, Hoffmeister F (eds): Cardiovascular Effects of Dihydropyridine-type Calcium Antagonists and Agonists. Berlin, Springer-Verlag, 1985, pp 259–269.

77. Cauvin C, Saida K, van Breemen C: Extracellular Ca dependence and diltiazem inhibition of contraction in rabbit conduit arteries and mesenteric resistance vessels. Blood Vessels 21:23–31, 1984.

78. Bevan JA, Bevan RD, Hwa JJ, et al: Calcium regulation in vascular smooth muscle: Is there a pattern to its variability within the arterial tree? J Cardiovasc Pharmacol 8(suppl 8):S71–S75, 1986.

Norman K. Hollenberg, M.D., Ph.D.
Gordon H. Williams, M.D.

2

The Kidney in Hypertension: Sodium Sensitivity and Renal and Adrenal Non-modulation

Recognition of the relationships between the kidney and hypertension has an extraordinary history. Although the usual attribution is to the classic work of Richard Bright, published from Guys Hospital in 1836, it is clear that many of the relationships were recognized in China thousands of years ago; The Yellow Emperors' classic of internal medicine pointed out that "The kidneys pass on the disease to the heart . . . when the pulse is abundant, but tense and hard and full like a cord, there are dropsical swellings . . . and an acute illness will develop, which is called convulsion."[1] They also recognized that "the heart rules over the kidneys . . .," perhaps an early statement on atrial natriuretic peptides! Bright related a full, hard pulse, the same index employed thousands of years earlier by the Chinese, to albuminuria in life, and contracted kidneys and left ventricular hypertrophy at necropsy. Although hypertension had not been recognized, the hard pulse was, and its meaning was clearly indicated in his conclusion that renal failure "affects the minute and capillary circulation to render greater action necessary towards blood through the distant subdivisions of the vascular system."[1]

By 1856, Traube[2] had come to understand the underlying mechanisms, arguing (to use modern parlance) that the responsible factors included an element of volume and vasoconstriction. His theory stated that the shrunken kidneys led to high blood pressure both through a reduction in the rate of blood flow from the arterial to the venous circulation (vasoconstriction) and a reduction in the volume of fluid excreted in the urine (volume). Left ventricular hypertrophy was attributed to these two factors.

By the mid-1870s the focus of the debate had shifted to a new question: Does evidence of hypertension occur in the absence of primary renal involvement? Mohamed concluded, on the basis of a long and careful study, that patients could show evidence of hypertension in the absence of obvious primary renal involvement.[1] It is of substantial historical interest that Mohamed made his observation at the same institution as did Bright (Guys Hospital), and that the first evidence that adrenal abnormalities could contribute to human disease was made by Addison in the same institution earlier in the 19th century.

Late in the 19th century, Tigerstedt and Bergman identified renin, a renal pressor substance, not only in tissue extracts from the renal cortex but also in the renal venous effluent. They recognized that the release of renin, a long-acting pressor substance, could provide the link between renal injury and the pathogenesis of hypertension. Shortly thereafter in 1904, Ambard and Beaujard proposed that hypertension reflected a failure of the individual to adapt to an excess of salt in the diet.[3] They did their seminal work while functioning as interns in the school of Vidal in Paris, where chloride balance was being measured for the first time. Indeed, they gave major emphasis to the chloride content of table salt, another suggestion that has new momentum.[4] Their clinical observations led them to another prescient observation: "It appears that there is cause here for distinguishing two categories of patients. The ones which, so to speak, accommodate themselves to the chloride . . .; the others whose chloride [sensitivity] . . . is revealed by a permanent hypertension . . . There is a non-adaptation to the saline saturation which is translated into a permanent hypertension or into a normotension.[11]

Only in the 1920s did a contribution begin to appear from the United States. Allen was the first to carry out careful dietary studies, which indicated that a severe reduction of salt in the diet would reduce blood pressure in about 60% of hypertensive patients.[5] Both Allen and his French predecessors believed that hypertension was due to an unknown renal defect with respect to the excretion of salt.

This essay, therefore, will attempt to deal with a series of questions, the most recent of which was first raised over 60 years ago. Who are the patients who have salt sensitive hypertension? What are the physiological factors responsible for salt sensitive hypertension? The term "sodium-sensitive hypertension" will be employed, because of its long usage, despite the fact that the accompanying union might be crucial.

The history of hypertension has involved the serial identification of a small subgroup of individuals with a specific pathogenesis, generally involving either the kidney or the adrenal. In this essay, we will attempt to describe with broad strokes a group of patients in whom there is an abnormality in the control of the renal circulation and the adrenal gland that leads to abnormalities in renal sodium handling, renin release, and to sodium-sensitive hypertension. Studies in progress raise the intriguing possibility that the abnormality is inherited and may be the most common cause of hypertension, it will also be appropriate to discuss, at least briefly, the implications of these observations for therapy. The observations have implications, we believe, for understanding the therapeutic effectiveness of two classes of vasodilator agent, the converting-enzyme inhibitors and the calcium channel blocking agents.

Sodium and Renal Vascular Responses to Angiotensin II

Lewis Dahl in his 1963 review of metabolism in hypertension was puzzled by five then-recent publications that described a paradoxical, natriuretic response to angiotensin II associated with a blunted or absent renal vascular response in some patients with essential hypertension.[6] He noted the parallel with hepatic cirrhosis.

Since then, the mechanism in cirrhosis has become clear[7]; the paradoxical natriuresis reflects the effects on renal sodium handling of the pressor response, when the renal vascular bed can no longer respond to angiotensin II because of angiotensin-mediated renal vasoconstriction.

During that time, two separate lines of investigation on disordered control of the renal blood supply[8] and adrenal aldosterone release[9] with shifts in the state of sodium balance led to the recognition that both abnormalities occur in the same patient.[10] This followed recognition of a highly predictable shift in renal vascular and adrenal responses to angiotensin II with changes in sodium intake; the renal vasculature is more sensitive to angiotensin II on a high salt diet, and adrenal aldosterone release is more sensitive with restriction of sodium intake.[11] Because the term "modulation" had been employed to describe such shifts in responsiveness in other endocrine systems, the inability of these individuals to change renal vascular and adrenal responsiveness to angiotensin II[12] was called "non-modulation."[13,14]

Several lines of evidence indicate that "non-modulation" is not part of a continuum, but rather represents a discrete subgroup present in about 45% of patients with normal renin and high renin essential hypertension.[8,9]

Sodium-sensitive Hypertension

The frequent sensitivity of hypertension to sodium intake has long been recognized. Allen in the 1920s demonstrated that a severe reduction of salt in the diet was effective in reducing blood pressure in about 60% of patients with hypertension.[4] Since that time, confirmation of the frequency of sodium-sensitive hypertension has come from estimates based on sodium intake as therapy,[15] the frequency of response to diuretics,[16] and careful metabolic balance studies;[17,18] these studies have confirmed a frequency of about 50 to 60%. The metabolic balance studies failed to identify a mechanism responsible for the blood pressure rise accompanying an increase in salt intake, but did demonstrate that individuals with salt-sensitive hypertension showed more positive sodium balance and gained more weight as their blood pressure rose.[17,18]

An abnormality involving the renal blood supply and adrenal aldosterone release, both crucial for sodium handling, suggested to us the intriguing possibility that the unidentified patients in the metabolic balance studies were the non-modulators. Indeed, that has turned out to be the case. Whether the pattern by which steady state external sodium balance is achieved when sodium intake is restricted[19] or the acute natriuretic response to a saline load is employed as the index[20] non-modulators show a clear inability to handle sodium. When the earlier metabolic balance study was replicated in a study in which external balance was first achieved on a restricted and then high-salt intake, the non-modulators showed more positive sodium balance as they gained more weight[19]; all of the sodium-sensitive hypertension that was identified occurred in that group.[21]

Control of the Renal Circulation

In addition to blunted renal vascular responses to angiotensin II, two other abnormalities in the control of the renal circulation occur in non-modulators that are germane both to renal vascular responses to angiotensin II and to renal sodium handling. Normal individuals display parallel changes in renal blood flow as they change salt intake: as they shift from a high-sodium to a low-sodium intake, renal blood flow falls; flow rises with an increase in salt intake.[8,12,14] Patients with essential hypertension who have intact modulation show similar changes, but renal blood flow is fixed with shifts in sodium intake in non-modulators (Fig. 1).[8,12,14,19−21] Again, this abnormality is not part of a continuum but rather reflects a discrete limitation reflected in a bimodal distribution.[19] To the extent that intrarenal physical forces and filtration fraction contribute to the ability of the kidney to handle sodium, the limited renal vascular response to changes in sodium intake could contribute to, and perhaps account for, the limited capacity of the kidney to handle sodium—described above.

A fixed renal blood supply in response to a physiological stimulus could reflect fixed, organic disease, so common as a by-product of hypertension. On the other hand, multiple lines of evidence suggest that in some patients there is a functional abnormality of the renal blood supply, vasoconstriction, that contributes to the reduced renal blood flow.[14] Angiotensin-converting enzyme (ACE) inhibition, long recognized as inducing a potentiated renal vasodilatation in essential hypertension,[22,23] is now recognized as producing preferential renal vasodilatation in the non-modulator: Indeed, only non-modulators display renal vasodilatation when an ACE inhibitor is administered on a high salt diet, with the renin system suppressed.[21]

ACE inhibition also restores renal vascular responsiveness to angiotensin II[21] and the capacity of the kidney to handle a sodium load (Fig. 2).[20] We believe that the restoration of the ability of the kidney to handle a sodium load represents a major factor by which ACE inhibitors are effective at achieving goal blood pressure in patients with essential hypertension who are ingesting a typical high-salt diet and

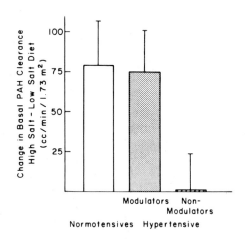

FIGURE 1. Change in renal plasma flow on a shift from a high-salt to a low-salt diet. Note the similar 20% change in renal plasma flow in normal subjects and in essential hypertensives in whom modulation was intact, and the absence of a change in renal plasma flow in the non-modulators. Reproduced with permission from Redgrave JE, Rabinowe SL, Hollenberg NK, Williams GH: J Clin Invest 75:1285-1290, 1985.

therefore have a suppressed circulating renin-angiotensin system. Similar arguments apply, we believe, to calcium channel blocking agents, as reviewed elsewhere in this monograph.

The restoration of the renal vascular response to angiotensin II following ACE inhibition also provides insight into mechanisms. If the renal vasodilatation reflected the accumulation of bradykinin because of reduced degradation, or prostaglandin release, the renal vasodilator response to ACE inhibition should have been associated with further blunting of renal vascular responsiveness to angiotensin II, since both prostaglandins and kinins share this characteristic.[24]

Renin Release and Non-modulation

Patients with non-modulation during the steady state have either a normal or elevated level of plasma renin activity,[10,12-14] but two abnormalities of renin release have been identified in non-modulators. In normal subjects on a low-salt diet, intravenous infusion of saline rapidly reduces plasma renin activity and plasma aldosterone concentration, but only about 50% of the patients with essential hypertension show this rapid fall.[25] The same patients that had a blunted renin response also had a reduced rate of sodium excretion and a transient pressor response to the saline infusion. These observations suggested the possibility that non-modulation was involved. Indeed, subsequent studies showed that it is the non-modulator that shows the delayed response to saline.[26]

The action of saline on the state of the renin-angiotensin system in the normal subjects did not involve simple plasma volume expansion, since the infusion of dextran in a volume to produce similar or more plasma volume expansion produced a delayed fall in plasma renin activity and plasma aldosterone concentration.[25] This observation made it possible to divide the stimulus into a "sodium sensitive" and a "volume sensitive" signal. The rate of fall of plasma renin activity in response to saline in non-modulators is identical to the normal response to dextran, the volume-sensitive signal. One attractive, but speculative, interpretation of these data is that non-modulators have a normal volume-sensing system but lack the ability to respond to the specific signal emitted by sodium.

A second evidence of disregulation of renin release involves the so-called "short feedback loop," by which angiotensin II reduces renin release. This response occurs within minutes, as opposed to the "long feedback loop," which involves aldosterone release and sodium retention. Patients with essential hypertension frequently do not show renin suppression with angiotensin II infusion,[27] an abnormality once again corrected by converting-enzyme inhibition.[28] Again, after identification of the non-modulating group, this abnormality was found to occur only in the non-modulator.[29]

Genetic Factors

A contribution of heredity to hypertension in many patients has long been recognized, but the precise factors inherited have been remarkably elusive. Information from renal transplantation, both in inbred animal models[30-32] and in man,[33,34] has suggested that the genetic information, at least some of the time, is coded in the kidney. Four lines of investigation have suggested that non-modulation is inherited.

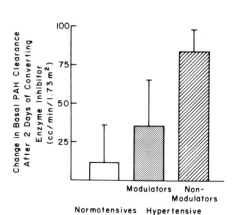

FIGURE 2. Change in renal plasma flow after two days of converting-enzyme inhibition in the same patients shown in Figure 1. The study was performed on a high sodium intake, so that the absence of a change in the normotensive subjects was anticipated. Note that the increase in renal plasma flow in non-modulators is essentially identical to the change in renal plasma flow with a shift in sodium intake in Figure 1. Reproduced with permission from Redgrave JE, Rabinowe SL, Hollenberg NK, Williams GH: J Clin Invest 75:1285–1290, 1985.

The first clue came from the frequency of a family history of hypertension in the parents of non-modulators.[19] In the neighborhood of 90% of the non-modulators in two studies where the family history could be evaluated had a parent with hypertension, as opposed to a rate of about 30% in essential hypertensives in whom modulation was intact. The second line of investigation is concerned with the identification of features identical to non-modulation in the offspring of hypertensives, involving both the adrenal gland and the kidney. In the case of the adrenal, plasma aldosterone concentration in the offspring of hypertensives on a low salt diet was substantially lower than the concentration in the offspring of normotensive parents, despite a similar level of plasma renin activity and plasma angiotensin II concentration.[35] In an elegant study on aldosterone release in response to angiotensin II infusion, performed by Beretta Piccoli and his co-workers, aldosterone release was shown to be blunted in the offspring of hypertensives.[36] Renal blood flow increased in response to captopril, not only in essential hypertensives but also in the normotensive offspring of hypertensives, but not in the normotensive offspring of normotensive parents.[34] This study was especially impressive because it was performed in Japan, where an ad libitum intake is especially rich in sodium chloride. We have confirmed that observation retrospectively in data for our earlier studies, and prospectively the calcium channel blockade increased renal blood flow preferentially in 50% of the offspring of hypertensives, but not in the control group made up of the normotensive offspring of normotensive parents.[32] Diltiazem blocked the action of angiotensin II on the renal blood supply in that study. The specificity of that response was confirmed by the observation that no difference could be identified in the renal vascular response to the vasodilator acetylcholine as a function of family history.

A third line of evidence involves red blood cell sodium:lithium countertransport. Lithium countertransport is increased not only in many hypertensives but also in their normotensive offspring.[38–40] There is a striking increase in the frequency with which increased lithium countertransport occurs in non-modulation.[41] Unfortunately, because of the number of confounding variables that influence lithium countertransport, that determination will be useful in identifying non-modulators only at the extremes of countertransport.

Finally, in a study still in progress involving multiple family members, renal plasma flow and its response to angiotensin have been found to aggregate significantly in families[39]. Although still preliminary, the available data are consistent with mendelian dominant inheritance. Sodium handling is altered significantly in the non-modulator.[19,20] There is evidence that sodium handling is also influenced by heredity and is modified by a family history of hypertension.[43] It will be intriguing to ascertain whether that genetic influence expressed itself through non-modulation.

Equally speculative, and equally intriguing, is the possibility that non-modulation has implications for the pathogenesis of renal disease. About one-third of patients with type 1 diabetes mellitus will develop nephropathy and two-thirds will not, despite an apparently identical severity and duration of disease. Studies in animal models have suggested a powerful role for renal hemodynamic factors but have not provided an explanation for the fact that 100% of rats but only 33% of people will progress in nephropathy. The information to indicate that the control of the renal circulation is altered not only in non-modulators but also in their normotensive offspring may be relevant. Patients with diabetes mellitus at risk of nephropathy display elevated red blood cell sodium, lithium countertransport, and a striking family history of hypertension,[44,45] features that they share with non-modulators. To the extent that non-modulators and their normotensive offspring act as though they have elevated intrarenal angiotensin II concentration—reflected in a blunted renal vascular response to angiotensin II, blunted renin release in response to saline and angiotensin II, and a potentiated renal vascular response to converting enzyme inhibition—the metabolic disarray of diabetes mellitus superimposed on a disordered control of the renal circulation could lead to glomerular hypertension and its consequences (reviewed in detail elsewhere in this monograph). The disordered control of the renal circulation, presumably angiotensin mediated, also appears to limit renal sodium handling—and reversal of the renal vasoconstriction by calcium antagonists and converting enzyme inhibitors improves renal sodium handling and thereby, we believe, the hypertension. If the goal of science is hypothesis generation, which in turn leads to new hypotheses that can be tested, then the thesis of non-modulation has met the goal.

References

1. Ruskin A: Classics in Arterial Hypertension. Springfield, IL, Charles C Thomas, 1956.

2. Gordon DB: Some early investigations of experimental hypertension. Tex Rep Biol Med 28:3, 1970.

3. Ambard L, Beaujard E: Causes de l'hypertension arterielle. Archives Gen Med 1:520–533, 1904.

4. Kurtz TW, Al-Bander HA, Morris RC Jr: "Salt-sensitive" essential hypertension in men: Is the sodium alone important? N Engl J Med 317:1043–1048, 1987.

5. Allen FM: Treatment of Kidney Disease and High Blood Pressure. Morristown, NJ, The Psychiatric Institute, 1925, p 206.

6. Dahl LK: Metabolic aspects of hypertension. Ann Rev Med 14:69–98, 1963.

7. Gutman RA, Forrey, AW, Flet WP, Cutler RE: Vasopressor-induced natriuresis and altered intrarenal haemodynamics in cirrhotic man. Clin Sci Mol Med 45:19–34, 1973.

8. Hollenberg NK, Merrill JP: Intrarenal perfusion in the young "essential" hypertensive: A subpopulation resistant to sodium restriction. Trans Assoc Am Physicians 83:93–101, 1970.

9. Williams GH, Rose LI, Dluhy RG, et al: Abnormal responsiveness of the renin-aldosterone system to acute stimulation in patients with essential hypertension. Ann Intern Med 72:317–326, 1970.

10. Williams GH, Tuck, ML, Sullivan JM, et al: Parallel adrenal and renal abnormalities in the young patient with essential hypertension. Am J Med 72:907-914, 1982.

11. Hollenberg NK, Chenitz WR, Adams DF, Williams GH: Reciprocal influence of salt intake on adrenal glomerulosa and renal vascular responses to angiotensin II in normal man. J Clin Invest 54:34–42, 1974.

12. Shoback DM, Williams GH, Hollenberg NK, et al: Endogenous angiotensin II as a determinant of sodium modulated changes in tissue responsiveness to angiotensin II in normal man. J Clin Endocrinol Metab 57:764–770, 1983.

13. Williams GH, Hollenberg NK: Abnormal adrenal and renal responses to angiotensin II in essential hypertension: Implications for pathogenesis. In Carey RM (ed): Clinical Endocrinology: Is Essential Hypertension an Endocrine Disease? England, Butterworth and Company, 1985, pp 184–211.

14. Hollenberg NK, Williams GH: Sensitivity to sodium and nonmodulation of renal and adrenal responsiveness to angiotensin II. Implications for the pathogenesis of essential hypertension. In Zanchetti A, and Tarazi RC (eds): Handbook of Hypertension, Vol 8. New York, Elsevier 1986 pp 520–552.

15. Chapman B: Some effects of the rice-fruit diet in patients with essential hypertension. In Bell ET (ed): Hypertension, A Symposium. Minneapolis, University of Minnesota, 1951, pp 504–516.

16. Freis E: Comparative effects of ticrynafen and hydrochlorothiazide in the treatment of hypertension (Veterans Administration Cooperative Study Group on Antihypertensive Agents). N Engl J Med 301:293–297, 1979.

17. Kawasaki T, Delea CS, Bartter FC, Smith H: The effect of high-sodium and low-sodium intakes on blood pressure and other related variables in human subjects with idiopathic hypertension. Am J Med 64:193–198, 1978.

18. Fujita T, Henry WL, Bartter FC, Lake CR, Delea CS: Factors influencing blood pressure in salt-sensitive patients with hypertension. Am J Med 69:334–344, 1980.

19. Hollenberg NK, Williams GH: Abnormal renal sodium handling in essential hypertension: Relation to failure to renal and adrenal modulation of responses to angiotensin II. Am J Med 81:412–418, 1986.

20. Rystedt LL, Williams GH, Hollenberg NK: The renal and endocrine response to saline infusion in essential hypertension. Hypertension 8:217–222, 1986.

21. Redgrave JE, Rabinowe SL, Hollenberg NK, Williams GH: Correction of abnormal renal blood flow response to angiotensin II by converting-enzyme inhibition in essential hypertensives. J Clin Invest 75:1285–1290, 1985.

22. Williams GH, Hollenberg NK: Accentuated vascular and endocrine responses to SQ 20881 in hypertension. N Engl J Med 297:184–188, 1977.

23. Hollenberg NK, Meggs LG, Williams GH, et al: Sodium intake and renal responses to captopril in normal man and in essential hypertension. Kidney 20:240–245, 1981.

24. Meggs LG, Katzberg RW, DeLeeuw P, Hollenberg NK: Specific desensitization of the canine renal vasculature to angiotensin II despite cyclo-oxygenase inhibition. Yale J Biol Med 58:453–458, 1985.

25. Tuck ML, Williams GH, Dluhy RG, et al: A delayed suppression of the renin-aldosterone axis following saline infusion in human hypertension. Circ Res 39:711-716, 1976.

26. Rabinowe SL, Redgrave JE, Rystedt LL, et al: Renin-suppression by saline is blunted in non-modulating essential hypertension. Hypertension 10:404–408, 1987.

27. Dluhy RG, Bavli SZ, Leung FK, et al: Abnormal adrenal responsiveness and angiotensin II dependency in high renin essential hypertension. J Clin Invest 64:1270–1276, 1979.

28. Leboff MS, Dluhy RG, Hollenberg NK, et al: Abnormal renin short feedback loop in essential hypertension is reversible with converting enzyme inhibition. J Clin Invest 70:335–341, 1982.

29. Seely EW, Moore TJ, Rogacz S, et al: Abnormal angiotensin II suppression of plasma renin activity in non-modulators is corrected with converting enzyme inhibition. Abstract from AHA 41st Annual Fall Conference and Scientific Sessions, New Orleans, LA, 1987.

30. Bianchi G, Fox U, DiFrancesco GF, et al: Blood pressure changes produced by kidney cross transplantation between spontaneously hypertensive rats (SHR) and normotensive rats (NR). Clin Sci Molec Med 47:435, 1974.

31 Dahl LK, Heine M: Primary role of renal homografts in setting blood pressure levels in rats. Circ Res 36:692, 1975.

32. Kawabe K, Watanabe TX, Shiono K, Sokabe H: Influence of blood pressure of renal isografts between spontaneously hypertensive and normotensive rats utilizing the F1 hybrids. Jpn Heart J 19:886, 1978.

33. Guidi E, Bianchi G, Dallosia V, et al: Influence of familial hypertension of the donor on the blood pressure and antihypertensive therapy of kidney graft recipients. Nephron 30:318, 1982.

34. Curtis JJ, Luke RG, Dustan HP, et al: Remission of essential hypertension after renal transplantation. N Engl J Med 309:1009, 1983.

35. Blackshear JL, Garnic D, Williams GH, Harrington DP, Hollenberg NK: Exaggerated renal vascular response to calcium entry blockade in first degree relatives of essential hypertensives: Possible role of intrarenal angiotensin II. Hypertension 9:384–389, 1987.

36. Beretta-Picolli C, Pusterla C, Stadler P, Weidmann P: Blunted aldosterone responsiveness to AII in normotensive subjects with familial predisposition to essential hypertension. J Hypertens 61:57–61, 1988.

37. Uneda S, Fukishima S, Fujika Y, et al: Renal hemodynamics and renin-angiotensin system in adolescents genetically predisposed to essential hypertension. J Hypertens 2 (suppl 3): 437-439, 1984.

38. Canessa M, Adranga N, Solomon H, et al: Increased sodium-lithium countertransport in red cells of patients with essential hypertension. N Engl J Med 302:772–776, 1980.

39. Cooper R, Miller T, Trevisan M, et al: Family history of hypertension and red cell cation transport in high school students. J Hypertens 1:145-152, 1983.

40. Clegg G, Morgan DB, Davidson C: The heterogeneity of essential hypertension: Relation between lithium efflux and sodium content of erythrocytes and a family history of hypertension. Lancet ii:891–894, 1982.

41. Redgrave JE, Canessa M, Williams GH, Hollenberg NK: Na-Li countertransport in non-modulating essential hypertensives. Abstract presented at 42nd annual fall conference and scientific sessions of the council for high blood pressure research. San Francisco, CA, 1988.

42. Dluhy RG, Hopkins P, Hollenberg NK, et al: Heritable abnormalities of the renin-angiotensin-aldosterone system in essential hypertension. J Cardiovasc Pharmacol (in press).

43. Luft FC, Rankin LI, Bloch R, et al: Cardiovascular and humoral responses to extremes of sodium intake in normal black and white men. Circulation 60:697-703, 1979.

44. Krolewski AS, Canessa M, Warram JH, et al: Predisposition to hypertension and susceptibility to renal disease in insulin-dependent diabetes mellitus. N Engl J Med 318: 140–145, 1988.

45. Mangill R, Bending JJ, Scott B, et al: Increased sodium-lithium countertransport activity in red cells of patients with insulin-dependent diabetes and nephropathy. N Engl J Med 318:146-150, 1988.

Rodger Loutzenhiser, Ph.D.
Murray Epstein, M.D.

3

The Renal Hemodynamic Effects
of Calcium Antagonists

In 1967, Albrecht Fleckenstein coined the term "calcium antagonist" to describe the actions of verapamil on the heart. As Fleckenstein correctly surmised, the negative inotropic activity of this agent derived from its ability to block the actions of extracellular calcium.[1] Since this initial observation, much progress has been made concerning the mechanisms of action and the physiologic effects of this important class of pharmacologic agents. Furthermore, substantial progress has been made in our understanding of vasoconstrictor mechanisms and the major role of calcium entry in the activation of vascular smooth muscle. In retrospect, it is not surprising that calcium antagonists are such potent vasodilators. The molecular targets of their pharmacologic actions, potential-dependent calcium channels, are entailed in excitation-contraction coupling of most blood vessels. The actions of calcium antagonists on these calcium channels underlies their effectiveness in preventing coronary vasospasm and their utility as antihypertensive agents.

The effects of calcium antagonists on renal vascular smooth muscle and their attendant effects on renal hemodynamics have only recently become an area of general interest. In diverse settings, calcium antagonists increase renal perfusion and may preserve renal function. Thus, the renal hemodynamic actions of these agents have important clinical applications. In addition, calcium antagonists represent unique investigative tools to elucidate the activating mechanisms and pharmacologic attributes of the renal microcirculation. Indeed, the manner in which calcium antagonists modify the renal responses to vasoconstrictors is complex and suggest a unique heterogeneity of smooth muscle activating mechanisms within the renal vascular bed.

This chapter examines the renal hemodynamic effects of calcium antagonists, highlights the distinctive features of the renal microcirculation that define the actions of these agents, and relates the renal effects to the settings in which calcium antagonists are administered. Findings with regard to the hemodynamic response of the isolated perfused kidney and the responsiveness of afferent and efferent arterioles to calcium antagonists are presented. Finally, the implications of the renal responses to calcium antagonists in diverse experimental settings are considered.

The Renal Hemodynamic Responses to Calcium Antagonists

Observations in Humans

Normotensive Subjects. Early studies in humans revealed marginal effects of calcium antagonists on renal hemodynamics in normal subjects.[2] Leonetti et al.[3] reported that single doses of either nifedipine (10 mg orally) or verapamil (160 mg orally) failed to alter glomerular filtration rate (GFR) in normal subjects. Similarly, Wallia et al.[4] observed that nitrendipine (5–10 mg orally) had no effect on GFR or renal blood flow (RBF). Van Schaik et al.[5] also found that nicardipine (60 mg orally) had no effect on GFR in normal subjects. In contrast, Yokoyama and Kaburagi[6] reported that intravenous administration of nifedipine (13 μg/min) produced a slight, albeit significant, increase in renal blood flow (2%) and GFR (6%) in normal volunteers.

Hypertensive Subjects. In an early study, Klutsch et al.[7] reported that nifedipine increased renal perfusion and GFR in a group of patients with essential hypertension (Fig. 1). More recently, several reports have also suggested that in contrast to the lack of effect in normal subjects, hypertensive subjects may exhibit an exaggerated renal hemodynamic response to calcium antagonists. Thus, whereas Yokoyama and Kaburagi[6] found that infusion of nifedipine produced only modest increases in RBF and GFR in normotensive subjects, the same dosage (13 μg/min) increased RBF and GFR by 45% and 46%, respectively, in hypertensive subjects. Sakurai et al.[8] also reported that diltiazem (60 mg orally) increased RBF and GFR by 11% and 15%, respectively, in hypertensive patients. Similarly, van Schaik et al.[5] reported that nicardipine produced an 11% increase in GFR of hypertensive subjects, whereas the same dosage (60 mg orally) had no effect in normotensive subjects. Finally, Blackshear et al.[9] reported that at least 50% of normotensive subjects with a family history of hypertension demonstrated an exaggereated renal vasodilatory response to diltiazem, suggesting an inherited abnormality of the renal vascular bed associated with hypertension.

Montanari et al.[9a] have recently extended these observations. They investigated nine young normotensive subjects with no family history of hypertension (F−) and nine age-matched normotensive subjects with one parent with essential hypertension (F+). They determined ERPF and GFR before and after the administration of a single 20-mg oral dose of nifedepine. Baseline renal function did not differ between the two groups. In contrast, nifedipine induced disparate renal hemodynamic and excretory responses. Whereas nifedipine did not alter ERPF of F(−) subjects, it produced an exaggerated renal vasodilater response in the F(+) group with a mean increase in ERPF of 31%. Concomitantly, GFR was unchanged. Collectively, the studies of Blackshear et al.[9] and Montanari et al.[9a] suggest an inherited trait associated with hypertension, manifested as an exaggerated response of calcium antagonists.

In contrast, Leonetti et al.[3] reported that the acute administration of verapamil and nifedipine (60 mg and 10 mg orally, respectively), had no effect on GFR in normotensive or hypertensive subjects. GFR was maintained in hypertensive patients, even though blood pressure fell 20–30%, suggesting a decrease in preglomerular vascular resistance. Sunderrajan et al.[10] found that diltiazem had no effect on the RBF or GFR of hypertensive patients whose basal GFR was above 80 ml/min/1.73 m^2, but caused an increase in GFR and RBF in hypertensive patients whose initial GFR was below this value. The filtration fraction was unchanged in these patients, and blood pressure decreased significantly. Reams et al.[11] found that nifedipine increased GFR in hypertensive subjects with normal (106 ± 19 ml/min/1.73 m^2) and impaired (68 ± 11 ml/min/1.73 m^2) initial GFR values.

Amodeo et al.[12] reported that in a group of patients with moderate hypertension (diastolic blood pressure of 90–120 mmHg), short-term administration of diltiazem (300 mg/day for 4 weeks) reduced blood pressure and increased RBF but had no effect on GFR, thereby reducing filtration fraction. In a follow-up study of the same patients after 1 year of treatment with diltiazem,[13] RBF remained elevated, GFR was unchanged, and filtration fraction decreased from $33 \pm 4\%$ to $18 \pm 10\%$, prompting these authors to suggest that diltiazem had a predominantly postglomerular effect in this group of patients.

The ability of calcium antagonists to augment renal hemodynamics may be diminished in the presence of an organic or "fixed" decrement in renal perfusion. Kutsch et al.[7] investigated the effects of nifedipine on a large group of patients with hypertension accompanied by varying degrees of renal functional impairment. They observed that patients with the highest basal inulin clearance manifested marked augmentation of renal hemodynamics, as assessed by increments in inulin and para-aminohippurate clearances. In contrast, patients with impaired renal function failed to manifest a renal vasodilatory response to nifedipine (Fig. 1). Presumably the group that responded to the calcium antagonists exhibited a greater renal vasodilatory capacity than the group with impaired renal function, in whom the decrement in renal perfusion may have been attributable to a "fixed" organic lesion.

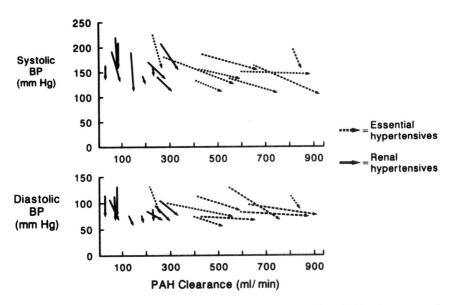

FIGURE 1. Effects of intravenous nifedipine (1 mg) on systolic and diastolic blood pressure and para-aminohippurate clearance (C_{PAH}) in 9 patients with esstential hypertension and 11 patients with "renal" hypertension. Nifedipine induced a significant increase in C_{PAH} in essential hypertensive patients. In contrast, "renal" hypertensive patients failed to augment C_{PAH} despite similar blood pressure reduction. Reproduced with permission from Klutsch et al., Artzneimittelforsch Drug Res, 1972.[7]

Renovascular Hypertension. Renovascular hypertension represents a clinical setting in which the unique renal vasodilatory actions of calcium antagonists may be of therapeutic importance (see Chapter 17). In a recent study, Ribstein et al.[14] compared the actions of nifedipine to those of captopril in patients with renal arterial stenosis. Captopril reduced the blood pressure level but caused a 23% fall in GFR, as would be anticipated based on previous reports.[15] In contrast, nifedipine produced a greater decrement in systemic blood pressure but induced a slight increase in GFR (13%) (see Fig. 5 in chapter 17). The authors suggest that the calcium antagonists reduced blood pressure while simultaneously preserving efferent arteriolar resistance.

Other Clinical Settings. Calcium antagonists may augment renal perfusion and preserve renal function in a number of clinical settings. The results of recent clinical trials using calcium antagonists in postcadaveric kidney transplantation and reports that these agents may prevent cyclosporine-induced nephrotoxicity (see Chapters 14 and 17) suggest that calcium antagonists may prevent or ameliorate acute renal vasoconstriction in humans.

Summary. The renal hemodynamic effects of calcium antagonists in humans vary, depending upon the setting in which they are administered. In normotensive, healthy subjects taking calcium antagonists orally, these agents have little effect on RBF or GFR. In contrast, hypertensive subjects usually manifest an increase in RBF. Accordingly, filtration fraction is reported to remain unaltered or in some studies to decrease. A preliminary report suggests that calcium antagonists increase GFR and filtration fraction in patients with renovascular hypertension, and thus they differ in this regard from converting enzyme inhibitors.[14] In concert, these findings suggest that if basal renal vascular tone is elevated by increased renal vasoconstriction, calcium antagonists tend to increase both GFR and RBF in humans, whereas if basal renal vascular tone is not enhanced, these agents have little effect on renal hemodynamics.

Observations in Animal Models

Reports of the in vivo effects of calcium antagonists in animal models have been inconsistent. Divergent findings can be attributed in part to differences in the animal models and experimental conditions employed. Because calcium antagonists elicit vasodilation by blocking specific postreceptor processes (see Chapter 1), it would be anticipated that the renal hemodynamic effects of these agents would depend largely on basal renal vascular resistance and on the nature of the renal vasoconstrictor hormones, autacoids, and neurotransmitters influencing the renal vasculature. An examination of the literature suggests, indeed, that the effects of calcium antagonists on the kidney vary according to the extrarenal conditions that exist at the time of study; however, several generalities may be drawn.

First, although calcium antagonists usually decrease renal vascular resistance, different experimental preparations exhibit markedly different sensitivities to these agents. In general, calcium antagonists exert a greater renal hemodynamic effect when administered directly into the renal artery than when administered systemically.[2] It is likely that the decrease in blood pressure accompanying systemic administration initiates compensatory reflexes that attenuate the renal vasodilator response. In support of this formulation, Brody et al.[16] reported that nisoldipine (10 μg/kg intravenously) reduced renal vascular resistance by 33% in conscious rats with sinoaortic baroreceptor denervation, whereas in baroreflex-intact rats, nisoldipine had no effect on renal resistance.

Second, it is apparent that the level of basal renal vascular resistance greatly affects the subsequent response to calcium antagonists. Experimental conditions associated with enhanced basal renal vascular tone predispose the renal vasculature to an enhanced vasodilatory response to calcium antagonists. Thus, calcium antagonists exert greater renal vasodilatory actions when administered during the infusion of exogenous vasoconstrictors. Several studies have demonstrated that the renal vasodilatory effects of calcium antagonists are markedly augmented by prior administration of angiotensin II (ANG II).[17-24]

Experimental conditions associated with an increase in endogenous vasoconstrictor stimuli also predispose the renal vasculature to the vasodilatory actions of calcium antagonists. Thus, administration of calcium antagonists to anesthetized animals produces a greater renal vasodilatation than that observed in conscious animals.[2] Presumably anesthesia and/or surgical trauma increase basal renal vascular tone, thereby favoring enhanced vasodilation.

Conversely, the renal hemodynamic effects of calcium antagonists are attenuated by conditions that reduce underlying vasoconstriction. Ishikawa et al.[25] demonstrated that, whereas infusion of diltiazem (3 μg/kg/min) into the renal artery of the anesthetized dog normally increased RBF by 13%, the response was reduced to 5% following ganglionic blockade with pentolinium tartrate. Similarly, the status of extracellular fluid volume may indirectly influence the renal hemodynamic effects of calcium antagonists by altering basal renal vascular tone. Bell and Lindner reported that in anesthetized dogs, volume expansion abolished the increase in RBF normally observed in response to infusion of verapamil.[17] Finally, Yamaguchi et al.[23] reported that suprarenal aortic clamping abolished the effects of diltiazem on GFR and RBF in the anesthetized dog. Presumably, reducing renal perfusion pressure by aortic clamping elicits a compensatory renal vasodilation, thereby eliminating the subsequent response to calcium antagonists.

Such observations stress the importance of the experimental conditions and basal renal vascular resistance as determinants of the renal hemodynamic response to calcium antagonists in vivo. The nature of the prevailing vasoconstrictor stimuli also influences the subsequent response to calcium antagonists. For example, reports in the literature consistently demonstrate that during ANG II-induced renal vasoconstriction, administration of calcium antagonists increase both GFR and RBF.[17-24] When calcium antagonists are administered during norepinephrine (NE)-induced renal vasoconstriction, the results do not demonstrate such consistency.[16,19,22,23,25,26]

Finally, studies with animal models of hypertension suggest that hypertension per se predisposes the renal vascular bed to the vasodilatory actions of calcium antagonists.[24-27] It is likely that this phenomenon represents an additional example of the dependency of the renal hemodynamic response to calcium antagonists on prevailing renal vascular tone. In a setting of increased renal perfusion pressure, myogenic renal vascular tone is enhanced.[95] Nevertheless, it is possible that hypertension may be associated with alterations in the renal vascular bed that selectively predispose the kidney to the vasodilatory actions of calcium antagonists. The study by Blackshear et al.[9] suggests that an enhanced renal vascular response to calcium antagonists is an inherited trait associated with hypertension. The observations by Steele et al.[28-31] demonstrating an exaggerated response of isolated kidneys obtained from hypertensive rats, are in accord with this formulation (see below).

Collectively, these findings delineate the problems encountered in interpreting the direct renal actions of calcium antagonists from data obtained solely from in vivo observations. Clearly, both the magnitude and the nature of underlying renal vasoconstriction exert a predominant influence on renal responsiveness to calcium antagonists. Furthermore, the renal effects of calcium antagonists are modified by the extrarenal reflexes triggered by the systemic actions of these agents.

The Effects of Calcium Antagonists On Renal Hemodynamics in the Isolated Perfused Kidney

Our laboratory and others have utilized the in vitro perfused rat kidney to determine the direct renal effects of calcium antagonists. This model circumvents the influence of extrarenal factors on the renal hemodynamic response to calcium antagonists. Furthermore, with the isolated perfused kidney, the vasoconstrictor stimuli affecting basal renal vascular tone can be accurately defined and controlled.

Characteristics on the Isolated Perfused Rat Kidney

The isolated perfused rat kidney model used in our laboratory has been described in detail[32,33] and is illustrated schematically in Figure 2. Typically, the kidney is perfused with an artificial cell-free medium that is recirculated. Renal perfusion pressure is measured within the renal artery and is maintained constant during the experiment.

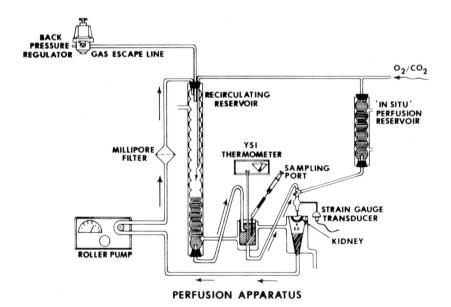

PERFUSION APPARATUS

FIGURE 2. Schematic diagram of perfusion apparatus used in isolated perfused kidney experiments. The kidney receives medium from a pressurized reservoir. Perfusion pressure is monitored at the level of the renal artery and controlled by adjusting the regulator in gas egress line. Perfusate flow is monitored with an electromagnetic flow meter. Reproduced with permission from Loutzenhiser et al. , J Pharmacol Exp Ther, 1985.[32]

The isolated perfused kidney has several advantages in the study of the direct renal actions of calcium antagonists: (1) extrarenal factors such as alterations in hormonal or neural stimuli are excluded; (2) renal perfusion pressure can be maintained constant; (3) the renal responses can be studied under conditions in which the vasoconstrictor stimuli are accurately controlled and defined; and (4) drug concentrations can be calculated accurately.

The interpretation of findings and extrapolations to in vivo settings, however, require knowledge of the characteristics of this model. When perfused with a cell-free medium, the isolated rat kidney exhibits abnormally high perfusate flow rates, primarily owing to the low viscosity of the perfusate compared with blood, but also reflecting the lack of extrinsic vasoconstrictor stimuli that is characteristic of this model.[34] Relatively normal glomerular filtration rates can be obtained with this preparation. Nevertheless, because of the high perfusate flow rates, filtration fraction is very low (<5%). Consequently, the oncotic pressure gradient along the glomerular capillary bed is nominal. Thus, GFR is relatively independent of glomerular flow.

The low viscosity of the perfusate may also alter the relationship between the magnitude of vasoconstriction at the level of the arteriole and the observed change in renal vascular resistance. The resistance (R) of a vascular segment is not only a function of the fourth power of the radius (r) and length of the segment (L), but is also directly proportional to the viscosity (v) of the perfusate ($R = 8 \, vl/\pi r^4$).[35] Accordingly, the first derivative of the change in resistance with respect to a change in radius (dR/dr) is directly proportional to viscosity ($dR/dr = -32 \, vl/\pi r^5$). Thus, the change in vascular resistance associated with a given change in vessel diameter is directly proporational to the viscosity of the perfusate. Such considerations may contribute to the impaired renovascular response to increased pressure, even though myogenic arteriolar vasoconstriction is well preserved (see below). Similarly, in the isolated perfused kidney afferent and efferent arterioles are perfused with fluid of the same viscosity, whereas in vivo the viscosity of the blood perfusing the efferent arteriole is elevated. This phenomenon tends to diminish the effect of efferent arteriolar vasoconstriction on efferent arteriolar resistance in the isolated perfused kidney.

Micropuncture studies indicate that sodium reabsorption is impaired in the loop of Henle of the isolated perfused kidney, causing an increased delivery of sodium to the distal segment.[35] Thus, tubuloglomerular feedback (TGF) should be maximally stimulated in this preparation; however, indirect evidence suggest that TGF is impaired. Calcium antagonists abolish TGF-induced vasoconstriction,[37] but do not alter basal perfusate flow or GFR in the isolated kidney (discussed below). To our knowledge a direct study of TGF has not been undertaken in the isolated perfused rat kidney.

Finally, the renin-ANG II system is uncoupled in the isolated perfused rat kidney. The kidney readily secretes renin in response to appropriate stimuli[38] and converts angiotensin I to ANG II.[39] Appropriate amounts of renin substrate appear to be lacking, however, as indicated by the marked vasoconstriction induced by the addition of angiotensinogen.[40] Thus, although recent data demonstrate the presence of intracellular angiotensinogen,[41] there is no evidence for endogenous ANG II-induced renal vasoconstriction, even though the renin concentration of the perfusate may attain very high levels.[38]

It is therefore apparent that differences exist between the isolated perfused kidney and the intact kidney. Nevertheless, the ability to control extrarenal factors offers a distinct advantage in the interpretation of observations in the isolated kidney. Similarly, the fact that certain intrarenal mechanisms are inoperative or impaired (i.e., renin-ANG II, TGF, filtration disequilibrium) actually facilitates the interpretation of

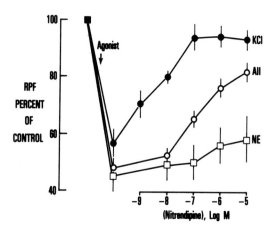

FIGURE 3. Summary of the effects of nitrendipine on renal perfusate flow (RPF) in the vaso-constricted kidney. Isolated perfused rat kidneys were treated with nitrendipine in the presence of KCL (closed circles), angiotensin II (AII, open circles), or norepinephrine (NE, open squares). Nitrendipine completely reversed KCl-induced vasoconstriction, but was less effective in revers-ing the response to NE. A component of the response to AII was also refractory to nitrendipine. Reproduced with permission from Loutzenhiser et al. , J Cardiovasc Pharmacol, 1987.[43]

the observed hemodynamic responses in this model. Although it may be argued that the isolated perfused kidney is an inappropriate model for the study of *normal* renal physiology, it is extremely useful for the study of the pharmacology of the renal vasculature. The novel information obtained with the isolated kidney preparation can be perceived as complementary to observations in intact animals. When interpreted in concert with the latter, additional inferences can be drawn about the direct actions of calcium antagonists on the kidney.

Effects of Calcium Antagonists on Renal Perfusate Flow

The isolated perfused rat kidney has little intrinsic vascular tone. As might be antic-ipated, calcium antagonists have little effect on renal hemodynamics when adminis-tered to this preparation in the absence of exogenous vasoconstrictor stimuli.[32,33,42] In contrast, if basal renal vascular tone is increased, a calcium antagonist-induced renal vasodilation is elicited. The response to calcium antagonists depends, however, on the type of vasoconstrictor stimuli used to establish basal renal vascular tone.

The different reponses to nitrendipine following renal ischemia induced by NE, ANG II, or potassium (KCl) are summarized in Figure 3. Each vasoconstrictor was administered at a concentration sufficient to produce a 50% decrease in renal per-fusate flow (RPF) (i.e., 3×10^{-7} M NE, 3×10^{-10} M ANG II, and 30 mM KCl). Nitrendipine was then administered in the continued presence of each agent. Nitrendipine was most potent and efficacious in reversing the renal vasoconstric-tion elicited by KCl-induced depolarization. At 0.1 μM, nitrendipine completely reversed the vasoconstriction induced by KCl. The contractile response to KCl is exclu-sively dependent on calcium entry through potential-dependent calcium channels. Inasmuch as this channel type is the primary molecular target for calcium antago-nists, it is not surprising that KCl-induced vasoconstriction is completely inhibited by calcium antagonists.

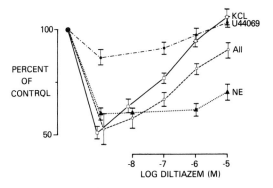

FIGURE 4. Summary of the effects of diltiazem on renal perfusate flow(RPF) of isolated perfused kidneys during vasoconstriction elicited by norepinephrine (triangles), angiotensin II (circles), and KCl (squares). Note that the pattern of response is similar to that depicted in Figure 3 for nitrendipine. Reproduced with permission from Loutzenhiser and Epstein, Am J Physiol, 1985.[2]

In contrast to KCl, the renal vasoconstrictions elicited by NE and ANG II were markedly less sensitive to nitrendipine. Nitrendipine only modestly reversed the renal vasoconstriction elicited by NE (Fig 3). Similar results have been obtained using other dihydropyridines (e.g., nifedipine and nisoldipine[44,45]). The same pattern of vasodilation is observed in response to the benzothiazepine calcium antagonist diltiazem (Fig. 4).

Note that with each calcium antagonist, the renal vasoconstriction elicited by ANG II is reversed to a greater degree than was that elicited by NE, suggesting that the renal vascular effects of these two agonists involve different mechanisms. Nevertheless, the ANG II-induced vasoconstriction was also much less sensitive to reversal by calcium antagonists than was the vasoconstriction elicited by KCl. Furthermore, as was observed with NE, a component of the ANG II-induced vasoconstriction was resistant to inhibition even at the highest concentration of calcium antagonist (i.e., 10 μM). Thus, in contrast to KCl, the renal vasoconstriction elicited by both NE and ANG II appear to involve complex mechanisms. A fraction of the renal vasoconstriction elicited by NE and ANG II is blocked by calcium antagonists, whereas another component is refractory.

Effects of Calcium Antagonists on Glomerular Filtration Rate

In the absence of renal vasoconstriction calcium antagonists exert little effect on GFR in vivo.[2] Similarly, in the isolated perfused kidney, calcium antagonists do not alter GFR unless exogenous vasoconstrictors are applied, or pressure-dependent renal vascular tone is induced.[32,33,42] Calcium antagonists do elicit striking effects on GFR of the isolated perfused kidney in many experimental settings. In the experiment depicted in Figure 5, NE was administered to establish basal renal vasoconstriction. The NE-induced vasoconstriction was associated with a marked decreased in GFR. In this setting, administration of nisoldipine only modestly increased RPF but returned GFR to control levels. This differential reversal of the actions of NE on GFR and RPF is further emphasized by the demonstration that the administration of phentolamine returns RPF to control values, but does not produce a further augmentation of GFR.

The preferential augmentation of GFR in the presence of NE-induced renal vasoconstriction is observed with each of the three classes of calcium antagonists,[28-33,45-46] but not with the inorganic calcium entry blocker manganese,[2,33] and is not mimicked by the removal of extracellular calcium.[46] Figure 6 summarizes the relative effects of a number of calcium antagonists and manganese on GFR and RPF of kidneys pretreated with NE. In contrast to the organic calcium antagonists, manganese exerted equal effects on RPF and GFR. This difference in selectivity reflects the differing actions of these two types of calcium entry blockers. Organic calcium antagonists act on specific channels (i.e., L-type calcium channels),[47-49] whereas inorganic cations block a wider variety of calcium translocating processes.[50-52] Since the preferential augmentation of GFR occurred only with the calcium antagonists, this action must reflect the consequence of selective blockade of the L-type calcium channels. It is the ability of calcium antagonists to affect specific calcium channels preferentially without altering other calcium entry processes that accounts for their unusual effects on GFR.

These observations suggest that calcium antagonists interact in an unusual fashion with the renal microcirculation. In evaluating the effects of calcium antagonists on renal vascular resistance, one must consider the unique architecture of the renal microcirculation. In the kidney, vascular resistance is determined by the summation of segmental resistances of the afferent and efferent arterioles. These two types of arterioles are arranged in series and therefore act in concert to regulate renal vascular resistance. Nevertheless, because the glomerular capillary bed is positioned between these two vessels, changes in level of vasoconstriction of the afferent and efferent arteriole result in diametrically opposing effects on glomerular capillary hydrostatic pressure. Consequently, a selective dilation of the afferent arteriole results in an increase in glomerular filtration pressure, particularly if efferent vasoconstriction is preserved.

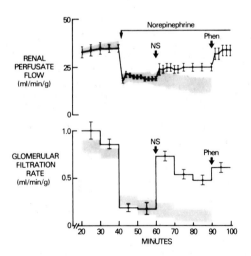

FIGURE 5. Effects of nisoldipine on RPF and GFR of isolated kidneys during norepinephrine-induced vasoconstriction. Norepinephrine (3×10^{-7}M) infusion decreased RPF and caused a reduction in GFR. Nisoldipine (NS, 10^{-7} M) administration returned GFR to control levels (shaded area), while producing only a modest increase in RPF. Phentolamine (Phen, 10^{-5} M) reversed the remaining effects on norepinephrine on RPF but produced no further increase in GFR. Modified with permission from Loutzenhiser et al., J Pharmacol Exp Ther, 1985.[32]

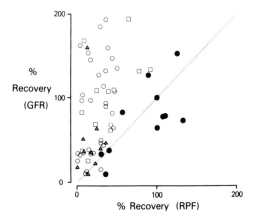

FIGURE 6. Comparison of the reversal by calcium antagonists of norepinephrine-induced decreases in GFR and RPF of isolated perfused rat kidneys. Each point represents a single study in which norepinephrine infusion was followed by administration of a calcium entry blocker. As indicated by open symbols, diltiazem (triangles), nisoldipine (squares), and nitrendipine (circles) exerted a preferential effect on GFR. In contrast, the inorganic calcium entry blocker manganese (closed circles) did not. Line represents unity. Reproduced with permission from Loutzenhiser and Epstein, Am J Physiol, 1985.[2]

We therefore proposed that the ability of calcium antagonists to augment GFR, during NE-induced vasoconstriction reflects a preferential action on preglomerular resistance vessels.[32] In our initial studies designed to test this hypothesis, we determined stop-flow (ureteral) pressure in isolated kidneys during the sequential administration of NE and nisoldipine.[32] Norepinephrine decreased stop-flow pressure from 33 ± 2 mmHg to 12 ± 2 mmHg. The subsequent administration of nisoldipine returned stop-flow pressure to 25 ± 2 mmHg (Fig. 7). Since RPF was affected only modestly, these data suggest a preferential action of the calcium antagonist on preglomerular vasoconstriction.

We have previously noted that the renal vasodilator response to calcium antagonists varies depending on the type of underlying vasoconstriction (Figs. 3 and 4). It would therefore be anticipated that the response of GFR to calcium antagonists would also depend on the type of vasoconstrictor stimuli used to set basal renal vascular tone. Indeed, this is the case.

Figure 8 illustrates the response of GFR to nitrendipine in the presence of identical degrees of vasoconstriction elicited by NE, ANG II and KCl. These data were obtained from the same studies in which the RPF response was previously assessed (Fig. 3). The effects on GFR differ in a number of ways. First, although the three vasoconstrictors elicited identical reductions in RPF, they produced dissimilar effects on GFR. Thus, 30 mM KCl reduced GFR to 3 ± 2% of control; whereas 3×10^{-7} M NE and 3×10^{-10} M ANG II reduced GFR to 24 ± 10% and 51 ± 15% of control, respectively. Such observations reflect different relative effects of these vasoconstrictors on afferent and efferent tone in addition to possible differences in the effects of these agents on the nonvascular determinants of GFR (e.g., K_f).

Second, nitrendipine exerted effects on GFR that were quantitatively dissociated from its effects on RPF. Thus, in the presence of ANG II and NE, nitrendipine elicited an augmentation of GFR (Fig. 8) that greatly exceeded its effects on RPF (Fig. 3). In contrast, this preferential augmentation of GFR was not observed with KCl. Rather,

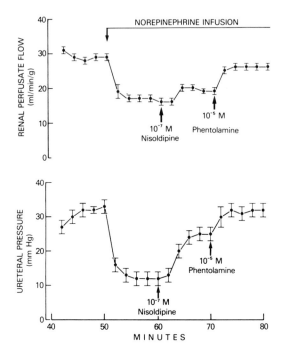

FIGURE 7. Effects of norepinephrine, nisoldipine, and phentolamine on RPF and "stop-flow" ureteral pressure in isolated kidneys, in which the ureters were attached to pressure transducers. Norepinephrine infusion (3×10^{-7} M) caused a decrease in ureteral pressure that was reversed by nisoldipine. As in the studies depicted in Figure 5, nisoldipine increased RPF only slightly, suggesting a preferential dilation of preglomerular vessels. Phentolamine reversed the remaining effects on norepinephrine. Modified with permission from Loutzenhiser et al., J Pharmacol Exp Ther, 1985.[32]

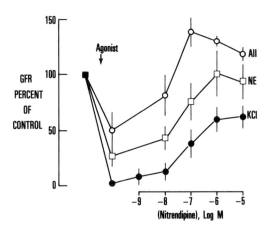

FIGURE 8. Summary of the effects of nitrendipine on glomerular filtration rate (GFR) in vaso-constricted kidneys. Isolated perfused rat kidneys were treated with nitrendipine in the presence of KCL (closed circles), angiotensin II (AII, open circles), or norepinephrine (NE, open squares). Nitrendipine completely reversed KCl-induced vasoconstriction, but was less effective in reversing the response to NE. A component of the response to AII was also refractory to nitrendipine. Reproduced with permission from Loutzenhiser et al., J Cardiovasc Pharmacl, 1987.[43]

in the presence of KCl, nitrendipine caused parallel increases in both GFR and RPF. Collectively, the above enumerated findings indicate that calcium antagonists have the potential to augment GFR and filtration fraction preferentially, but do so only in the presence of certain vasoconstrictor stimuli (e.g., NE and ANG II).

In order to understand such observations, it is necessary to consider the concept of regional heterogeneity of smooth muscle-activiating mechanisms. Receptor-linked activating mechanisms may exhibit different characteristics in different regions of the circulation. Thus, a single agonist such as NE may initiate vasoconstriction by different mechanisms in different blood vessels.[53] In contrast to the mechanisms linking receptor occupation to vasoconstriction, the mechanism of KCl-induced vasoconstriction does not exhibit regional heterogeneity.[47,53] Accordingly, vessels that demonstrate dissimilar sensitivities to calcium antagonists when activated by NE exhibit similar sensitivities when activated by KCl.[47,53]

We therefore proposed that the selective augmentation of GFR by calcium antagonists requires the presence of an agonist that acts upon afferent and efferent resistance vessels by different activating mechanisms. [2,32] Such agonists may elicit membrane depolarization and activate potential-dependent calcium channels in afferent but not efferent arteriolar smooth muscle. Because organic calcium antagonists selectively inhibit the function of this channel type, they increase GFR by preferentially attenuating afferent arteriolar tone.

Effects of Calcium Antagonists on Kidneys Isolated from Hypertensive Animals

Several investigators have reported that the administration of calcium antagonists to hypertensive animals elicits an exaggerated renal hemodynamic response.[2,24-27] Steele and coworkers have investigated the actions of calcium antagonists on perfused kidneys isolated from hypertensive animals.[28-31] As described in Chapter 4, these investigators have found that the preferential augmentation of GFR during NE-induced renal vasoconstriction is exaggerated in kidneys from spontaneously hypertensive rats (SHR) [28] and salt-sensitive Dahl rats.[29-30]

More recently, Steele et al.[31] have reported that the renal vasoconstrictor response to a calcium channel agonist (Bay K 8644) is enhanced in kidneys isolated from prehypertensive salt-sensitive Dahl rats, and augmented further in kidneys from animals in which salt-dependent hypertension was induced. Accordingly, Steele has proposed that a genetically conferred abnormality in calcium channel function may exist in the renal vasculature of this specific animal model, and that cellular events associated with exposure to hypertension may further influence calcium channel activity. The observation by Rusch and Hermsmeyer[54] that cultured smooth muscle cells from SHR have a greater proportion of "L"-type calcium channels than those from their normotensive controls (Wistar-Kyoto rats) supports this formulation.

Effects of Calcium Antagonists on the Renal Microcirculation as Assessed in vivo

Inferences from Micropuncture Studies

Normal Rats. To our knowledge, only two studies have been conducted with normal kidneys (i.e., Munich Wistar rats) to assess directly the microvascular actions of calcium antagonists by using micropuncture techniques to measure the determinants of glomerular hemodynamics. Ichikawa et al.[21] examined the effects of the calcium antagonist verapamil on glomerular hemodynamics in control conditions and during ANG II–induced renal vasoconstriction. In the control setting, intravenously administered verapamil (20 μg/kg/min) caused a significant increase in whole kidney GFR (from 1.20 $\pm$ 0.12 to 1.33 $\pm$ 0.10 ml/min) and single nephron GFR (from 46.5 $\pm$ 3.6 to 52.3 $\pm$ 4.0 nl/min). Verapamil decreased afferent resistance (R_a, from 2.2 $\pm$ 0.3 to 1.8 $\pm$ 0.3 10^{-10} dynes sec cm^5) and tended to decrease efferent resistance (R_e, from 1.7 $\pm$ 0.2 to 1.4 $\pm$ 0.1 10^{-10} dynes sec cm^{-5}, although the latter effect was not statistically significant. Verapamil had no effect on the ultrafiltration coefficient (K_f).

In parallel studies, Ichikawa et al.[21] examined the interaction of ANG II and verapamil. In the absence of verapamil, ANG II infusion (0.2 μg/kg/min) caused a striking increase in both R_a (from 2.1 $\pm$ 0.2 to 3.0 $\pm$ 0.3 10^{-10} dynes sec cm^{-5}) and R_e (from 1.7 $\pm$ 0.1 to 3.0 $\pm$ 0.1 10^{-10} dynes sec cm^{-5}), increased glomerular capillary hydrostatic pressure (P_{GC}) (from 49.1 $\pm$ 0.9 to 59.9 $\pm$ 1.5 mmHg), and reduced K_f (From 0.091 $\pm$ 0.009 to 0.040 $\pm$ 0.005 nl sec^{-1} mm^{-1}). The subsequent administration of verapamil completely reversed all glomerular actions of ANG II. Furthermore, when ANG II was infused following pretreatment with verapamil, the calcium antagonist completely prevented the glomerular hemodynamic actions of ANG II.

Pelayo[55] examined the effects of verapamil and nifedipine on the alterations in glomerular hemodynamics associated with renal nerve stimulation. In the absence of calcium antagonists, renal nerve stimulation (3 Hz) increased R_a and R_e by 85% and 35%, respectively, and decreased P_{GC} and GFR. A second group of animals were pretreated with verapamil (20 μg/kg/min, intravenously) or nifedipine (2.5 μg/kg/min, intravenously). In the animals treated with calcium antagonists (data were combined), basal R_a was significantly lower (1.35 $\pm$ 0.09 10^{-10} dynes sec cm^{-5}) than that of the control group (1.89 $\pm$ 0.20 10^{-10} dynes sec cm^{-5}, p < 0.025). The GFR, P_{GC}, K_f, and R_e did not differ significantly between control and calcium antagonists-treated animals. Pretreatment with calcium antagonists greatly attenuated the effects of nerve stimulation on both R_a and R_e. Thus, in the presence of the calcium antagonist R_a and R_e increased only 29% and 16%, respectively (only the increase in R_a was significant, p >0.01). The decrements in GFR and P_{GC} induced by renal nerve stimulation were also blunted by pretreatment with calcium antagonists.

Models of Chronic Renal Failure.   Additional micropuncture studies have recently been conducted with the remnant kidney model to determine if calcium antagonists are beneficial in attenuating the progression of renal insufficiency in this model of chronic renal failure. In a preliminary study, Anderson et al.[56] examined the effects of calcium antagonists in Munich Wistar rats 4 weeks after 5/6ths nephrectomy. They reported that the acute administration of verapamil (15 μg/kg/min, intravenously) or diltiazem (50 μg/kg/min, intravenously) lowered P_{GC} from a control value of 69 $\pm$ 3 mmHg to 52 $\pm$ 2 and 49 $\pm$ 2 mmHg (p < 0.05), respectively. In this setting, administration of a calcium antagonist was also associated with a decrease in single nephron GFR.

In a recent comprehensive study, Yoshioka et al.[57] examined the acute effects of verapamil on glomerular hemodynamics in subtotal (5/6ths) nephrectomized Munich Wistar rats. At 4–6 weeks after nephrectomy, P_{GC} was elevated (65 $\pm$ 3 vs. 45 $\pm$ 1 mmHg, controls), owing to a decrease in R_a (0.156 $\pm$ 0.010 vs. 0.275 $\pm$ 0.020 mmHg min/nl, control) and an increase in R_e (0.143 $\pm$ 0.009 vs. 0.115 $\pm$ 0.009/mmHg min, control). Verapamil (50 μg/kg/min, intravenously) reduced both R_a (to 0.074

$\pm$ 0.004 mmHg min/nl) and R_e (to 0.064 $\pm$ 0.004 mmHg min/nl), normalized P_{GC} (45 $\pm$ 3 mmHg), and lowered single nephron GFR. The authors observed that single-nephron protein filtration was elevated in normal glomeruli, and verapamil reduced protein filtration to normal levels. The authors suggested that glomerular hypertension is associated with an increase in glomerular pore size and that this abnormality is corrected by verapamil.

Pelayo et al.[58] observed different effects of verapamil on glomerular hemodynamics in Munich Wistar rats with 5/6ths nephrectomy, following chronic treatment (oral) with the calcium antagonist. At 4 weeks after surgery, P_{GC} was similar in verapamil-treated and control rats (58.0 $\pm$ 0.8 vs. 59.3 $\pm$ 1.3 mmHg, respectively). Furthermore, verapamil did not appear to alter R_a or R_e. Both resistances were significantly lower in the partially nephrectomized rats than controls. The authors suggested that verapamil decreased filtration pressure by causing an increase in pressure within Bowman's capsule. The mechanisms mediating such a proposed effect are not readily apparent. In attempting to interpret their findings, it is disturbing to note that verapamil did not attenuate the development of hypertension in their study, as would be anticipated. Such a failure raises the possibility that therapeutic levels of the calcium antagonists may not have been attained, confounding interpretation of their data.

Dworkin[59] reported that in another model of chronic renal failure, the DOCA-salt rat, nifedipine (chronic oral administration) normalized blood pressure without lowering P_{GC} or single nephron GFR. Dworkin concluded that nifedipine reduced R_a in this setting, and suggested that the protective actions of this agent are due to non-hemodynamic actions (see Chapter 8).

Summary. The few available micropunture studies seem to suggest that calcium antagonists act on both R_a and R_e. In normal kidneys, verapamil abolished the ANG II-induced increments in both resistances.[21] This finding is not in accordance with the observation that calcium antagonists preferentially increase GFRand filtration fraction during ANG II-induced renal vasoconstriction.[17-24] Verapamil and nifedipine blocked the effects of renal nerve stimulation of R_a and R_e, although nerve stimulation predominantly altered R_a.[55]

In the remnant kidney, the effects of calcium antagonists appear controversial. When administered intravenously, calcium antagonists are reported to reduce P_{GC} [56,57] whereas oral administration is reported to have no effect on P_{GC}.[58] In the DOCA-salt model, P_{GC} was not altered even though blood pressure was lowered, suggesting a predominant effect on R_a.[59]

In attempting to reconcile these findings with other reports that indicate a preferential action of calcium antagonists on preglomerular resistance, a number of caveats should be considered. Although not generally appreciated, it is clear that at high concentrations individual calcium antagonists exhibit vasodilatory actions that are independent of the "class" effects of these agents on calcium channels. This is particularly true with verapamil, which has been demonstrated to directly interfere with agonist-binding to receptors in the micromolar range.[60,61] Diltiazem has also been demonstrated to interfere with intracellular calcium mobilization, and with myofilament activation at high concentrations.[62,63] It is important to separate these non-class actions of individual agents from effects directly mediated by the blockade of L-type calcium channels. Thus, it is necessary to determine the dose-dependent effects of less specific agents such as verapamil on R_a and R_e. In this regard, it would be of interest to compare the actions of verapamil with those of a more potent dihydropyridine such as isradipine, since the concentration of isradipine required to modulate calcium channel activity differs from that subtending its actions by several orders of magnitude.[64]

Finally, the effects of calcium antagonists on the K_f are not completely defined. Micropuncture studies demonstrate that verapamil, nifedipine, and diltiazem increase K_f in some experimental settings.[21,58] When administered under basal conditions to hydrated normal rats, however, verapamil is reported to have no effect on K_f.[21,55] It is likely that the actions of calcium antagonists on K_f may also depend on the intrinsic factors influencing this parameter and may therefore vary depending on experimental or clinical setting.

Direct in Vivo Observations in the Hydronephrotic Kidney

The ability to observe the vasoconstrictor responses of intact renal microvessels directly would obviously facilitate an investigation into the renal hemodynamic actions of calcium antagonists. Unfortunately, the vascular pole of the glomerulus is not accessible to direct intravital microscopic observation. An early attempt to circumvent this problem involved transplantation of glomeruli into the hamster cheek pouch and subsequent observation following revascularization of these structures.[65] To our knowledge, this technique has not been directly applied to the study of the renal microvascular actions of calcium antagonists.

Steinhausen et al.[66] introduced a novel technique for direct observation of the in vivo response of renal microvessels. These investigators noted that chronic unilateral hydronephrosis, attained by ureteral ligation, results in a marked atrophy of renal tubular elements, thereby allowing visual access to the microcirculatory network of the kidney. Previous workers had observed that the tubular atrophy associated with hydronephrosis is accompanied by relatively minor pathologic changes in the blood vessels.[67,68]

Steinhausen and coworkers have utilized the hydronephrotic rat kidney to visualize vascular responses within the renal microcirculation in situ. Rats with unilateral hydronephrosis are prepared by complete ligation of one ureter, followed by clamping of the renal artery of the affected kidney for 60 minutes.[66] After 8–12 weeks, the animals are studied by exteriorizing the kidney and splitting it along the greater curvature with a cautery knife. One-half of the kidney, with its corporeal circulation intact, is transilluminated and observed with videomicroscopy.

Using this preparation Fleming et al.[69] directly assessed the effects of diltiazem on afferent and efferent arterioles in vivo. Calcium antagonists were added topically to the surface of the kidney, thereby reaching the arteriolar smooth muscle cells from the interstitial space. This approach circumvents systemic effects of calcium antagonists, allowing a direct assessment of the renal actions of these agents in an intact in vivo setting. Figure 9 illustrates the effects of diltiazem on the diameters of the resistance vessels of in situ hydronephrotic kidneys. As depicted, the calcium antagonist exerted a preferential dilation of preglomerular vessels, increasing the diameters of segments of the arcuate, interlobular (cortical radial artery), and afferent arterioles. In contrast, diltiazem elicited little vasodilation of postglomerular vessels (i.e., efferent arterioles near glomeruli and at the "welling point"). The lack of postglomerular vasodilation was not due to an inability of these vessels to respond, as is evident from the marked vasodilation that could be subsequently elicited by acetylcholine (Fig. 9). In the same study, Fleming and coworkers[69] observed similar effects of nitrendipine.

Of interest, however, the dihydropyridine elicited a more heterogeneous pattern of vasodilation among preglomerular vessels. The authors suggested that there may be slight differences in the microvascular responses to calcium antagonists but also proposed that the vehicle used to administer dihydropyridines have significant actions at high concentrations.

Fleming et al.[70] compared the renal microvascular effects of nitrendipine with those of hydralazine in rats with unilateral hydronephrosis. When applied topically to the surface of the hydronephrotic kidney, nitrendipine and hydralazine both preferentially dilated preglomerular vessels. At all concentrations between 0.01 μM and 1.0 μM, nitrendipine elicited a greater increase in afferent arteriolar diameter (30–50%) than did hydralazine 6–30%. The authors concluded that the glomerular actions of the calcium antagonist were greater than those of hydralazine following topical application. In contrast, when these agents were administered systemically (0.3 –3.0 mg/kg, intravenously), hydralazine and nitrendipine produced equivalent vasodilatory responses in the afferent arteriole. In this setting, both agents caused marked decrements in blood pressure (30–50%), confounding an interpretation of the microvascular responses. The authors noted that a simultaneous renal autoregulatory response (see below) may have contributed to the afferent response to systemic administration of hydralazine, although a possible biotransformation of hydralazine to a more active metabolite may have participated in its enhanced effects this setting.

Finally, in a study described in more detail below, Steinhausen et al.[71] found that aortic clamping produces an afferent arteriolar vasodilation that is attenuated by pretreatment with nitrendipine. Although this may appear paradoxical, the interpretation of this observation is that nitrendipine abolished pressure-dependent (i. e., "myogenic") afferent arteriolar tone. Accordingly, whereas the normal response to aortic clamping was an afferent arteriolar vasodilation, pretreatment with nitrendipine abolished normal myogenic tone, thereby attenuating the vasodilatory response to a reduction in renal arterial pressure (see section on renal autoregulation, below).

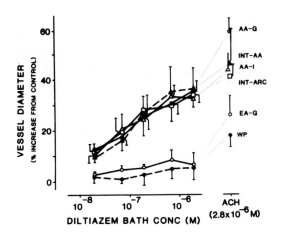

FIGURE 9. Changes in the diameter of pre- and postglomerular vessels of the hydronephrotic kidney of anesthetized rat following topical application of diltiazem and acetylcholine (ACH). AA-G and AA-I represent afferent arteries near glomerulus and intralobular artery, respectively. INT-ARC and INT-AA represent intralobular artery near arcuate artery and afferent arteriole, respectively. EA-G and WP represent efferent arteriole near glomerulus and at welling point, respectively. Reproduced with permission from Fleming et al. , Am J Physiol, 1987.[69]

The results of these initial studies assessing the effects of calcium antagonists on the renal microcirculation in vivo indicate that these agents act preferentially on preglomerular vessels, including the afferent arteriole, but do not vasodilate the efferent arteriole.

As was emphasized earlier, the renal effects of calcium antagonists depend on the underlying renal vasoconstriction. Accordingly, in order to interpret appropriately the actions of calcium antagonists in this model it is necessary to assess the determinants of renal tone in anesthetized rats with unilateral hydronephrosis. Steinhausen and co-workers have demonstrated that in Inactin-anesthetized rats, the renal microvessels of the situ hydronephrotic kidney do not respond to phentolamine[72] but dilate in response to saralasin.[73] In conjunction with the finding that aortic clamping also results in vasodilation,[71] these observations imply that a combination of "myogenic" or pressure-dependent tone, and ANG II-induced renal vasoconstriction contribute to basal vascular tone of the afferent and efferent arterioles in this model.

Effects of Calcium Antagonists on the Renal Microcirculation as Assessed In Vitro

A direct evaluation of the effects of calcium antagonists on the renal microvascular response to diverse vasoconstrictor stimuli is required to understand fully the renal hemodynamic actions of these agents. In order to eliminate the numerous extrarenal effects of calcium antagonists, and at the same time define the underlying vasoconstrictor stimuli, it is necessary to utilize in vitro models of renal microvessels. Recently, a number of such models have been developed, including isolated resistance vessels, the blood perfused juxtamedullary nephron preparation, and the isolated perfused hydronephrotic kidney. To date, relatively few studies have been undertaken to assess directly the actions of calcium antagonists using in vitro approaches.

Isolated Renal Resistance Vessels

Over the past few years, Edwards and coworkers have applied the microperfusion techniques developed for the study of isolated renal tubules to the study of microdissected, pressurized, isolated afferent and efferent arterioles.[74–76] Although this model offers promise, few other laboratories have been successful in utilizing this approach, and to our knowledge there have been no published reports of the actions of calcium antagonists on this preparation.

Harder et al.[77] have examined the effects of verapamil on the myogenic response of isolated pressurized interlobular arteries (cortical radial arteries) of the dog. The effects of altering transmural pressure (20–120 mmHg) on membrane electrical activity and vessel diameter were ascertained in isolated vessels (approximately 100–130 μm in diameter). Increasing pressure caused a progressive depolarization of the smooth muscle membrane Although the usual response was a graded depolarization, spontaneous action potentials were observed in some preparations. These were most prominent near vessel bifurcations. Vessel diameter was relatively unchanged over this pressure range. In contrast, when the vessels were treated with verapamil (1.0 μm), increasing pressure caused a passive increase in vessel diameter. These studies suggest that the pressure-induced activation of the cortical radial artery is mediated by an electrical depolarization and subsequent activiation of potential-dependent calcium channels.

The Blood-perfused Juxtamedullary Nephron

Casellas and Navar recently developed a novel in vitro model for direct observation of the renal microvessels of juxtamedullary nephrons in the rat kidney.[78] This approach takes advantage of the anatomic position of a population of glomeruli located on the surface of the renal cortex in a region normally covered by the pelvic mucosa. The afferent arterioles of these glomeruli arise directly from the arcuate artery, and can be observed following partial dissection of the kidney, retraction of the papilla, and exposure of the inner cortical surface. The methodology involves in situ perfusion of the kidney, followed by excision of the perfused kidney, dissection and subsequent perfusion of the area under observation with whole blood.

Using this model, Carmines and Navar[79] recently studied the effects of calcium antagonists on basal renal vascular tone, and on the microvascular responses to ANG II. Under basal conditions, verapamil (10–50 μM) and diltiazem (10 μM) dilated the afferent arteriole by 17 $\pm$ 3% and 22 $\pm$ 8%, respectively. This high concentration of verapamil also caused a modest, albeit significant efferent arteriolar vasodilation (9 $\pm$ 4%, p $<$ 0.05), which was not observed with diltiazem. The authors attributed the efferent vasodilatory actions of verapamil to an effect that does not involve calcium channel antagonism.

Carmines and Navar[79] observed that ANG II (0.1 nM) caused a 17 $\pm$ 2% decrease in afferent arteriolar diameter and a 15 $\pm$ 3% decrease in efferent arteriolar diameter. Both verapamil (10–50 μM) and diltiazem (13 μM) blocked the afferent arteriolar response to ANG II. In contrast, both calcium antagonists had no effect on the efferent arteriolar response to the peptide. Thus, in this setting the calcium antagonists clearly exerted a preferential action on the preglomerular vessel.

The Isolated Perfused Hydronephrotic Kidney

Recently, our laboratory developed a model that allows direct assessment of the renal microvascular responses under controlled in vitro conditions, without the necessity of extensive microdissection.[80] We combined the approach pioneered by Steinhausen and coworkers (discussed previously) with the isolated kidney perfusion technique. Using this approach, the vasoconstrictor responses of the afferent and efferent arterioles of the hydronephrotic kidney can be directly assessed under conditions identical to those used in studies of the hemodynamic response of the isolated perfused normal kidney. A recent study of the renal hemodynamic and microvascular responses to atrial natriuretic peptide has confirmed the utility and attributes of this model.[80]

Figure 10 is a schematic representation of the isolated perfused hydronephrotic kidney preparation. Kidney donors with unilateral hydronephrosis are prepared by ligation of the right ureter. After 8–10 weeks, the right renal artery is cannulated in situ as described in detail elsewhere.[32,33] The right kidney is then excised, and placed on the stage of an inverted microscope. The kidney is perfused with an artificial cell-free medium identical in composition to that used in the normal isolated kidney studies described above. Renal arterial pressure is measured at the level of the renal artery and adjusted by manipulating the pressure in the perfusate reservoir (Fig. 10). Perfusate flow to the kidney is monitored by an electromagnetic flow probe, while the renal microvascular responses are video-recorded for later analysis. The video recordings are subsequently transmitted to an IBM computer equipped with a video acquisition board. Microvascular diameters are measured by custom-designed automated software.

This model offers several advantages. First, because microdissection is not required, this model avoids the alterations in vascular responsiveness associated with surgical trauma. Furthermore, the responses of the afferent and efferent arterioles can be determined without altering their anatomic relationship and can be ascertained in settings in which the basal tone of the vessels is determined by a single vasoconstrictor stimuli. For example, pressure is under direct experimental control, and the microvascular response to alterations in perfusion pressure can be directly ascertained. Alternatively, perfusion pressures can be chosen in which pressure-dependent tone is minimal, thereby allowing the study of other vasoconstrictor stimuli in a setting in which the contribution of a myogenic component of renal vascular tone is eliminated. Finally, pharmacologic probes can be utilized with this in vitro model that cannot be applied to in vivo models.

Effects of Calcium Antagonists on Angiotensin II-induced Vasoconstriction. As described in previous sections of this chapter, the actions of calcium antagonists on the kidney during ANG II-induced renal vasoconstriction have been studied extensively. We have therefore elected to consider ANG II as a paradigm of agonist-induced vasoconstriction in the isolated perfused kidney.[81]

In normal kidneys, 0.3 nM ANG II causes a marked vasoconstriction and reduces GFR. In this setting, calcium antagonists preferentially increase GFR (Figs. 3 and 8). Thus, diltiazem returned RPF to 82% of control, but increased GFR to 174% of control.[81] In hydronephrotic kidneys perfused in vitro under identical conditions, 0.3 nM ANG II reduced afferent and efferent arteriolar diameters by 24% and 20%, respectively. In this setting, diltiazem reversed the ANG II-induced afferent arteriolar vasoconstriction with an IC_{50} of 0.16 μM, but was ineffective in reversing the ANG II-induced efferent arteriolar vasoconstriction ($IC_{50} > 10$ μM). Figure 11 depicts a representative tracing that illustrates the effects of ANG II and nifedipine on an afferent arteriole and its adjacent efferent arteriole. Note that ANG II constricts both vessels, and that nifedipine preferentially reverses the afferent arteriolar response to ANG II.

These findings with the isolated perfused hydronephrotic kidney are consistent with the results of Carmines and Navar[79] in the blood-perfused juxtamedullary nephron. They are also in accord with the observations of Fleming et al.[69] in the in vivo hydronephrotic kidney, a model in which basal renal vascular tone appears to be predominantly influenced by ANG II.[73] In each of these models, under conditions in which basal renal vascular tone was set by ANG II, calcium antagonists elicited a preferential vasodilation of the afferent arteriole but did not dilate the efferent arteriole.

These direct observations offer a plausible explanation for the hemodynamic actions of calcium antagonists obtained when the agents are administered under conditions in which ANG II is the predominant renal vasoconstrictor stimulus. We previously described the preferential augmentation of GFR in the isolated kidney during ANG II-induced vasoconstriction (Figs. 3 and 8). Numerous studies indicate that calcium antagonists exert similar effects on GFR and filtration fraction when these agents are administered during infusion of ANG II in vivo.[17,24] A recent study by Navar et al.[82] also suggested a postglomerular action of ANG II that is insensitive to calcium antagonists. Navar et al. observed that calcium antagonists produced a renal vasodilator response in anesthetized dogs subjected to an autoregulatory challenge that appeared to be predominantly preglomerular in character. With this model, captopril produced a vasodilation that was additive to that elicited by calcium antagonists

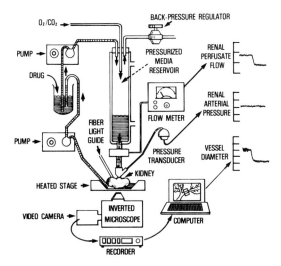

FIGURE 10. Schematic diagram of apparatus used in our laboratory to study microvessels in the isolated perfused hydronephrotic kidney. Kidneys are excised and perfused with artificial medium on the stage of an inverted microscope. Perfusate enters the renal artery from a pressurized reservoir and is returned to the reservoir with roller pumps. Renal arterial presure is maintained constant by adjusting the pressure within the perfusate reservoir, by means of the back-pressure type regulator in the gas escape line. Perfusate flow is monitored with an electromagnetic flow meter, and video images of the renal microcirculation are recorded during the experimental manipulation. Video images are then transmitted to a microcomputer, and changes in vessel diameter are determined by automated software. Reproduced with permission from Loutzenhiser et al. , J Pharmacol Exp Ther, 1988.[80]

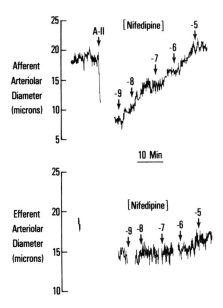

FIGURE 11. Original tracings depicting the effects of angiotensin II (AII, 0.3 nM) and nifedipine (concentrations in log M units) on the diameter of an afferent arteriole and its adjoining efferent arteriole in an isolated perfused hydronephrotic kidney. AII elicits a vasoconstriction in both vessels. Nifedipine reverses the afferent arteriolar vasoconstriction but has no effect on the efferent arteriole.

and this action was reversed by ANG II, indirectly suggesting a calcium antagonist-insensitive, ANG II-dependent efferent vasoconstriction.

Preliminary findings suggest that calcium antagonists preserve or increase GFR when administered to humans with renovascular hypertension,[14] a clinical setting in which ANG II-induced renovascular tone may be elevated (See Fig . 5, Chapter 17). In concert, these observations suggest that the preferential attenuation of preglomerular ANG II-induced vasoconstriction by calcium antagonists occurs in vivo.

In summary, calcium antagonists preferentially attenuate ANG II-induced afferent arteriolar vasoconstriction in the isolated perfused hydronephrotic kidney. This preferential vasodilation of preglomerular vessels explains the marked augmentation of GFR observed in normal kidneys perfused under identical conditions.

Vasoconstrictor Response to KCl.   One possible explanation for the differing effects of calcium antagonists on afferent and efferent arterioles may be a regional variation in the distribution of potential-dependent calcium channels within the renal microcirculatory bed. Thus, the afferent arteriole may exhibit a greater density of potential-dependent calcium channels and therefore may be more sensitive to calcium antagonists. Because these calcium channels respond to membrane electrical potential and are directly activated by KCl-induced depolarization, one prediction of this hypothesis is that the afferent and efferent arteriole should differ with regard to their sensitivity to KCl.

In order to assess this prediction directly, we have examined the microvascular response of the isolated perfused hydronephrotic kidney to KCl.[83] Figure 12 summarizes our findings on the ability of 30 mM KCl to constrict afferent and efferent arterioles, and the reversal by nifedipine of this vasoconstriction. As depicted, KCl preferentially constricted the afferent arteriole. Thus, KCl reduced afferent arteriolar diameter by $38 \pm 6\%$ (i.e., from 20.7 ± 1.5 μm to 13.0 ± 1.8 μm, $p < 0.005$), whereas it reduced efferent arteriolar diameter by only $12 \pm 4\%$ (i.e., from 15.8 ± 1.6 μm to 13.8 ± 1.4 μm, $p = 0.05$). As anticipated, nifedipine returned afferent arteriolar diameter to control levels ($IC_{50} = 41 \pm 2$ nM).[83]

The preferential constriction of the afferent arteriole elicited by KCl corresponds to a preferential decrement in GFR in normal kidneys. As discussed above, we have compared the effects of NE, ANG II, and KCl on the RPF and GFR of isolated perfused normal kidneys (Figs. 3 and 8). For example, 30 mM KCl and 0.3 nM ANG·II decreased RPF of normal kidneys by $44 \pm 5\%$ and $53 \pm 3\%$, respectively. Whereas these two vasoconstrictors produced similar decrements in RPF, KCl caused a $97 \pm 2\%$ reduction in GFR, and ANG II-administration reduced GFR by only $49 \pm 15\%$.

The relative effects of these two vasoconstrictors on GFR and RPF reflect, at least in part, the disparate actions of these two agents on afferent and efferent arterioles (Fig. 12, lower panel). Thus, as described above, KCl elicited a preferential vasoconstriction of afferent arterioles and caused a more marked decrement in GFR, whereas ANG II elicited similar vasoconstrictor responses in afferent and efferent arterioles, and reduced GFR to a lesser extent.

In concert with the observations described above concerning the preferential actions of calcium antagonists on the afferent arteriole, the recent finding that KCl elicits a predominant afferent arteriolar vasoconstriction is compelling indirect evidence of the regional heterogeneity of the renal microcirculation. These observations indicate that potential-dependent calcium channels play a prominent role in the vasoconstrictor responses of the afferent arteriole. As reviewed recently,[83] such channels may either be sparsely distributed or physiologically silent in the efferent arteriole.

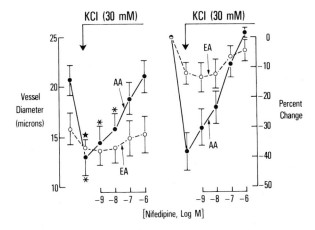

FIGURE 12.   The effects of KCl and nifedipine on the afferent (closed circles) and efferent (open circles) arterioles of isolated perfused hydronephrotic kidneys. Primary data (vessel diameters) are depicted on the left, and percent changes in vessel diameters are depicted on the right. KCl elicited a 38 ± 6% decrease in the diameter of the afferent arteriole (p < 0.005), but reduced efferent arteriolar diameter by only 12 ± 4% (p = 0.05). The administration of nifedipine returned the diameters of both vessels to control values, in a dose-dependent manner. Asterisks and star indicate p < 0.01 and p = 0.05, respectively, compared to pre-KCl (primary data only, left panel). Reproduced with permission from Loutzenhiser et al., Am J Physiol, 1989.[83]

Implications of the Heterogeneous Actions of Calcium Antagonists on the Renal Microcirculation

An intriguing development derived from investigations of the renal hemodynamic and microvascular actions of calcium antagonists concerns the implications of the heterogeneous nature of the renal microvascular smooth muscle. In addition to their importance as therapeutic agents, calcium antagonists have a novel utility as pharmacologic probes in the investigation of smooth muscle activation mechanisms. Since calcium antagonists act on a specific class of calcium channels (i.e., "L"-type channels), they can be used to delineate the involvement of such channels in the vascular responses to vasoconstrictor stimuli.

The differing sensitivities of the afferent and efferent arterioles to calcium antagonists imply intrinsic differences in mechanisms whereby vasoconstrictor stimuli affect smooth muscle contractile tone in these two vessels. The smooth muscle cells of pre-glomerular vessels have been demonstrated to exhibit membrane depolarization in response to diverse stimuli such as elevated pressure[77] and the application of ANG II, vasopressin, and catecholamines.[84] It is likely that the sensitivity of these vessels to calcium antagonists reflects a predominance of depolarization-induced activation of potential-dependent calcium channels in response to vasoconstrictor stimuli (i.e., electromechanical coupling). In contrast, the lack of sensitivity of the efferent arteriole to the vasodilatory actions of calcium antagonists and the reduced vasoconstrictor response of this vessel to KCl-induced depolarization are indicative of a minor role for electromechanical coupling in this vessel.

In recent years additional evidence has accrued that the pharmacologic attributes of vascular smooth muscle vary within other regions of the circulation. Indeed, calcium antagonists exhibit differing potencies on different types of conduit arteries.[47,85]

Furthermore, within the mesenteric circulation, calcium antagonists inhibit agonist-induced contractions more effectively in small resistance vessels than in larger conduit vessels.[86]

In many regards, however, the heterogeneity exhibited by the renal microcirculation is unique. Unlike the mesenteric circulation, differing responses to calcium antagonists are observed in renal vessels of the same caliber. Furthermore the smooth muscle cells comprising the afferent and efferent arterioles exhibit distinct morphologic differences. The cells of the afferent arteriole have the typical "spindle-shape" morphology that is characteristic of other vascular smooth muscle cells.[87] In contrast, efferent arteriolar smooth muscle cells lack this typical bipolar cell shape and are more irregular in appearance.[87] Finally, because the afferent and efferent arterioles play distinct roles in regulating glomerular capillary hydrostatic pressure and GFR, the impact of the differing pharmacologic responsiveness of these vessels is of particular importance. The characterization of the cellular events mediating vasoconstriction in these two vessel types represents a singular challenge. Such an undertaking is required, however, in order to understand the pharmacologic attributes of the renal microcirculation.

Effects of Calcium Antagonists on Renal Autoregulation

The kidney exhibits a remarkable ability to maintain a constant blood flow and GFR in the face of alterations in renal perfusion pressure. This complex renal autoregulatory response is modulated by renal autacoids and involves both tubuloglomerular feedback and pressure-dependent renal vascular tone.[88,89] Calcium antagonists attenuate the renal autoregulatory response to pressure. Recent evidence has accrued indicating the calcium antagonists directly inhibit the intrinsic ability of preglomerular resistance vessels to constrict in response to elevated transmural pressure (i. e. , "myogenic" vasoconstriction). Additional sites at which calcium antagonists could conceivably affect renal autoregulation include the tubuloglomerular feedback response (see Chapter 8), and an inhibition of the actions of renal autacoids (e. g. , adenosine, ANG II).

In Vivo Observations

Navar et al.[82] recently demonstrated that the intrarenal arterial infusion of verapamil (5-7 μg/kg/min) abolished autoregulation of renal blood flow in the anesthetized dog (Fig. 13). Furthermore, in the presence of the calcium antagonist, autoregulation of GFR was impaired, suggesting an inhibition of preglomerular vasoconstriction (Fig. 13). More recently, Lin and Young[90] reported that verapamil (4 μg/kg/min, intravenously) abolishes the autoregulation of GFR in anesthetized rabbits.

Steinhausen et al.[71] obtained indirect evidence suggesting that nitrendipine inhibits the autoregulatory response of preglomerular resistance vessels in vivo. These authors used suprarenal aortic clamping to reduce renal arterial pressure and elicit an autoregulatory renal vasodilation. A reduction of renal arterial pressure from 120 mmHg to 80 mmHg vasodilated arcuate arteries, interlobular arteries (cortical radial arteries), and afferent arterioles. Nitrendipine (applied topically to the kidney) dilated these vessels and abolished further vasodilation in response to aortic clamping.

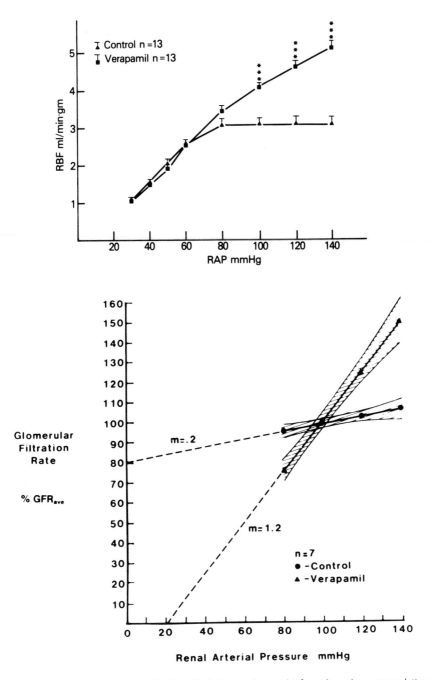

FIGURE 13. Effects of verapamil (5–7 μg/kg/min, renal arterial infusion) on the autoregulation of renal blood flow (RBF, top) and glomerular filtration rate (GFR bottom) in anesthetized dogs. In the presence of the calcium antagonist (triangles) the autoregulatory responses of RBF and GFR were abolished. Reproduced with permission from Navar et al., Circ Res, 1986.[82]

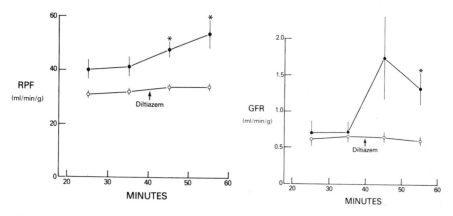

FIGURE 14. Perfusion pressure as a determinant of the renal hemodynamic effects of diltiazem in the isolated perfused rat kidney. Diltiazem had no effect on RPF (left) or GFR (right) of kidneys perfused at 100 mmHg(open circles). In contrast, diltiazem increased RPF and GFR of kidneys perfused at 150 mmHg(closed circles). Reproduced with permission from reference Loutzenhiser et al. , Am J Cardiol, 1987.[93]

Effects on the Response of the Isolated Perfused Kidney to Pressure

The early studies by Ono et al.[91] and Cohen and Fray [92] demonstrated the ability of calcium antagonists to inhibit autoregulation in isolated kidneys. Recent studies from our laboratory have demonstrated that perfusion pressure is an important determinant of the response of the isolated kidney to calcium antagonists.[93] Thus, as illustrated by Figure 14, the administration of diltiazem to kidneys perfused at 100 mmHg does not alter either perfusate flow or GFR, reflecting the lack of intrinsic renal vascular tone in this preparation. In contrast, a vasodilation associated with a striking increase in GFR is observed when the calcium antagonist is administered to kidneys perfused at 150 mmHg.

Effects on Pressure-induced Contractions of Renal Resistance Vessels

In the isolated perfused hydronephrotic kidney, acute alterations in perfusion pressure elicit direct changes in afferent arteriolar caliber that are also sensitive to inhibition by calcium antagonists.[93-96] Figure 15 depicts a representative study illustrating the renal microvascular response obtained when the pressure within the renal artery is altered over a range of 80 to 180 mmHg. As illustrated, pressure-induced vasoconstriction is elicited in the afferent arteriole, whereas the efferent arteriole does not respond to this stimulus. This observation is in accord with the concept that pre-glomerular vasoconstriction is an important mediator of the autoregulatory control of GFR and renal blood flow during elevations in renal perfusion pressure. Furthermore, these findings agree with early observations using glomeruli transplanted into the hamster cheek pouch,[97] and more recent observations by Edwards[74] and Steinhausen et al.[71] that myogenic tone is restricted to preglomerular vessels.

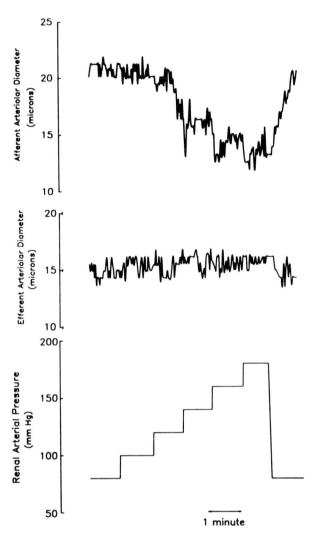

FIGURE 15. Representative tracings depicting the response of the afferent arteriole and efferent arteriole of isolated perfused hydronephrotic kidney to alterations in renal arterial pressure. Increasing pressure in the renal artery (bottom) elicited a vasoconstriction of the afferent arteriole (top), but not of the efferent arteriole (center).

Calcium antagonists reverse pressure-induced afferent arteriolar vasoconstriction in the isolated perfused hydronephrotic kidney. The photomicrographs depicted in Figure 16 demonstrate vividly the ability of calcium antagonists to dilate the afferent arteriole of a hydronephrotic kidney when administered at an elevated renal arterial pressure. As illustrated, diltiazem increased renal perfusate flow when administered to a kidney perfused at 140 mmHg (lower panel). Photomicrographs of the microcirculation, depicted in the upper panel of Figure 16, illustrate the vasodilation of the

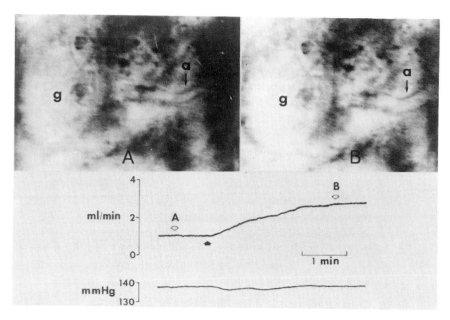

FIGURE 16. Photomicrographs of a hydronephrotic kidney perfused in vitro at 140 mmHg. Tracing of renal arterial pressure and perfusate flow to the kidney are depicted on the lower panel. Afferent arteriole (a) and adjoining glomerulus (g) are identified in video images obtained before (A) and after administration of diltiazem (solid arrow). A vasodilation of the afferent arteriole is clearly discernible. Reproduced with permission from Loutzenhiser et al., Am J Cardiol, 1987.[93]

afferent arteriole that occurred during this manipulation. The diameter of the afferent arteriole ("a") in the image obtained following the administration of diltiazem ("B", right panel) is clearly greater that that observed before the calcium antagonists ("A", left panel).

Our laboratory reported that isolated hydronephrotic kidneys from hypertensive animals exhibit unimpaired afferent arteriolar responsiveness to pressure.[95,96] Maximal activation occurred at perfusion pressures that were within the range of blood pressures measured in the donor animals, suggesting that pressure-dependent afferent arteriolar tone might contribute to basal renal vascular tone in these animals.[98] Nifedipine completely inhibited the myogenic response of afferent arterioles from both SHR and WKY[95,96] (Figs. 17 and 18). The ability of calcium antagonists to inhibit pressure-induced afferent arteriolar vasoconstriction may provide an explanation for the observation that the renal hemodynamic response to calcium antagonists is often elevated in the setting of systemic hypertension.[2]

Finally, as discussed above, Harder et al.[77] demonstrated that verapamil abolishes pressure-induced vascular tone in isolated interlobular arteries from the dog. The ability of calcium antagonists to inhibit this type of vasoconstriction suggests that potential-dependent calcium channels are activated in response to pressure. Indeed, Harder and co-workers have demonstrated that elevated transmural pressure elicits a membrane depolarization in resistance vessels from the kidney and brain.[77,99,100] In pial arteries, this "myogenic" response to pressure is abolished by removal of the endothelium, suggesting that the response of these vessels to pressure involves an endothelial-derived factor.[100]

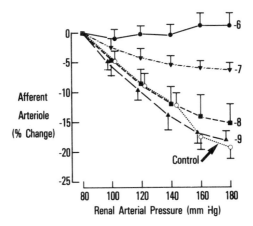

FIGURE 17. Inhibition by nifedipine of pressure-induced afferent arteriolar vasoconstriction in isolated perfused hydronephrotic kidneys. Open circles represent changes in vessel diameters in response to graded increases in renal arterial pressure observed in the absence of calcium antagonists. Closed symbols represent the responses obtained after pretreatment with nifedipine (concentrations indicated as log M values on right). Note that nifedipine produced a dose-dependent inhibition of pressure-induced vasoconstriction. Reproduced with permission from Hayashi et al. , Circ Res, 1989.[95]

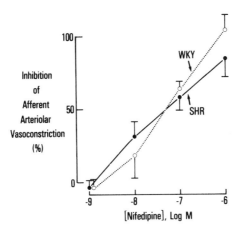

FIGURE 18. Dose-response curves subtending the reversal by nifedipine of pressure-induced afferent arteriolar vasoconstriction in isolated perfused hydronephrotic kidneys obtained from normotensive (WKY) and hypertensive (SHR) rats. Note that nifedipine was equipotent in inhibiting pressure-induced afferent arteriolar vasoconstriction in these two models. Reproduced with permission from Hayashi et al. , Circ Res, 1989. [95]

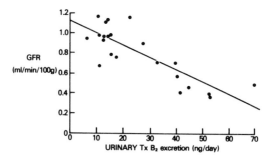

FIGURE 19.   Correlation between glomerular filtration rate and urinary thromboxane B_2 excretion in rats treated with cyclosporin A (40 mg/kg/48 hr) (R = -0.82; p < 0. 01; n = 22). Reproduced with permission from Perico et al., Am J Physiol, 1986.[105]

Summary.   In summary, evidence from a wide variety of experimental approaches indicates that pressure-dependent tone in preglomerular resistance vessels is abolished by calcium antagonists. It is likely that the response of these vessels to pressure is mediated by a depolarization-induced activation of potential-dependent calcium channels.

Reversal by Calcium Antagonists of the Renal Effects of Thromboxane A₂

Thromboxane A₂ as a Potential Mediator of Renal Dysfunction

In the preceding sections, we have examined the effects of calcium antagonists on the renal response to vasoconstrictor stimuli that are considered to mediate normal renal vascular tone (i.e., NE, ANG II, neural stimulation, pressure). In this final section, we consider the effects of these agents on the renal actions of thromboxane A_2, a vasoconstrictor thought to mediate the deranged renal hemodynamics associated with a number of clinical disorders.

Thromboxane A_2 (TBX) has been implicated in the alterations in renal hemo-dynamics associated with a number of experimental models of renal insufficiency, including glycerol-induced renal failure,[101] nephrotoxic serum nephritis,[102] renal venous constriction,[103] and ureteral obstruction.[104] In addition, a potential role of TBX in the development of cyclosporine A-induced nephrotoxicity has been proposed (Fig. 19)[105]. Finally, it has been suggested that TBX may be involved in the reduced postgraft function of transplanted kidneys.[106,107] Accordingly, the actions of calcium antagonists on the renal response to thromboxane A_2 may have important clinical implications.

Reversal of the Renal Effects of Thromboxane Mimetic U44069

The unstable chemical nature of thromboxane A_2 precludes direct investigations into the renal effects of this agent. The chemical half life of the prostanoid is approximately 30 sec.[108] This problem can be circumvented, however, by the use of stable prostanoid derivatives that mimic the biological actions of thromboxane A_2, such as the epoxymethano-derivatives of PGH_2, U44069, and U46119.[109] These compounds are potent vasoconstrictors,[110] reduce GFR when administered in vivo,[111,112] and have been shown to elicit contraction in cultured mesangial cells.[113]

Our laboratory has demonstrated that calcium antagonists completely reverse the decrement in GFR that is induced by U44069.[114] Figure 20 illustrates the striking effects of U44069 on GFR of the isolated perfused kidney. In this preparation, U44069 reduced GFR by $82 \pm 3\%$, but reduced RPF by only $13 \pm 8\%$. Diltiazem completely restored GFR (Fig. 20) with a dose-dependency that corresponded precisely with that subtending its inhibitory actions on U44069-induced tension development and ^{45}Ca uptake in isolated vascular smooth muscle.[114] In contrast, we observed that diltiazem did not inhibit U44069-induced contraction in isolated glomeruli.[114]

In a preliminary report, we recently demonstrated that U44069 elicited a predominantly afferent arteriolar vasocontriction in the isolated perfused hydronephrotic kidney that was reversed by diltiazem.[115] Thus, 1.0 μM U44069 caused a 28% decrement in afferent arteriolar diameter (i. e. from 18.4 to 13.2 μm), but elicited only a 7% decrement in efferent arteriolar diameter (i.e., from 15. 5 to 14. 4 μm). This preferential afferent effect of U44069 may explain its striking ability to reduce GFR (Fig. 20). Diltiazem reversed the U44069-induced afferent arteriolar vasoconstriction with a dose-dependency identical to that subtending its reversal of the U44069-induced decrement in GFR of normal kidneys perfused under identical in vitro conditions.[115]

The ability of calcium antagonists to reverse U44069-induced afferent arteriolar vasoconstriction is graphically illustrated by the photomicrographs depicted in Figure 21. In this instance, nifedipine completely returned afferent arteriolar diameter to control levels in the presence of the thromboxane mimetic. In parallel studies, nifedipine was demonstrated to also reverse the U44069-induced decrement in GFR of normal perfused kidneys.[44]

In concert, these observations suggest that thromboxane A_2 is a potent renal vasoconstrictor that acts predominantly on preglomerular vessels. Furthermore, calcium antagonists represent an effective means of reversing thromboxane A_2- induced afferent arteriolar vasoconstriction. Through this mechanism, calcium antagonists augment GFR in the presence of thromboxane-induced vasoconstriction. A thromboxane A_2- induced mesangial contraction and a corresponding decrement in K_f have also been proposed to mediate the detrimental actions of thromboxane on the kidney.[113,116] The actions of calcium antagonists on this mechanism have not been fully ascertained. Nevertheless, the ability of calcium antagonists to reverse the microvascular and hemodynamic actions of thromboxane are intriguing. Further studies are required to delineate clinical implications of these findings (see Chapter 17).

Summary and Synthesis

In the preceding sections, we have reviewed the renal hemodynamic effects of calcium antagonists as assessed by observations in both in vivo and in vitro models. It is apparent that the renal effects of these agents vary considerably, depending on the experimental model and the setting in which they are administered. In general, the data obtained with in vitro techniques complement observations made in vivo. Thus, a number of inferences and generalizations may be drawn.

Basal Renal Vascular Resistance Is the Primary Determinant of the Renal Vasodilatory Response to Calcium Antagonists.   The magnitude of the renal vasodilation observed in response to calcium antagonist administration depends predominantly

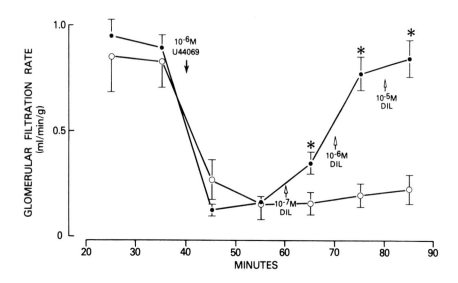

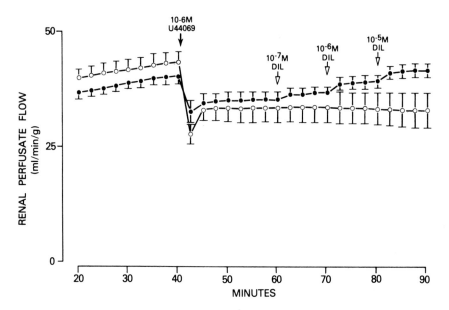

FIGURE 20. Reversal by diltiazem of the effects of the thromboxane A$_2$ mimetic U44069 on the isolated perfused rat kidney. U44069 (1 μM, open circles and solid circles) caused a striking decrease in GFR (upper panel) accompanied by a modest decrease in RPF (lower panel). Diltiazem (DIL, solid circles) completely reversed these effects in a dose-dependent manner. Reproduced with permission from Loutzenhiser et al., Am J Physiol, 1986.[114]

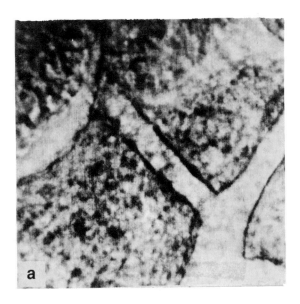

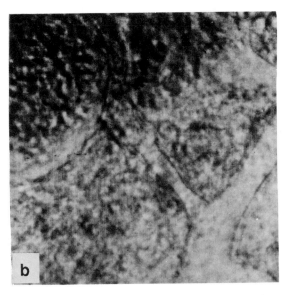

FIGURE 21. Photomicrographs of an isolated perfused hydronephrotic kidney during control perfusion (*A*), and the administration of the thromboxane A_2 mimetic U44069 (1.0 μM) *B*), followed by the administration of 1.0 μM nifedipine (*C*). U44069 caused an afferent arteriolar vasoconstriction (arrow) that was completely reversed by nifedipine. Reproduced with permission from Loutzenhiser and Epstein, Am J Nephrol, 1987.[44]

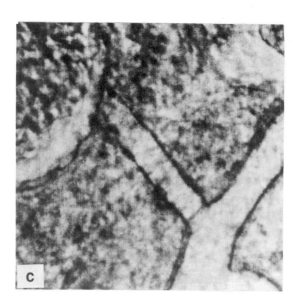

FIGURE 21 Continued.

on the level of underlying renal vascular tone. In the absence of renal vasoconstriction, calcium antagonists cause little change in renal hemodynamics. This is anticipated, since calcium antagonists promote vasodilation by countervailing vasoconstrictor mechanisms.

The above formulation may have important implications for understanding the nature of "basal" renal vascular tone. Since calcium antagonists have little effect on renal vascular resistance when they are administered to normotensive, well hydrated subjects,[2] it would appear that basal renal vascular tone is very low in this setting. Alternatively, it is possible that the vasoconstrictor mechanisms mediating normal basal renal vascular resistance are insensitive to the inhibitory actions of calcium antagonists, at least at therapeutic concentrations. In vitro studies indicate, however, that preglomerular vasoconstriction induced by pressure,[71,77,93,95] NE,[32] renal nerve stimulation,[55,118] ANG II,[79,81] and adenosine[118] are all inhibited by these agents.

The Nature of the Underlying Renal Vasoconstriction is a Primary Determinant of the Effects of Calcium Antagonists on GFR and Filtration Fraction. When administered to the vasoconstricted kidney, calcium antagonists predictably reduce renal vascular resistance, but exert variable effects on GFR and filtration fraction depending on the nature of the vasoconstrictor stimuli. In settings characterized by elevated efferent arteriolar tone, calcium antagonists increase filtration fraction. Thus, GFR is preferentially augmented when these agents are administered during ANG II-induced renal vasoconstriction.[24,17,43] In vitro studies suggest that this property derives from the ability of these agents to dilate preglomerular vessels selectively, while preserving efferent arteriolar tone (Fig. 22).

In contrast, this *preferential* effect on GFR is not observed in settings in which increased renal vascular resistance is predominantly afferent in nature (e.g. , U44069, KCl). In the isolated kidney, calcium antagonists exert equivalent effects on GFR and RPF in

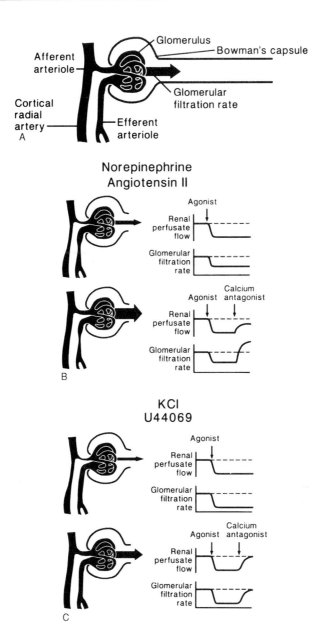

FIGURE 22. Schematic model (A) contrasting the effects of calcium antagonists in the presence of vasocontrictors that act on both afferent and efferent arterioles (B norepinephrine, angiotensin II) and vasoconstrictors that act primarily on the afferent arteriole (C KCl, U44069). When renal vasoconstriction is elicited by agents that act on both afferent and efferent arterioles, calcium antagonists preferentially dilate preglomerular vessels and augment GFR to control values or greater. In contrast renal perfusate flow (RPF) is only partially restored. When renal vasoconstriction is elicited by agents that act exclusively on the pre-glomerular vessels, calcium antagonists restore GFR and RPF in a parallel fashion.

such settings. Such considerations could conceivably contribute to the renal hemodynamic actions of calcium antagonists in hypertension, since it has been suggested that afferent arteriolar resistance is preferentially increased in hypertensives.[119]

Although we have proposed that the magnitude of renal vasoconstriction and the ratio of afferent to efferent resistances are *primary* determinants of the renal hemodynamic actions of calcium antagonists, other contributing factors must be considered. As discussed above, calcium antagonists increase K_f in some experimental settings. The sites mediating the effects of calcium antagonists on K_f and the determinants of the nonvascular effects of calcium antagonists on GFR require further clarification.

Calcium Antagonists Preferentially Act on Preglomerular Vessels.   As detailed above, indirect evidence suggests that calcium antagonists preferentially reduce preglomerular vascular resistance. Recent direct observations of the microvascular responses to calcium antagonists, utilizing the hydronephrotic kidney, and the perfused juxtamedullary nephron, confirm this postulate.[69,79,81] Thus, direct visualization utilizing these techniques has demonstrated that calcium antagonists completely reverse afferent arteriolar vasoconstriction but fail to reverse efferent arteriolar vasoconstriction.

In contrast, calculated segmental resistances based on data obtained from micropuncture studies suggest that calcium antagonists also exert an effect on efferent resistance.[21,55,57] The reasons for this ostensible discrepancy are not readily apparent, and further studies are required to address this issue.

Importance of Extrarenal Effects.   Finally, a caveat is in order. Although we have focused on the direct effects of calcium antagonists on the kidney, it must be emphasized that the net renal hemodynamic effects of these agents must also reflect extrarenal events. Clearly, the systemic actions of calcium antagonists and the attendant compensatory responses may contribute to the response of the kidney to the systemic administration of these agents. Such factors confound the interpretation of in vivo studies designed to investigate the renal actions of these agents. These considerations are important, however, in predicting the renal actions of these agents in clinical settings. Clearly, calcium antagonists are not renal-selective vasodilators, and the hypotensive actions of these agents can exert secondary effects on renal vascular tone and renal function.

Conclusions

It has been more than two decades since Fleckenstein and coworkers first demonstrated the "calcium antagonistic" actions of verapamil.[1] Within a relatively short span of time, this important class of vasodilators has been catapulted into the forefront of clinical pharmacology. Nevertheless, it is only recently that attention has been directed toward the renal actions of these agents. Although it is clear that calcium antagonists have major renal hemodynamic effects, the determinants and scope of these actions have not been completely defined. We believe that investigations during the next several years in this field will be enlightening. Future studies directed toward delineating the intrarenal sites of action of calcium antagonists and the determinants of their intrarenal actions will lead to a greater understanding of the renal hemodynamic effects of these agents. Final resolution of the pharmacologic basis for the renal hemodynamic actions of calcium antagonists requires a more complete understanding of the divergent mechanisms utilized to activate the microvasculature of the kidney.

References

1. Fleckenstein A, Kammermeier H, Doring HJ, Freund HJ: Zum wirjungsmechanismus neuartiger koronardilatoren mit gleichzeitig sauerstoff-einsparenden myokard-effeckten, prenylamin und iropveratril. Z Kreislaufforsch 56:716–744, 1967.

2. Loutzenhiser R, Epstein M: Effects of calcium antagonists on renal hemodynamics. Am J Physiol 249:F616–F629, 1985.

3. Leonetti G, Cuspidi C, Sampieri L, et al: Comparison of cardiovascular, renal and humeral effects of acute administration of two calcium channel blockers in normotensive and hypertensive subjects. J Cardiovasc Pharmacol 4:S319–S324, 1982.

4. Wallia R, Greenberg A, Puschett JB: Renal hemodynamic and tubular transport effects of nitrendipine. J Lab Clin Med 105:498–503, 1985.

5. Van Schaik BAM, Van Nistelrooy AEJ, Geyskes GG: Antihypertensive and renal effects of nicardipine. J Lab Clin Med 105:498–503, 1985.

6. Yokoyama S, Kaburagi T: Clinical effects of intravenous nifedipine on renal function. J Cardiovasc Pharmacol 5:67–71, 1983.

7. Klutsch K, Schmidt P, Grosswendt J: Der einfluss von BAY a 1040 auf die Nierenfunktion des Hypertonikers. Arztneimittelforsch 22:377–380, 1972.

8. Sakurai T, Kurita T, Nagano S, Sonoda T: Antihypertensive vasodilating and sodium diuretic actions of D-cis isomer of benzothiazepine derivative (CRD-401) Acta Urol Jpn 18:695–701, 1972.

9. Blackshear JL, Garnic D, Williams GH: Exaggerated renal vasodilator response to calcium entry blockade in first-degree relatives of essential hypertensive subjects. Hypertension 9:384–389, 1987.

9a. Montanari A, Vallisa D, Ragni G, et al.: Abnormal renal responses to calcium entry blockade in normotensive offspring of hypertensive parents. Hypertension 12:498–505, 1988.

10. Sunderrajan S, Reams G, Bauer J: Renal effects of diltiazem in primary hypertension. Hypertension 8:238–242, 1986.

11. Reams GP, Hamory A, Lau A, Bauer JH: Effect of nifedipine on renal function in patients with essential hypertension. Hypertension 11:452–456, 1988.

12. Amodeo C, Kobrin I, Ventura HO, et al: Immediate and short-term hemodynamic effects of diltiazem in patients with hypertension. Circulation 73:108–113, 1986.

13. Isshiki T, Amodeo C, Messerli FH, et. al: Diltiazem maintains renal vasodilation without hyperfiltration: Studies in essential hypertensive man and the spontaneously hypertensive rats. Cardiovasc Drugs Ther 1:359–366, 1987.

14. Ribstein J, Mourad G, Mimran A: Contrasting acute effects of captopril and nifedipine on renal function in renovascular hypertension. Am J Hypertens 1:239–244, 1988.

15. Blythe WB: Captopril and renal autoregulation. N Engl J Med 308:390–391, 1983.

16. Brody MJ, Barron KW, Faber JE, et al: Effects of nitrendipine and nisoldipine on arterial pressure and regional hemodynamics in the conscious rat. In Scriabine A, Vanov S, Deck K (eds): Nitrendipine. Baltimore and Munich, Urban & Schwarzenberg, 1984, pp 271–279.

17. Bell AJ, Lindner A: Effects of verapamil and nifedipine on renal function and hemodynamics in the dog. Renal Physiol 7:329–343, 1984.

18. Abe Y, Okahara T, Yamamoto K: Effect of D-3-acetoxy-2-3-dihydro-5-2-(dimethylamino)ethyl-2-(p-methoxyphenyl)-1-5-benzothiazepin-4(5H)-one-hydrochloride (CRD) on renal function in the dog. Jpn Circ J 36:1002–1003, 1972.

19. Goldberg JP, Schrier RW: Effects of calcium membrane blockers on in vivo vasoconstrictor properties of norepinephrine, angiotensin II and vasopresin. Miner Electrolyte Metab 10:178–183, 1984.

20. Hof RP: The calcium antagonists PY 108-068 and verapamil diminish the effects of angiotensin II: Sites of interaction in the peripheral circulation of anesthetized cats. Br J Pharmacol 82:51–60, 1984.

21. Ichikawa I, Miele JF, Brenner BM: Reversal of renal cortical actions of angiotensin II by verapamil and manganese. Kidney Int 16:137–147, 1979.

22. Seino M, Abe K, Ito S, et al: Effects of nifedipine on renal vascular responses to vasoactive agents in rabbits. Tohoku J Exp Med 142:67–76, 1984.

23. Yamaguchi I, Ikezawa K, Takada T, Kiyomoto A: Studies on a new 1,5-benzothiazepine derivative (CRD-401). VI. Effects on renal blood flow and renal function. Jpn J Pharmacol 24:511–522, 1974.

24. Huelsemann JL, Sterzel B, McKenzie DE, Wilcox CS: Effects of a calcium entry blocker on blood pressure and renal function during angiotensin-induced hypertension. Hypertension 7:374–379, 1985.

25. Ishikawa H; Matsushima M, Matsui H, et al: Effects of diltiazem hydrochloride (CRD-401) on renal hemodynamics of dogs. Arzneim Forsch/Drug Res 28:402–406, 1978.

26. Maclaughlin M, De Mello Aires M, Malnic G: Verapamil effect on renal function of normotensive and hypertensive rats. Renal Physiol 8:112–119, 1985.

27. Bolt GR, Saxene PR: Acute systemic and regional effects of felodipine, a new calcium antagonist, in conscious renal hypertensive rabbits. J Cardiovasc Pharmacol 6:707–712, 1984.

28. Steele TH, Challoner-Hue L: Glomerular response to verapamil by isolated spontaneously hypertensive rat kidney. Am J Physiol 248:F668–F673, 1985.

29. Steele TH, Challoner-Hue L: Response of isolated Dahl rat kidney to calcium antagonists. Kidney Int 31:941–945, 1987.

30. Steele Th, Challoner-Hue L: Influence of salt on response to nitrendipine by Dahl rat kidney. Am J Physiol 252:F487–F490, 1987.

31. Steele Th, Challoner-Hue L: Increased response to calcium channel agonist by Dahl S rat kidney Am J Physiol 254:F533–F539, 1988.

32. Loutzenhiser R, Epstein M, Horton C, Sonke P: Reversal by the calcium antagonists nisoldipine of norepinephrine-induced reduction of GFR: Evidence for preferential antagonism of preglomerular vasoconstriction. J Pharmacol Exp Ther 232:382–387, 1985.

33. Loutzenhiser R, Horton C, Epstein M: Effects of diltiazem and manganese on real hemodynamics: Studies in the isolated perfused rat kidney. Nephron 39:382–388, 1985.

34. Maack T: Physiological evaluation of the isolated perfused rat kidney. Am J Physiol 238:F71–F78, 1980.

35. Poiseuille JLM: Recherches experimentales sur le mouvement des liquides dans les tubes de tres-petits diametres, Memoires Presentes par divers savants, a L'Acad Sci de L'Institut de France 9:433–448, 1846.

36. DeMello G, Maack T: Nephron function of the isolated perfused rat kidney. Am J Physiol 231:1699–1707, 1976.

37. Bell PD: Calcium antagonists and intrarenal regulation of glomerular filtration rate. Am J Nephrol 7 (suppl 1):24–31, 1987.

38. Epstein M, Flamenbaum W, Loutzenhiser R: Characterization of the renin-angiotensin system in the isolated perfused rat kidney. Renal Physiol 2:244–256, 1979.

39. Hofbauer KG, Zschiedrich H, Rauh W, et al: Conversion of angiotensin I into angiotensin II in the isolated perfused rat kidney. Clin Sci 44:447–456, 1973.

40. Haufbauer KG, Zschiedrich H, Rauh W, et al: Reaction of endogenous renin with exogenous renin substrate within the isolated perfused rat kidney. Proc Soc Exp Biol Med 142:796–799, 1973.

41. Dzau VJ: Circulating verses local renin- angiotensin system in cardiovascular homeostasis. Circulation 77 (suppl I):4–13, 1986.

42. Marre M, Misumi J, De Raemsch K, et al: Diuretic and natriuretic effect of nifedipine on isolated perfused rat kidney. J Pharmacol Exp Ther 223:263–270, 1982.

43. Loutzenhiser R, Epstein M, Horton, C: Modification by dihydropyridine type calcium antagonists of the renal hemodynamic response to vasoconstrictors. J Cardiovasc Pharmacol 9 (suppl 1):S70–S75, 1987.

44. Loutzenhiser R, Epstein M: Modification by calcium antagonists of the renal hemodynamic response to vasoconstrictors. Am J Nephrol 7(suppl 1):7–16, 1987.

45. Loutzenhiser R, Epstein M, Hayashi K: Renal hemodynamic effects of calcium antagonists. Am J Cardiol 64 (suppl): Sept 1989 (in press).

46. Steele TH, Challoner-Hue L: Renal interactions between norepinephrine and calcium antagonists. Kidney Int 26:719–724, 1984.

47. Cauvin C, Loutzenhiser R, van Breemen C: Mechanisms of calcium antagonist-induced vasodilation. Annu Rev Pharmacol 23:373–396, 1983.

48. Meisheri K, Hwang O, van Breemen C: Evidence for two separate Ca^{+2} pathways in smooth muscle plasmalemma. J Membr Biol 59:19–25, 1981.

49. Hess P, Lansman JB, Tsein RW: Different modes of Ca channel gating behavior favored by dihydropyridine Ca agonists and antagonists. Nature 311:538–544, 1984.

50. van Breemen C: Blockade of membrane calcium fluxes by lanthanum in relation to vascular smooth muscle contractility. Int Arch Physiol Biochem 77:710–717, 1969.

51. Deth D, Lynch C: Inhibition of alpha-receptor induced Ca^{+2} release and Ca^{+2} influx by Mn^{+2} and La^{+3}. Eur J Pharmacol 71:1–11, 1981.

52. Hagiwara S, Byerly L: Calcium channel. Annu Rev Neurosci 4:69–125, 1981.

53. Cauvin C, van Breemen C: Effects of Ca^{+2} antagonists on isolated rabbit mesenteric resistance vessels as compared to rabbit aorta. In Fleckenstein, van Breemen, Gross, Hoffmeister (eds): Cardiovascular Effects of Dihydropyridine-type Calcium Antagonists and Agonists. Berline, Springer-Verlag, 1985, pp 259–269.

54. Rusch NJ, Hermsmeyer K: Calcium currents are altered in the vascular muscle cell membrane of spontaneously hypertensive rats. Circ Res 63:997–1002, 1988.

55. Pelayo JC: Modulation of renal adrenergic effector mechanisms by calcium entry blockers. Am J Physiol 252:F613–F620, 1987.

56. Anderson S, Clarey LE, Riley SL, Troy JL: Acute infusion of calcium blockers (CCB) reduces glomerular capillary pressure (P_{GC} in rats with reduced renal mass. Kidney Int 33:370 (abs), 1988.

57. Yoshioka T, Shiraga H, Yoshida Y, et al: "Intact nephrons" as the primary origin of proteinuria in chronic renal disease. Study in the rat model of subtotal nephrectomy. J Clin Invest 82:1614–1623, 1988.

58. Pelayo JC, Harris DCH, Shanley PF, et al: Glomerular hemodynamic adaptations in remnant nephrons: Effects of verapamil. Am J Physiol 254:F425–F431, 1988.

59. Dworkin LD, Benstein J, Feiner HD, Parker M: Nifedipine prevents glomerular injury without reducing glomerular pressure (P_{GC}) in rats with desoxycorticosterone-salt (DOC-SALT) hypertension. Kidney Int 33:374 (abs), 1988.

60. Motulsky HJ, Snavely MD, Hughes RJ, Insel PA: Interaction of verapamil and other calcium channel blockers with a1- and a2-adrenergic receptors. Circ Res 52:226–231, 1983.

61. Triggle DJ, Swamy VC: Calcium antagonists: some chemical-pharmacologic aspects. Circ Res 52 (suppl I):17–28, 1983.

62. Saida K, van Breemen C: Inhibiting effect of diltiazem on intracellular Ca^{+2} release in vascular smooth muscle. Blood Vessels 20:105–108, 1983.

63. Saida K, van Breemen C: Mechanism of Ca^{++} antagonist-induced vasodilation. Intracellular actions. Circ Res 52:137–142, 1983.

64. Hof R, Scholtysik G, Loutzenhiser R, et. al: PN 200–110, A new calcium antagonist: Electrophysiological ino- and chromotropic effects on guinea pig myocardial tissue and effects on contraction and calcium uptake of rabbit aorta. J Cardiovasc Pharmacol 6:399–406, 1984.

65. Click R, Gilmore JP, Joyner WL: Direct affect of norepinephrine and angiotensin II on afferent and efferent arterioles of renal allografts in hamster. Fed Proc 35:1381, 1976.

66. Steinhausen M, Snoei H, Parekh N, et al: Hydronephrosis: A new method to visualize vas afference, efferens, and glomerular network. Kidney Int 23:794–806, 1983.

67. Altschul R; Fedor S: Vascular changes in hydronephrosis. Am Hear J 46:291–295, 1953.

68. Rao NR, Heptinstall RH: Experimental hydronephrosis: A microangiographic study. Invest Urol 6:183–204, 1968.

69. Fleming JT, Parekh N, Steinhausen M: Calcium antagonists preferentially dilate pre-glomerular vessels of hydronephrotic kidney. Am J Physiol 253:F1157–F1163, 1987.

70. Fleming JT, Garthoff B, Mayer D, et. al: Comparison of the effects of antihypertensive drugs on pre- and postglomerular vessels of the hydronephrotic kidney. J Cardiovasc Pharmacol 10 (suppl 10):S149–S153, 1987.

71. Steinhausen M, Fleming JT, Holtz FG, Parekh N: Nitrendipine and the pressure-dependent vasodilation of vessels in the hydronephrotic kidney. J Cardiovasc Pharmacol 9 (suppl I):39–43, 1987.

72. Steinhausen M, Weis S, Fleming J, et al: Responses of in vivo renal microvessels to dopamine. Kidney Int 30:361–370, 1986a.

73. Steinhausen M, Kucherer H, Parekh N, et al: Angiotensin II control of the renal microcirculation: Effect of blockade by saralasin. Kidney Int 30:56–61, 1986.

74. Edwards RM: Segmental effects of norepinephrine and angiotensin II on isolated renal microvessels. Am J Physiol 244:F526–F534, 1983.

75. Edwards RM, Weidley EF: Lack of effect of atriopeptin II on rabbit glomerular arterioles in vitro. Am J Physiol 252:F317–F321, 1987.

76. Edwards RM, Trizna W: Characterization of alpha-adrenoceptors on isolated rabbit arterioles. Am J Physiol 254:F178–F183, 1988.

77. Harder DR, Gilbert R, Lombard JH: Vascular muscle cell depolarization and activation in renal arteries on elevation of transmural pressure. Am J Physiol 253:F778–F781, 1987.

78. Casellas D, Navar LG: In vitro perfusion of juxtamedullary nephrons in rats. Am J Physiol 246:F349–F358, 1984.

79. Carmines PK, Navar LG: Desparate effects of calcium channel blockade on afferent and efferent arteriolar responses to angiotensin. Am J Physiol, 1989, (in press).

80. Loutzenhiser R, Hayashi K, Epstein, M: Atrial natriuretic peptide reverses afferent arteriolar vasoconstriction and promotes efferent arteriolar vasoconstriction in the isolated perfused rat kidney. J Pharmacol Exp Ther 246:522–528, 1988.

81. Loutzenhiser R, Hayashi K, Epstein M: Calcium antagonists augment glomerular filtration rate of angiotensin II-vasoconstricted isolated perfused rat kidneys by dilating afferent but not efferent arterioles. J Cardiovasc Pharmacol S149, 1988.

82. Navar LG, Champion WJ, Thomas CE: Effects of calcium channel blockade on renal vascular resistance responses to changes in perfusion pressure and angiotensin-converting enzyme inhibition in dogs. Circ Res 58:874–881, 1986.

83. Loutzenhiser R, Hayashi K, Epstein M: Divergent effects of KCl- induced depolarization of afferent and efferent arterioles. Am J Physiol, 1989 (in press).

84. Buhrle CP, Nobiling R, Taugner R: Intracellular recordings from renin-positive cells of the afferent glomerular arteriole. Am J Physiol 249:F272–F281, 1985.

85. Bevan JA, Bevan RD, Hwa JJ, et al: Calcium regulation in vascular smooth muscle: Is there a pattern to its variability within the arterial tree: J Cardiovasc Pharmacol 8(suppl 8):S71–S75, 1986.

86. Cauvin C, Saida K, van Breemen C: Extracellular Ca^{+2} dependence and diltiazem inhibition of contraction in rabbit conduit arteries and mesenteric resistance vessels. Blood Vessels 21:23–31, 1984.

87. Gattone VH, Luft FC, Evan AP: Renal afferent and efferent arterioles of the rabbit. Am J Physiol 247:F219–F228, 1984.

88. Navar LG: Renal autoregulation: Perspectives from whole kidney and single nephron studies. Am J Physiol 234:F357–F370, 1978.

89. Navar GL, Rosivall L: Contribution of the renin-angiotensin system to the control on intrarenal hemodynamics. Kidney Int 25:857–868, 1984.

90. Lin H, Young DB: Verapamil alters the relationship between renal perfusion pressure and glomerular filtration rate and renin release: The mechanism of the antihypertensive effect. J Cardiovasc Pharmacol 12 (suppl 6):S57–S59, 1988.

91. Ono H, Kokubun H, Hashimoto K: Abolition by calcium antagonists of the autoregulation of renal blood flow. Naunyn Schmiedebergs Arch Pharmacol 285:201–207, 1974.

92. Cohen AJ, Fray JCS: Calcium ion dependence of myogenic renal plasma flow autoregulation: Evidence from the isolated perfused rat kidney. J Physiol (Lond) 330:449–460, 1982.

93. Loutzenhiser R, Epstein M, Horton C: Inhibition by diltiazem of pressure-induced afferent vasoconstriction of the isolated perfused rat kidney. Am J Cardiol 59:72A–75A, 1987.

94. Loutzenhiser R, Epstein M: Calcium antagonists and the renal hemodynamic response to vasoconstrictors. Ann NY Acad Sci 522:771–784, 1988.

95. Hayashi K, Epstein M, Loutzenhiser R: Pressure-induced vasoconstriction of renal microvessels in normotensive and hypertensive rats: Studies in the isolated perfused hydronephrotic kidney. Circ Res 1989, (in press).

96. Loutzenhiser R, Hayashi K, Epstein M: Effects of nifedipine on pressure-induced affer-

ent arteriolar vasoconstriction in isolated perfused hydronephrotic kidneys from normotensive and hypertensive rats. Blood Vessels 25:40 (abs), 1988.

97. Gilmore JP, Cornish KG, Rogers SD, Joyner WL: Direct evidence for myogenic autoregulation of the renal microcirculation in the hamster. Circ Res 47:226–230, 1980.

98. Arendshorst WJ, Beierwaltes WH: Renal and nephron hemodynamics in spontaneously hypertensive rats. Am J Physiol 236:F246–F251, 1979.

99. Harder DR: Pressure dependent membrane depolarization in cat middle cerebral artery. Circ Res 47:226–230, 1984.

100. Harder DR: Pressure-induced myogenic activation of cat cerebral arteries is dependent on intact endothelium. Circ Res 60:102–107, 1987.

101. Benabe JE, Klahr S, Hoffman MH, Morrison AR: Production of thromboxane A_2 by the kidney in glycerol-induced acute renal failure. Prostaglandins 19:333–347, 1980.

102. Lianos EA, Andres GA, Dunn MJ: Glomerular prostaglandin and thromboxane synthesis in rat nephrotoxic serum nephritis. J Clin Invest 72:1439–1448, 1983.

103. Zipser R, Meyers S, Needleman P: Exaggerated prostaglandin and thromboxane synthesis in the rabbit with renal vein constriction. Circ Res 47:231–237, 1980.

104. Morrison AR, Nishikawa K, Needleman P: Thromboxane A_2 biosynthesis in the ureter obstructed isolated perfused kidney of the rabbit. J Pharmacol Exp Ther 205:1–8, 1978.

105. Perico N, Benigni A, Zoja C, et al: Functional significance of exaggerated renal thromboxane A_2 synthesis induced by cyclosporine A. Am J Physiol 251:F581–F587, 1986.

106. Coffman TM, Yarger WE, Klotman PE: Functional role of thromboxane production by acutely rejecting renal allografts in rats. J Clin Invest 75:1242–1248, 1985.

107. Mangino MJ, Brunt EM, von Doersten P, Anderson CB: Effects of the thromboxane synthesis inhibitor CGS-12970 on experimental acute renal allograft rejection. J Pharmacol Exp Ther 248:23–28, 1989.

108. Hamberg M, Svensson J, Samuelsson B: Thromboxanes: a new group of biologically active compounds derived from prostaglandin endoperoxides. Proc Natl Acad Sci 72:2994–2998, 1975.

109. Malmsten C: Some biological effects of prostaglandin endoperoxide analogs. Life Sci 18:169–176, 1976.

110. Loutzenhiser R, van Breemen C: Mechanism of activation of isolated rabbit aorta by PGH_2 analogue U–44069. Am J Physiol 241:C243-C249, 1981.

111. Gerber JG, Ellis E, Hollified J, Neis A: Effect of prostaglandin endoperoxide analogue on canine renal function, hemodynamics and renin release. Eur J Pharmacol 53:239–246, 1979.

112. Feigen L, Chapnick BM, Flemming JE, et al: Renal vascular effects of endoperoxide analogs, prostaglandins, and arachidonic acid. Am J Physiol 233:H573–H579, 1977.

113. Mene P, Dunn MJ: Contractile effects of TXA_2 and endoperoxide analogues on cultured rat glomerular mesangial cells. Am J Physiol 251:F1029–F1035, 1986.

114. Loutzenhiser R, Epstein M, Horton C, Sonke P: Reversal of renal and smooth muscle actions of the thromboxane mimetic U-44069 by diltiazem. Am J Physiol 250:F619–F626, 1986.

115. Epstein M, Hayashi K, Loutzenhiser R: Direct evidence that thromboxane mimetic U44069 preferentially constricts the afferent arteriole. Kidney Int 35:291 (abs), 1989.

116. Scharschmidt LA, Lianos E, Dunn MJ: Arachidonate metabolites and the control of glomerular function. Fed Proc 42:3058–3063, 1983.

117. Mejia G, Challoner-Hue L, Steele TH: Calcium in neural control of renal circulation. Am J Physiol 247:F739–F745, 1984.

118. Rossi N, Churchill P, Ellis V, Amore B: Mechanism of adenosine receptor-induced renal vasoconstriction in rats. Am J Physiol 255:H885–H890, 1988.

119. Gothberg G, Lundin S, Richsten S, Folkow B: Apparent and true vascular resistances to flow in SHR and NCR kidneys as related to the pre/postglomerular resistance ratio. Acta Physiol Scand 105:282–294, 1979.

Thomas H. Steele, M.D.

4

Renal Responses to Calcium-Entry Modulators: Alteration by Genetic Hypertension and Dietary Salt

Calcium Entry and Salt in Genetic Hypertension

Calcium channel blockers are efficacious in reducing blood pressure exceptionally well in certain hypertensive patients. Data are available suggesting that patients most responsive to calcium channel blockers often manifest subtle abnormalities of calcium metabolism, suggesting a relative calcium deficiency state.[1-3] In addition, their hypertension is more likely to be exacerbated by a high NaCl intake.[4] Nevertheless the "calcium deficiency hypothesis" of hypertension has come under criticism because dietary calcium supplementation in hypertensives has produced variable results and only modest decrements in blood pressure.[5] Also, the elevation of cytosol calcium in vascular smooth muscle during calcium supplementation presumably would further augment vascular tone—a situation that would promote rather than alleviate hypertension. However the removal of calcium that is bound to cell membranes of vascular smooth muscle can result in increased contractility secondary to an increase in calcium influx *via* specific membrane calcium channels.[6,7] Presumably these calcium channels remain in the "closed" or "inactivated" state a greater fraction of the time when the amount of membrane-bound calcium is normal or increased. When membrane-bound calcium is depleted, the calcium channels would spend a greater fraction of time in the "open" state, thereby promoting calcium influx and vascular contractility.

Pathophysiology of Salt-sensitive Hypertension

What mechanisms could foster the development of a calcium deficiency state in salt-sensitive hypertension? Inbred salt-sensitive hypertensive Dahl rats (DS) of the Rapp strain manifested hypercalciuria when compared to their salt-resistant (DR) counterparts, but only in early life.[8] The DS rat kidneys also contained diminished parathyroid hormone-stimulated adenylate cyclase, an abnormality that could contribute to hypercalciuria. Although not yet explored in detail, there is little direct evidence that calcium deficiency or hypercalciuria is consistently present in any subgroup of human hypertensives.[9] Calcium supplementation has been reported to lower blood pressure in the DS rat *via* a neural mechanism, not because of altered vascular reactivity *per se*.[10] The neural mechanism underlying the hypotensive action of calcium probably is extrarenal, because current evidence suggests that renal denervation has little effect on DS rat hypertension.[11] Transplantation studies suggest that salt-dependent hypertension in the DS rat is caused by the kidneys, in that the genetic kidney-type determines the degree of susceptibility of the blood pressure to dietary NaCl.[12] Isolated perfused DS rat kidneys excrete sodium sluggishly compared to their DR kidney counterparts,[13,14] although the amount of sodium retained by the intact DS rat during acute volume expansion appears to be modest.[15] The isolated perfused Kyoto spontaneously hypertensive rat (SHR) kidney also excretes less sodium at any given perfusion pressure than its Wistar-Kyoto (WKY) counterpart.[16] Transplantation studies utilizing the F_1 hybrid progeny of SHR-WKY matings have indicated that the kidneys are likely to be at least partially responsible for SHR hypertension.[17] Hypertension in the Kyoto SHR is only partially salt dependent, in that increased dietary NaCl superimposes an additional increment upon already elevated SHR blood pressure.[18]

It seems plausible that calcium channel antagonists and agonists might affect kidney function uniquely in experimental hypertension if abnormal membrane calcium flux regulation is present. Furthermore, experimental hypertension models in which the kidneys play a key role in pathogenesis would likely manifest aberrant *renal* responses to calcium channel modulators.

Kidney Function in Hypertension Models

In order to study kidney function in animal hypertension models without the risk of concomitant changes in extrarenal humoral, neural and circulatory factors, we made use of an oxygenated isolated perfused rat kidney preparation that allows precise control of the perfusion pressure, temperature, and pH.[19] We employed a recirculating cell-free perfusate containing albumin as an oncotic agent, with glucose and amino acids as metabolic fuels. Its electrolyte composition approximates that of normal extracellular fluid in the rat.

The same protocol was used for all the isolated kidney calcium antagonist studies. During the initial control phase, we measured the glomerular filtration rate (GFR), renal vascular resistance (RVR), and sodium excretion. Next, sufficient norepinephrine was infused to increase the RVR by 50% over the original control value. This also decreased the GFR by more than 50%.[20] A calcium antagonist was then superimposed upon norepinephrine and final measurements of GFR, RVR and sodium excretion made. The renal perfusion pressure was maintained constant throughout these maneuvers.

Initially, we studied kidneys isolated from normal male Sprague-Dawley rats.[20] The addition of verapamil or diltiazem to perfusates of kidneys previously vasoconstricted by norepinephrine evoked large increases in GFR—with the values rebounding to levels significantly exceeding the original control levels prior to norepinephrine.[20] Sodium excretion tended to change in parallel with the GFR. When administered in the absence of vasoconstrictors, these calcium antagonists did not elicit significant changes in hemodynamics or function of other isolated kidneys. The RVR did not return entirely to control during calcium antagonist superimposition upon norepinephrine, an observation also noted by investigators in other laboratories.[21] Adding the calcium channel blockers prior to norepinephrine in "reverse order" also produced similar increases in GFR during the final phase.[20]

These glomerular responses to calcium antagonists by the isolated kidney can be reproduced in the intact rat.[22] We measured the renal blood flow and GFR of anesthetized rats before and during the infusion of sufficient nisoldipine, a dihydropyridine calcium channel blocker, to decrease the renal perfusion pressure by 20 mmHg. The perfusion pressure then was returned to control by partially occluding the superior mesenteric artery and infrarenal aorta with vascular snares.[23] Renal blood flow returned to control, but the GFR and filtration fraction increased significantly, by more than 20% over their original control values.[22] The aortic and mesenteric arterial snares then were released. Mean arterial pressure promptly fell by 20 mmHg, indicating a persistent action of nisoldipine. Therefore, when the perfusion pressure remains constant, the intact rat manifests renal responses to calcium entry blockers that are qualitatively similar to those of the isolated kidney preparation.[20]

Experiments then were done utilizing isolated perfused SHR kidneys and kidneys from normotensive WKY controls.[24] Each group was perfused at two different perfusion pressures (Fig. 1). Control GFR values of SHR kidneys were significantly less than those of WKY kidneys perfused at similar pressures. Following the superimposition of

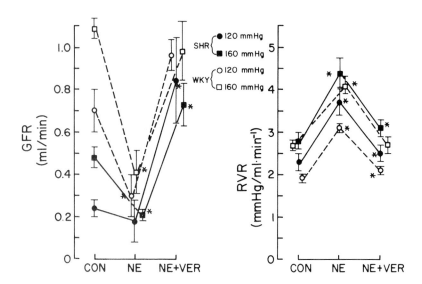

FIGURE 1. Partial reversal of norepinephrine (NE) vasoconstriction during verapamil (VER) superimposition. During the control (CON) phase, GFR of WKY kidneys exceeded those of SHR kidneys. After the addition of verapamil, GFR of SHR kidneys rebounded to values similar to those of WKY kidneys. Asterisks indicate significant difference from control (p < 0.05). RVR remained residually increased. Constant perfusion pressures of 120 or 160 mmHg were maintained (data from ref. 24).

verapamil upon norepinephrine, the GFR of SHR kidneys rebounded to levels similar to the control GFR values of the WKY kidneys.[24] The WKY kidneys responded to verapamil with return of their GFR values to control levels only (Fig. 1). Thus the GFR of SHR kidneys responded to verapamil in an exaggerated manner compared to kidneys from their WKY counterparts. Again, RVR values during verapamil superimposition did not revert to control levels, a result similar to experiments with normal rat kidneys.[20]

The magnified glomerular responses of SHR kidneys to verapamil, compared to WKY kidneys, might have occurred secondary to prior hypertensive damage rather than as a consequence of genetic predilection to development of hypertension. It was important to determine whether kidneys from genetically hypertension-prone rats would exhibit magnified glomerular responses to calcium antagonists in the absence of antecedent hypertension. The DS rat seemed ideal for this purpose. We already alluded to the observation that the blood pressures of DS rats increase dramatically only during NaCl feeding, whereas blood pressures of DR counterparts remain unchanged and normal in the face of a high NaCl intake.[25]

The same protocol was followed for kidneys isolated from male DS and DR rats maintained on a low NaCl regimen.[26] After control measurements, sufficient norepinephrine was infused to increase the RVR by 50%. Following measurements during norepinephrine administration alone, either nitrendipine or verapamil was superimposed upon norepinephrine (Fig. 2). The GFR of the DS rat kidneys during nitrendipine or verapamil increased to values substantially greater than the original control level (Fig. 2). The DR rat kidneys responded to calcium antagonist superimposition with significantly less "GFR rebound" than the DS kidneys.[26] Nevertheless,

Accentuation of DS/DR Differences in Sodium Excretion by Ca-Antagonists

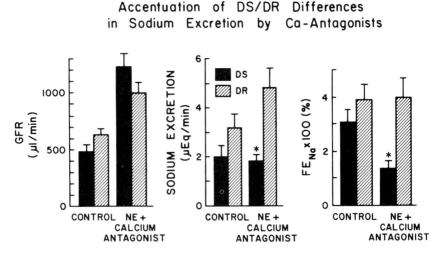

FIGURE 2. Nitrendipine or verapmil superimposition on norepinephrine (NE) vasoconstriction in Dahl rat kidneys (data from ref. 26). Although the "GFR rebound" of DS kidneys was greater than that of DR kidneys after calcium antagonist superimposition, DS kidney sodium excretion failed to increase. FE_{Na} = fractional sodium excretion. Reproduced from Steele TH, Challoner-Hue L: Dihydropyridine calcium antagonists and agonists in the isolated perfused Dahl rat kidney. Reproduced with permisssion from J Cardiovasc Pharmacol 9(suppl 1):S44–S48, 1987.

in spite of the large GFR rebound by the DS kidneys during nitrendipine or verapamil, sodium excretion returned only to control levels (Fig. 2). The large rebound increase in GFR of these DS rat kidneys was insufficient to elicit a natriuresis.[26] In contrast, DR rat kidneys manifested a brisk natriuresis during calcium antagonist superimposition (Fig. 2). Nitrendipine or verapamil alone did not affect Dahl rat kidney hemodynamics or function. [26]

Since the DS rat responds to a high dietary NaCl by increasing its blood pressure, we repeated the experiments using male Dahl rats exposed to high and low NaCl intakes.[27] After 1 month, mean arterial pressures of the high NaCl DS rats were significantly increased compared with high NaCl DR rats as well as with low NaCl DS and DR rats. In isolated kidney studies, DS kidneys manifested greater sensitivity to norepinephrine than DR kidneys, and the low NaCl kidneys were more sensitive than corresponding high NaCl kidneys. Again, the increase in RVR elicited by norepinephrine was partially reversed by nitrendipine superimposition (Fig. 3). Dietary NaCl modification had little effect on the extent of DS kidney GFR rebound during nitrendipine (Fig. 4). However NaCl loading markedly blunted or eliminated DR kidney GFR rebound.[27] The GFR after nitrendipine superimposition was significantly greater than control in every group except the high NaCl DR kidneys (Fig. 4).

These observations did not reflect an anomalous response of the DR kidneys to nitrendipine.[28] NaCl loading also decreased or eliminated the GFR rebound during nitrendipine of normal Sprague-Dawley rat kidneys (Fig. 4). Therefore, persistence of the exaggerated glomerular response to the calcium antagonist by the DS kidneys after salt–loading appeared to be the aberrant response. The DS rat kidney failed to modulate its glomerular response to the calcium entry blocker in spite of a normal modulating stimulus—the ingestion of large amounts of NaCl. In spite of increased

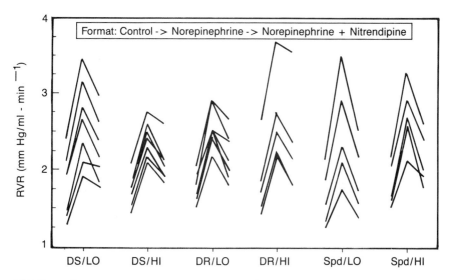

FIGURE 3. Renal vascular resistance in Dahl and Sprague-Dawley (SpD) rats. Each panel depicts a three-phase experiment. Sufficient norepinephrine was infused to increase RVR by 50%. Nitrendipine superimposition only partially reversed the increase in RVR. HI = high NaCl intake; LO = low NaCl intake (data from refs. 27 and 28).

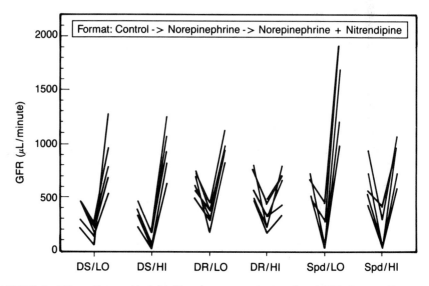

FIGURE 4. Effect of low and high NaCl intake on nitrendipine-induced GFR changes. Format is the same as Figure 3. NaCl loading ameliorated the "glomerular rebound" responses of all high NaCl kidneys except high NaCl DS kidneys. Reproduced with permission from Steele.[28]

GFR rebound by DS kidneys during nitrendipine superimposition, sodium excretion modulate its glomerular response to the calcium entry blocker in spite of a normal modulating stimulus—the ingestion of large amounts of NaCl. In spite of increased GFR rebound by DS kidneys during nitrendipine superimposition, sodium excretion tended to remain less than control values (Fig. 5). This may have reflected greater sensitivity of tubular sodium reabsorption to norepinephrine in the DS kidney.

Studies with Bay-K-8644

Nitrendipine, which blocks membrane calcium fluxes, elicited accentuated glomerular responses in our prehypertensive and hypertensive DS rat kidneys. Therefore, one might expect that a structurally similar agent that *increases* calcium fluxes would produce the opposite functional changes. Bay-k-8644 is a substituted dihydropyridine derivative with a chemical structure somewhat resembling that of nitrendipine. However bay-k-8644 *facilitates* the entry of calcium into cells.[29] Bay-k-8644 binds at the same dihydropyridine receptor as nitrendipine, although presumably during a different state of calcium channel electrical activity.[30] The two agents also exhibit competitive binding properties.[29]

Bay-k-8644 elicited the largest increments in the RVR of high NaCl DS rat kidneys and significantly smaller increases in the RVR of low NaCl DS rat kidneys.[31] At the same concentration (100 μM), bay-k-8644 did not increase the RVR of DR rat kidneys—either the high or low NaCl variety (Fig. 6). The GFR decreased during bay-k-8644 in all four groups of kidneys, but to a significantly greater degree in high NaCl DS kidneys than in low NaCl DS kidneys (Fig. 7). Decrements in the GFR after bay-k-8644 did not differ significantly between high and low NaCl DR kidneys.[31]

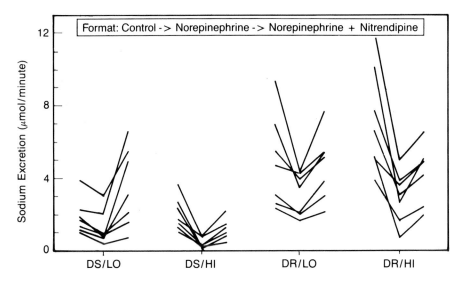

FIGURE 5. Sodium excretion in Dahl rat kidney experiments of Figures 3 and 4 (data from ref. 27). Despite greater nitrendipine-induced "GFR rebound" by DS kidneys (Fig. 4), sodium excretion during nitrendipine superimposition increased to a similar degreee in DS and DR rat kidneys.

Bay-k-8644 normally functions as a calcium channel agonist, but the compound is actually a racemic mixture of two isomers with opposing pharmacological activities.[32] The "minus" isomer functions as a pure calcium channel agonist, whereas the "plus" isomer operates as a pure calcium antagonist. We tested the isomers of bay-k-8644 on high and low NaCl DS and DR isolated rat kidneys over a wide range of concentrations.[31] The results largely agreed with the experiments employing the racemate. The high NaCl DS kidneys exhibited the greatest sensitivity of RVR to the

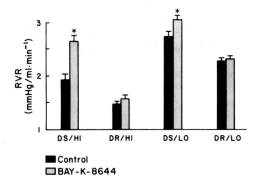

FIGURE 6. Effect of calcium channel agonist, bay-k-8644, on RVR of Dahl rat kidneys from animals stabilized on low or high NaCl intakes. Abbreviations are the same as previously, with asterisks indicating significant changes from paired control values ($p < 0.05$). Bay-k-8644 significantly increased the RVR of DS rat kidneys only, and significantly more in those from DS rats receiving a high NaCl regimen. Reproduced with permission from Steele and Challoner-Hue.[31]

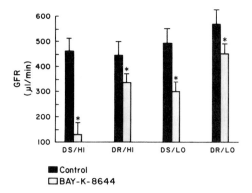

FIGURE 7. Changes in GFR during bay-k-8644 in the experiments of Figure 6. Bay-k-8644 decreased the GFR in all groups, but more in DS than in DR kidneys and more in high than in low NaCl kidneys (by analysis of variance). Reproduced with permission from Steel and Challoner-Hue.[31]

agonist isomer, followed by the low NaCl DS kidneys, and then followed by the high and low NaCl DR kidneys, respectively. Once vasoconstricted by the agonist isomer, however, no differential predilection to vasoconstriction reversal by the antagonist isomer of bay-k-8644 could be distinguished for the different groups.[31,33]

The results of the bay-k-8644 experiments[31] are consistent with the nitrendipine experiments[27] in that DS kidneys manifested greater responses to both nitrendipine and bay-k-8644 than DR kidneys. These differential responses were amplified further by NaCl loading. Thus the magnitude of responses to both nitrendipine and bay-k-8644 was contingent on the amount of dietary salt, but in a manner varying with the genetic Dahl S or R status of the isolated kidney. Whereas the nitrendipine studies involved blockade of receptor-operated calcium channels activated by norepinephrine, the bay-k-8644 studies probably involved opening

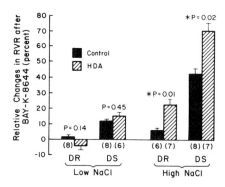

FIGURE 8. Effect of 6-hydroxydopamine (HDA) "chemical sympathectomy" on bay-k-8664—induced increments in RVR. Although DS kidneys were more sensitive to bay-k-8644 than DR kidneys, "chemical sympathectomy" increased renovascular sensitivity to bay-k-8644 equivalently in the high NaCl DS and DR groups. HDA did not affect the sensitivity to bay-k-8644 of the low NacI groups. Reproduced with permission from Steele and Challoner-Hue.[31]

of voltage-operated channels. In order to further delineate the nature of the calcium channels opened in the bay-k-8644 experiments, we examined the effect of "chemical sympathectomy" on the increments in RVR produced by bay-k-8644. Chemical sympathectomy was produced by prior injection of six-hydroxydopamine intraperitoneally.[31] Six-hydroxydopamine renders isolated kidneys refractory to electrical stimulation[34] and also prevents the development of hypertension in the NaCl-loaded DS rat.[35]

Six-hydroxydopamine significantly augmented the increments in RVR produced by bay-k-8644 in *high NaCl* Dahl rat kidneys, irrespective of their S or R status, compared to "nonsympathectomized" counterpart kidneys (Fig. 8). However Six-hydroxy dopamine did not affect the increments in RVR produced by bay-k-8644 in low NaCl Dahl rat kidneys, whether DS or DR (Fig. 8). 6-hydroxydopamine increases the numbers of adrenergic receptors and dihydropyridine calcium channels.[36] If the dihydropyridine channels up-regulated by chemical sympathectomy are those associated with up-regulated adrenergic receptors, then dihydropyridine calcium channels could be involved in cell calcium translocations initiated by the binding of adrenergic agents. However such speculation requires further documentation.

Summary

To summarize these studies, calcium channel antagonists increased the GFR of DS rat kidneys to a greater degree than DR rat kidneys, and increased the GFR of SHR kidneys to a greater degree than WKY kidneys. This effect was *blunted* by a high dietary NaCl intake in DR rat kidneys, similarly to kidneys from normal NaCl-loaded Sprague-Dawley rats. After NaCl loading, the DS rat kidneys failed to decrease their glomerular response to calcium channel blockade normally. A calcium channel agonist reduced the GFR and increased the RVR to a greater extent in DS than in DR rat kidneys. This effect was *magnified* by a high dietary NaCl intake to a greater extent in the DS than in DR rat kidneys. Chemical sympathectomy by 6-hydroxydopamine intensified these effects of the calcium channel agonist equivalently in DS and DR rat kidneys, but only after dietary NaCl loading.

Abnormalities of cell calcium regulation have been implicated repeatedly in the pathogenesis of hypertension.[1-4] We have shown that renal vascular and glomerular responses to calcium channel agonists and antagonists are modulated by genetic susceptibility to the development of hypertension, and also by dietary NaCl in a manner depending on genetic susceptibility. The results are consistent with the hypothesis that derangements of vascular and glomerular calcium-entry modulation may be critical determinants of altered renal hemodynamics in salt-sensitive hypertension. One possibility is that calcium channel-active pharmacologic probes may interact with vascular smooth muscle and other tissues at specific sites where genetic predilection to the development of hypertension is specifically expressed, i.e., the calcium channel. Results reported by other laboratories have indicated that glomerular hemodynamic actions of calcium antagonists most likely result from a relatively selective afferent arteriolar vasodilation (see also Chapter 1).[37,38] Conceivably, abnormalities of afferent arteriolar function may be key factors in the pathogenesis of renally dependent genetic salt-sensitive hypertension. It is therefore tempting to speculate that agents interfering with cell calcium influx may offer us the therapeutic potential to interdict the hypertensive process at sites critical to pathogenesis—at least in the case of salt-sensitive hypertension.

Acknowledgments. Work from the author's laboratory was supported by grants from the National Institutes of Health (HL.29001), the American Heart Association of Wisconsin, the University of Wisconsin Graduate School Research Committee, and the University of Wisconsin Department of Medicine Research & Development Fund.

References

1. Karanja N, McCarron DA: Calcium and hypertension. Ann Rev Nutr 6:475–494, 1986.

2. McCarron DA, Morris CD: The calcium deficiency hypothesis of hypertension. Ann Intern Med 107:919–922, 1987.

3. Resnick LM, Miller FB, Laragh JH: Calcium-regulating hormones in essential hypertension. Ann Intern Med 105:649–654, 1986.

4. Resnick LM, Nicholson JP, Laragh JH: Calcium, the renin-aldosterone system, and the hypotensive response to nifedipine. Hypertension 10:254–258, 1987.

5. Kaplan NM, Meese RB: The calcium deficiency hypothesis of hypertension: A critique. Ann Intern Med 105:947–955, 1986.

6. Bohr DF: Actions of calcium on smooth muscle: Historical overview. Ann NY Acad Sci 522:210–215, 1988.

7. Khalil R, Lodge N, Saida K, van Breemen C: Mechanism of calcium activation in vascular smooth muscle. J Hypertens 5(suppl 4):S5–S15, 1987.

8. Umemura, S, Smyth DD, Nicar M, et al: Altered calcium homeostasis in Dahl hypertensive rats: Physiological and biochemical studies. J Hypertens 4:19–26, 1986.

9. Heath H III: Calcium tablets for hypertension? Ann Intern Med 103:946–947, 1985.

10. Peuler JD, Morgan DA, Mark AL: High calcium diet reduces blood pressure in Dahl salt-sensitive rats by neural mechanisms. Hypertension 9(suppl III):III159–III165, 1987.

11. Wyss JM, Sripairojthikoon W, Oparil S: Failure of renal denervation to attenuate hypertension in Dahl NaCl-sensitive rats. Can J Physiol Pharmacol 65:2428–2432, 1987.

12. Rapp JP: Dahl salt-susceptible and salt-resistant rats; a review. Hypertension 4:753–763, 1982.

13. Maude DL, Kao-Lo G: Salt excretion and vascular resistance of perfused kidneys of Dahl rats. Hypertension 4:532–537, 1982.

14. Girardin E, Caverzasio J, Iwai J, et al: Pressure natriuresis in isolated kidneys from hypertension-prone and hypertension-resistant rats (Dahl rats). Kidney Int 18:10–19, 1980.

15. Roman RJ, Osborn JL: Renal function and sodium balance in conscious Dahl S and R rats. Am J Physiol 252:R833–R841, 1987.

16. Steele TH, Challoner-Hue L, Gottstein JH: Function of arachidonate-deficient spontaneously hypertensive rat kidney. Miner Electrolyte Metab 10:5–11, 1984.

17. Kawabe K, Watanabe TX, Shiono K, Sokabe H: Influence on blood pressure of renal isografts between spontaneously hypertensive and normotensive rats, utilizing the F_1 hybrids. Jpn Heart Jl 20:886–894, 1979.

18. Chen Y-F, Meng Q, Wys JM, et al: High NaCl diet reduces hypothalamic norepinephrine turnover in hypertensive rats. Hypertension 11:55–62, 1988.

19. Steele TH, Gottstein JH, Challoner-Hue L: Function of the isolated spontaneously hypertensive rat kidney after blood pressure reduction. Renal Physiol (Basel) 8:65–72, 1985.

20. Steele TH, Challoner-Hue L: Renal interactions between norepinephrine and calcium antagonists. Kidney Int 26:719–724, 1984.

21. Loutzenhiser R, Epstein M: Effects of calcium antagonists on renal hemodynamics. Am J Physiol 249:F619–F629, 1985.

22. Steele TH: Calcium entry modulation and renal hemodynamics in the hypertensive kidney. Am J Nephrol 7(suppl 1):17–23, 1987.

23. Roman RJ, Cowley AW Jr: Characterization of a new model for the study of pressure-natriuresis in the rat. Am J Physiol 248:F190–F198, 1985.

24. Steele TH, Challoner-Hue L: Glomerular response to verapamil by isolated spontaneously hypertensive rat kidney. Am J Physiol 248:F668–F673, 1985.

25. Rapp JP: Dahl salt-susceptible and salt-resistant rats; a review. Hypertension 4:753–763, 1982.

26. Steele TH, Challoner-Hue L: Response of isolated Dahl rat kidney to calcium antagonists. Kidney Int 31:941–945, 1987.

27. Steele TH, Challoner-Hue L: Influence of salt on response to nitrendipine by Dahl rat kidney. Am J Physiol 252:F487–F490, 1987.

28. Steele TH: Function of the hypertensive kidney during calcium flux manipulation. Am J Cardiol 62: 74G-78G, 1988.

29. Schramm M, Thomas G, Toward R, Franckowiak G: Novel dihydropyridines with positive inotropic action through activation of Ca^{2+} channels. Nature 303:535–537, 1983.

30. Bean BP, Sturek M, Puga A, Hermsmeyer K: Calcium channels in muscle cells isolated from rat mesenteric arteries: Modulation by dihydropyridine drugs. Circ Res 59:229–235, 1986.

31. Steele TH, Challoner-Hue L: Increased response to calcium channel agonist by Dahl S rat kidney. Am J Physiol 254:F533–F539, 1988.

32. Franckowiak G, Bechem M, Schramm M, Thomas G: The optical isomers of the 1,4-dihydropyridine bay-k-8644 show opposite effects on calcium channels. Eur J Pharmacol 114:223–226, 1985.

33. Steele TH, Challoner-Hue L: Exaggerated Dahl salt sensitive kidney response to calcium channel agonist isomer of bay-K-8644, but not to calcium channel antagonist isomer of bay-K-8644. J Hypertens 4(suppl 6):S136–S137, 1986.

34. Mejia G, Challoner-Hue L, Steele, TH: Calcium in neural control of renal circulation. Am J Physiol 247:F739–F745, 1984.

35. Takeshita A, Mark A, Brody MJ: Prevention of salt-induced hypertension in the Dahl strain by 6-hydroxydopamine. Am J Physiol 236:H48–H52, 1979.

36. Skattebøl A, Triggle DJ: 6-Hydroxydopamine treatment increases β-adrenoceptors and Ca^{2+} channels in rat heart. Eur J Pharmacol 127:287–289, 1986.

37. Fleming JT, Parekh N, Steinhausen M: Calcium antagonists preferentially dilate preglomerular vessels of hydronephrotic kidney. Am J Physiol 253:F1157–F1163, 1987.

38. Loutzenhiser R, Epstein M, Horton C: Inhibition by diltiazem of pressure-induced afferent vasoconstriction in the isolated perfused rat kidney. Am J Cardiol 59:72A–75A, 1987.

Joseph V. Bonventre, M.D., Ph.D.

5

Calcium and the Renal Mesangial Cell

The ability to maintain renal mesangial cells in culture has provided an experimental system to examine the characteristics of this important glomerular cell. The mesangial cell in culture contracts[1] and produces cyclooxygenase and lipoxygenase products of arachidonic acid,[2,3] interleukin-1, neutral proteases, and collagens. The rate of growth of the mesangial cell in culture is altered by a number of different agents. Each of these cellular responses may play an important regulatory role in vivo in the intact glomerulus. Because of the proposed critical role that mesangial cell contraction, eicosanoid production, and proliferation play in renal function and dysfunction, and since Ca^{2+} has been implicated in each of these functions, there is a great deal of interest in defining the role of Ca^{2+} in the mesangial cell.

Cytosolic Free Ca^{2+} Concentration ($[Ca^{2+}]_f$)

Under normal conditions we have measured $[Ca^{2+}]_f$ to be 102 ± 3 nM (n = 154) or 82 ± 4 nM (n = 34) using two intracellular fluorescent probes, quin2 and fura-2, respectively.[4] Other laboratories have since found similar results with these and other (Indo-1) dyes.[5-8] Baseline levels of $[Ca^{2+}]_f$ are regulated by plasma membrane Ca^{2+} transport process, such as the Ca^{2+}-ATPase, and likely a Na^+/Ca^{2+} exchange process as well as intracellular nonmitochondrial storage sites.[9] When digitonin is added to a suspension of mesangial cells the bath $[Ca^{2+}]$ equilibrates at approximately 300 nM. Under these cell-permeant conditions, the cytosol is in equilibrium with the bath. Ruthenium red, which blocks the Ca^{2+} uniporter of the mitochondria and results in Ca^{2+} release from Ca^{2+}-loaded mitochondria,[10] has no effect on the permeabilized cells. This suggests that a nonmitochondrial compartment (e.g., a subfraction of endoplasmic reticulum called calciosomes)[11] serves to regulate $[Ca^{2+}]_f$ at a level of approximately 300 nM under these conditions when the plasma membrane transport properties are not able to contribute. At higher levels of $[Ca^{2+}]_f$ the mitochondria became more important as a buffering compartment (unpublished observation).

Hormone and Growth Factor/Cytokine-Induced Increases in [Ca²⁺]$_f$

The first hormones that we found to produce changes in mesangial cell $[Ca^{2+}]_f$ were angiotensin II (ANG II) and arginine vasopressin (AVP).[4] The increase in $[Ca^{2+}]_f$ with AVP was observed independent of the culture passage whereas the increase observed with ANG II was seen only in early passages (<6th). After addition of AVP or ANG II, $[Ca^{2+}]_f$ reached a peak value within 10 sec. In one set of experiments (n = 17) $[Ca^{2+}]_f$ increased from 74 ± 7 nM to 578 ± 39 nM and then rapidly returned toward the baseline (Fig. 1). After 115 sec of exposure to AVP, $[Ca^{2+}]_f$ was 125 ± 9 nM, which was significantly higher than time-matched controls. The increase in $[Ca^{2+}]_f$ observed with AVP was prevented by prior treatment of the cells with the 2-0-methyltyrosine 4-valine AVP, a V_1 receptor analogue.

To determine whether the increase in $[Ca^{2+}]_f$ was dependent upon entry of Ca^{2+} from the extracellular milieu, we determined whether large amounts of extracellular EGTA (4 mM), which resulted in a reduction of extracellular $[Ca^{2+}]$ to below 10 nM, prevented the AVP-induced increase in $[Ca^{2+}]_f$. This experimental maneuver did not eliminate the rapid increase in $[Ca^{2+}]_f$ observed with AVP, although it did reduce the peak level somewhat. The $[Ca^{2+}]_f$ increased from 61 ± 5 nM to 340 ± 36 nM (Fig. 2). In contrast to the results without EGTA, $[Ca^{2+}]_f$ returned to values indistinguishable from control values in 70 sec after addition of AVP.

Thus, the $[Ca^{2+}]_f$ response to AVP could be separated into two components, an

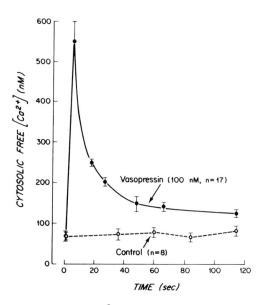

FIGURE 1. Effect of vasopressin on $[Ca^2]_f$ in mesangial cells loaded with the flourescent dye, fura-2. In vasopressin-treated cells $[Ca^{2+}]_f$ remained statistically higher than time-matched controls at 115 sec after addition of the agonist (p < .025). *n* = number of experiments. Reproduced with permission from Bonventre et al.[4]

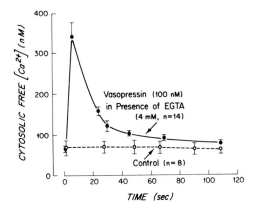

FIGURE 2. Effect of EGTA on the vasopressin-induced change in $[Ca^{2+}]_f$ in mesangial cells. Cells were loaded with fura-2. The $[Ca^{2+}]_f$ returned to values not statistically different from control values at 70 sec after vasopressin addition. Control cells were also exposed to 4mM EGTA. n = number of experiments. Reproduced with permission from Bonventre et al. [4]

initial response that was, in large part, independent of Ca^{2+} entry, and a sustained increase that was dependent upon the presence of physiological levels of extracellular $[Ca^{2+}]$. The initial phase was due to Ca^{2+} release from nonmitochondrial intracellular stores, likely secondary to the action of inositol trisphosphate, which was produced by AVP-induced phospholipase C activation (see below) (Fig. 3). The sustained increase in $[Ca^{2+}]_f$ was subsequently shown to be associated with Ca^{2+} entry across the plasma membrane from the extracellular milieu.

Since these initial observations a number of other hormones and growth factors have been found to alter $[Ca^{2+}]_f$. These are listed in Table 1, which may be "out of date" when this chapter is published since progress in this area is very rapid. With the exception of atrial natriuretic factor (ANF), all substances listed in Table 1 have been found to increase $[Ca^{2+}]_f$. Hassid has reported that atriopeptins decrease basal

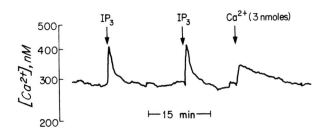

FIGURE 3. Mobilization of Ca^{2+} from intracellular storage sites by inositol 1,4,5-trisphosphate (IP_3). Mesangial cells were suspended in a medium whose composition approximated that of the normal intracellular milieu. They were made permeable with digitonin. A Ca^{2+}-sensitive electrode was used to monitor the Ca^{2+} concentration of the bath. Addition of IP_3 (final concentration, $5\mu M$) resulted in release of Ca^{2+} from the intracellular stores, raising the $[Ca^{2+}]$ of the bath. Reproduced with permission from Bonventre et al. [9]

$[Ca^{2+}]_f$ by up to 30% and can also reduce the ANG II- and AVP-induced increases in $[Ca^{2+}]_f$. Meyer-Lehnert et al.[16] found no effect of atriopeptin III on basal $[Ca^{2+}]_f$ but found that atriopeptin III decreased the peak level that $[Ca^{2+}]_f$ reached in response to AVP. There is tachyphylaxis to agents such as ANG II and AVP but no cross-tachyphylaxis to these agents.[7]

An interesting feature of the $[Ca^{2+}]_f$ response that has received little attention is the kinetics of the response. In the reported studies, the response has been determined in the 5–10 second-to-minutes time scale. Recent studies by Exton in liver cells would suggest that early time kinetics (msec time scale) are necessary in order to better define relationships between phospholipase activation (vide infra) and $[Ca^{2+}]_f$ changes.[21]

We have compared the time response of $[Ca^{2+}]_f$ to three different agonists: AVP, platelet activating factor (PAF), and platelet derived growth factor (PDGF).[4,9] While AVP and PAF increased $[Ca^{2+}]_f$ to peak values in less than 10 sec, the response to PDGF was much more prolonged, with peak values of $[Ca^{2+}]_f$ observed at approximately 60 sec after addition of the agonist. This different time response may reflect fundamental differences in cell activation patterns (see below).

Phospholipases, Arachidonic Acid and Eicosanoids

Phospholipase C.   Many external stimuli are believed to exert their action upon cells via intracellular second messengers produced by a surface receptor-coupled activation of phospholipase C. The coupling between receptor and phospholipase C may involve a guanine nucleotide binding protein. Phospholipase C acts upon phosphatidylinositol-bis-phosphate, cleaving this membrane phospholipid into two parts, diacylglycerol and inositol trisphosphate. Troyer and colleagues demonstrated that IP$_3$ and diacylglycerol were increased after 45 sec of AVP exposure.[22] The IP$_3$ is released into the cytosol and acts upon nonmitochondrial calcium storage sites to release Ca^{2+} and increase $[Ca^{2+}]_f$. By analogy to the neutrophil the source of the released Ca^{2+} may be a subpopulation of endoplasmic reticulum, which Lew and colleagues have called calciosomes.[11]

What is the evidence for GTP binding protein (G protein) involvement in the coupling between receptor and phospholipase C in the mesangial cell? We found that AVP, when added to permeabilized cells in the presence of a nonhydrolyzable GTP analog, GTPγS, resulted in an increase in diacylglycerol levels.[23] Pfeilschifter and Bauer[24] reported that the ANG II-induced stimulation of phospholipase C was inhibited by pertussis toxin, which ADP-ribosylates the G$_i$ binding protein, inactivating it. Thus it could be concluded that G$_i$ was involved in the coupling of the ANG II receptor to phospholipase C, acting in an inhibitory manner. Schlondorff et al.[25] examined the

TABLE I.   Substances Found to Alter $[Ca^{2+}]_f$ in Glomerular Mesangial Cells

Angiotensin II[4,7,12]	PGF$_{2\alpha}$[6]
Bradykinin[5]	PGE$_2$[6]
Endothelin[8,13]	U-46619[6]
Platelet Derived Growth Factor[9,14]	Vasopressin[4,7,16]
Platelet Activating Factor[9,15]	Atrial Natriuretic Factor*[17-20]

*Atrial natriuretic factor decreases $[Ca^{2+}]_f$. Each of the other agents has been reported to increase $[Ca^{2+}]_f$.

sensitivity of ANG II-induced PGE_2 production in mesangial cells to varying doses of pertussis toxin. PGE_2 production is the result of activation of phospholipase C and phospholipase A_2. These investigators found that pertussis toxin could be inhibitory or stimulatory for PGE_2 synthesis, depending upon the dose used and the resultant degree of ADP-ribosylation.

The diacylglycerol generated as a result of phospholipase C activation can be expected to activate protein kinase C. Orita and colleagues[26] and Pfeilschifter[27] fractionated the 100,000 xg supernatant of mesangial cells by DEAE-cellulose ion-exchange chromatography and demonstrated a peak of protein kinase activity, which they identified as protein kinase C due to the activation of this activity with phospholipid, diacylglycerol, and Ca^{2+}. Pfeilschifter[28] demonstrated that pretreatment of mesangial cells with activators of protein kinase C inhibited the subsequent activation of phospholipase C with ANG II. He later demonstrated that inhibition of protein kinase C with either H-7 (1-(5- isoquinolinesulfonyl)-2-methylpiperazine), sphingosine or cytotoxin 1, prevented the homologous desensitization observed with ANG II. Thus it appears that this homologous desensitization is mediated via protein kinase C.[27] Furthermore it was proposed that this inhibition of activation due to protein kinase C was due to an effect on G-protein, perhaps due to inhibition of the dissociation of the $\beta\gamma$ subunit.[29]

Phospholipase A_2. Human and rat mesangial cells produce cyclooxygenase as well as lipoxygenase products. The cyclooxygenase products include PGE_2, $PGF_{2\alpha}$, 6-keto $PGF_{1\alpha}$, and PGI_2.[4,30−33] Rat mesangial cells have been found to produce the lipoxygenase product, 12-hydroxyeicosatetraenoic acid.[34] The precursor for all these products is arachidonic acid. The control of cellular production of cyclooxygenase or lipoxygenase products depends upon levels of arachidonic acid. The regulation of arachidonic acid levels is multifaceted. Probably the primary determinant of arachidonic acid levels in the cell is the activity of phospholipase A_2, which cleaves phospholipids at the sn-2 position, resulting in release of free fatty acids and the residual lysophospholipids. Since arachidonic acid is enriched at the sn-2 position, phospholipase A_2 activation increases cellular levels of arachidonate, which can then be acted upon by cyclooxygenases, lipoxygenases, and p450 mixed-function oxidases. Another regulatory process may be the sequential effects of phospholipase C followed by diacylglycerol lipase. Schlondorff and colleagues,[35] however, found that little arachidonate is generated from mono- or diacylglycerols in the mesangial cell. An additional potential pathway is phospholipase D forming phosphatidic acid, followed by phospholipase A_2. Finally regulation might occur to some degree at the level of reacylation of the arachidonate. In spite of the myriad of possibilities for arachidonate regulation, phospholipase A_2 appears to be the most important regulatory enzyme.

Calcium is central to the activation of many forms of phospholipase A_2 in many different systems. Most of the experiments, however, that have demonstrated Ca^{2+} sensitivity of phospholipase A_2 have been performed using very high Ca^{2+} concentrations, frequently in the millimolar concentration range.[36,37] Clearly the enzyme may never be exposed to Ca^{2+} concentrations of this magnitude under physiological conditions, since the $[Ca^{2+}]_f$ in intact mesangial cells probably never gets much higher than 1 to 10 μM and then only under very stimulated conditions. To evaluate the Ca^{2+} dependence of prostaglandin synthesis, we initially examined whether AVP-induced PGE_2 production was dependent upon extracellular Ca^{2+}. We found

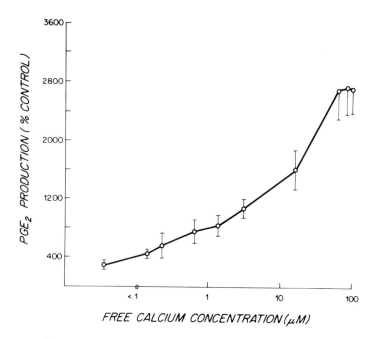

FIGURE 4. Ca^{2+} sensitivity of PGE_2 production in mesangial cells. Cells were rendered permeable with digitonin in a buffer designed to mimic the intracellular milieu. PGE_2 production was then determined after 10 min of exposure to varying concentrations of $Ca.^{2+}$ Each data point represents the mean ± 1 SE of 4–10 experiments. Modified from Bonventre and Swidler.[23]

that it was not, indicating that the initial release of Ca^{2+} from intracellular stores, perhaps together with other cellular mediators activated by AVP, was sufficient to result in the PGE_2 production we found with AVP in cells bathed with physiological levels of extracellular Ca^{2+}.[23]

We then performed experiments on cells made permeable with digitonin and exposed to a wide range of Ca^{2+} concentrations. We found that the production of prostaglandin E_2 (PGE_2) was Ca^{2+}-dependent (Fig. 4). Importantly, this $[Ca^{2+}]$ dependency was observed over the range of change in $[Ca^{2+}]_f$ measured physiologically. To establish that the Ca^{2+} dependency of PGE_2 production was correlated with acylhydrolase activity, we examined the release of arachidonate from cells exposed to digitonin in the presence of varying levels of media $[Ca^{2+}]$. Similar to PGE_2 production, there was increased arachidonate release with increasing levels of Ca^{2+}. This enhanced acylhydrolase activity was inhibited by N-(6-aminohexyl-l-naphthelene sulfonamide) (W-7), an inhibitor of calmodulin. This inhibition with W-7 was similar to the inhibition of PGE_2 production demonstrated with other calmodulin antagonists. Arachidonate release was markedly inhibited by dibucaine and mepacrine, two phospholipase A_2 inhibitors. Thus, the phospholipase A_2 activity of the mesangial cell was Ca^{2+} dependent over the range of $[Ca^{2+}]_f$ measured in these cells. The activity also appeared to be calmodulin enhanced.

Calcium alone, however, could not explain the total PGE_2 production seen after the addition of AVP.[4] Using phorbol myristate acetate (PMA) to stimulate protein

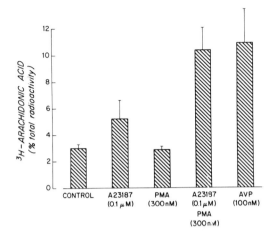

FIGURE 5. Levels of free ^{3}H-arachidonic acid after 10 min of stimulation of nonpermeabilized, intact mesangial cells previously labelled with ^{3}H-arachidonic acid and stimulated with various agonists. PMA alone had no effect on ^{3}H-arachidonic acid release but acted synergistically with A23187 to increase ^{3}H-arachidonic acid release to levels observed with vasopressin alone. Each data bar represents the mean ± SEM of six to eight experiments. Reproduced with permission from Bonventre and Swidler.[23]

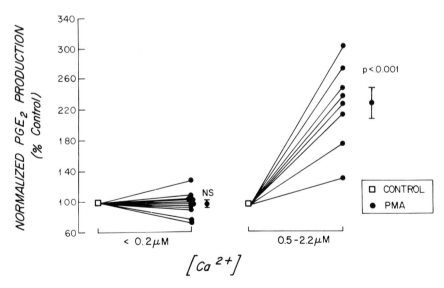

FIGURE 6. Effects of phorbol myristate acetate (PMA) on PGE_2 synthesis in mesangial cells made permeable with digitonin at two different ranges of ambient $[Ca^{2+}]$. PMA enhances PGE_2 production only when Ca^{2+} is elevated into the range of cytosolic free Ca^{2+} concentration observed with an agonist such as vasopressin. Reproduced with permission from Bonventre and Swidler.[23]

kinase C activity in intact mesangial cells, we demonstrated that the activation of protein kinase C functions synergistically with a calcium ionophore (A23187)-induced increase in $[Ca^{2+}]_f$, to generate arachidonic acid release (Fig. 5). A cell permeant diacylglycerol analogue, 1-oleoyl 2-acetylglycerol (OAG), also acted synergistically with A23187 in the intact mesangial cell to enhance arachidonate release.

We examined the effects of protein kinase C activation on PGE_2 production in permeabilized cells where Ca^{2+} was fixed at two different levels: resting cell ($[Ca^{2+}]_f$ < 0.2μM), and in the range achieved in AVP-stimulated cells (0.5 − 2.2μM). At the resting levels of $[Ca^{2+}]_f$ there was no effect of phorbol esters on PGE_2 production. At the higher concentrations of Ca^{2+}, however, phorbol myristate acetate significantly enhanced PGE_2 production (Fig. 6).

Thus, the AVP-induced stimulation of PGE_2 production in mesangial cells is the product of activation of two intracellular mediators, $[Ca^{2+}]_f$ and DAG, whose increase is related to phospholipase C activation. DAG in the presence of Ca^{2+} and phospholipid stimulates protein kinase C. The enhanced PGE_2 production induced by protein kinase C activation may be due to a modification of the phospholipase A_2 enzyme directly or modification of a phospholipase A_2 modulatory protein.[38,39] Lipocortins are a recently described class of compounds that are proposed to be endogenous phospholipase A_2 inhibitors. It has been postulated that, upon phosphorylation, lipocortins have less of an inhibitory effect on the enzyme, thereby resulting in activation of phospholipase A_2.[38] In collaboration with Dr. B. Pepinsky of Biogen Corporation, we found 35 and 36 kD proteins in the mesangial cell,[40] which react with antibodies specific to proteins that have been isolated, cloned, and identified as lipocortin I and lipocortin II by Pepinsky's group.[41] There is, however, some concern that these particular proteins may not be endogenous modulators of phospholipase A_2, since they may interact with the phospholipid substrates for the enzyme rather than the enzyme itself.[42]

In order to evaluate whether there is a stable modification of the enzymatic activity, we measured phospholipase A_2 activity directly in cell-free extracts of mesangial cells that were stimulated with AVP or PMA.[43] The enzymatic activity was assayed by the release of labelled arachidonic acid from phosphatidylcholine under saturating conditions of calcium concentration in the assay buffer. The phospholipase A_2 activity was enhanced in extracts from cells previously stimulated with either agonist. The ability to recover stimulated activity in the cell-free extract suggests that the enzyme has undergone stable modification as a result of cell activation by the agonist. This might take the form of phosphorylation of the enzyme itself, or a modulatory protein by protein kinase C, which would be activated by both PMA as well as AVP.

Under the conditions in which these experiments were performed, the enzymatic activity was localized to the high-speed supernatant. This indicates that the enzyme is not an integral membrane enzyme. Our data further suggested that the enzyme is bound to membranes in a Ca^{2+}-dependent manner. The enzymatic activity is released from the membranes in the presence of EGTA, which markedly reduces media free $[Ca^{2+}]$. The stimulated activity was eluted as a single peak from DEAE-cellulose anion exchange columns and FPLC Superose 12 gel filtration columns. The same elution pattern was seen with extracts from AVP- or PMA-treated cells. The enzyme had an absolute requirement for calcium when phosphatidylcholine was used as substrate and had optimal activity at slightly alkaline pH.

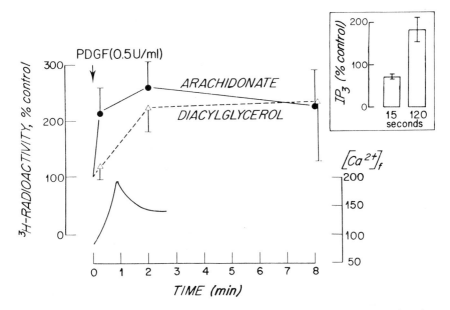

FIGURE 7. Effects of PDGF on release of free arachidonate, diacylglycerol, and inositol trisphosphate from mesangial cells. Cells were prelabelled with either ^{3}H-arachidonic acid or ^{3}H-inositol. For comparison the time course of response of $[Ca^{2+}]_f$ to PDGF is drawn on the same timescale. The $[Ca^{2+}]_f$ is presented in nM concentration units. Note that arachidonate release precedes diacylglycerol and inositol trisphosphate elevation. The $[Ca^{2+}]_f$ response to PDGF is significantly slower than that observed with vasopressin (see Fig. 1). Modified from Bonventre et al.[9]

In addition to stimulation of phospholipase A_2 associated with phospholipase C activation, there may be other mechanisms independent of phospholipase C in the mesangial cell by which agonists activate phospholipase A_2. In experiments performed with PDGF as an agonist,[9] we have found that the peak increase in $[Ca^{2+}]_f$ is delayed compared to that seen with AVP or PAF. PDGF stimulates phospholipase C as does AVP. However, when inositol phosphates were measured 15 sec after PDGF activation, there was no increase in IP_3 or inositol bisphosphate (IP_2) levels. By 2 min, however, there was a statistically significant increase in IP_2 and IP_3 (Fig. 7). Although there was no increase in IP_3 or diglyceride levels by 15 sec, there was an increase in free arachidonic acid. This suggests that there may be a mechanism for stimulation of phospholipase A_2 independent of phospholipase C or DAG lipase. Possible explanations would include a change in membrane potential.[44] Furthermore, Sweatt and colleagues found in platelets that ADP and epinephrine increase phospholipase A_2 activity prior to phospholipase C activation.[45] In fact they found that a cyclooxygenase product was necessary to mediate the phospholipase C activation. Also, G proteins may play an important role in activation of phospholipase A_2.[46,47]

Another potential role played by phospholipase A_2 and Ca^{2+} in the mesangial cells is in PAF biosynthesis. Lianos and Zanglis[48] have demonstrated that A23187 enhances the formation and release of PAF with concomitant decreases in intracellular

1-0-alkyl-2-acyl-GPC and lyso-PAF levels. Although the authors used A23187 as a phospholipase A_2 agonist and these experiments demonstrate a role for Ca^{2+} in PAF production, they do not prove that Ca^{2+} is acting through phospholipase A_2 to exert this effect on PAF production. Further studies of the Ca^{2+} sensitivities of other enzymes in the biosynthetic pathways for PAF would be useful.

Contraction

It has long been appreciated that blood flow through glomeruli can be altered in response to vasoactive substances.[49,50] The first direct evidence for contraction within the mammalian glomerulus was reported by Bernik,[51] who noted contraction of human glomeruli in culture. Bernik suggested that the rhythmic contractions she noted emanated from the mesangium. Mesangial cells in vivo and in vitro in culture contain bundles of microfilaments and actomyosin.[52–54] Early studies of mesangial cell contraction focused on the shape change observed when cells adherent to a glass or plastic support were exposed to vasoactive agents.[1,55,56] It was concluded by some investigators, however, that appreciation of mesangial cell contraction might be hampered by the strong adherence of cells to the glass or plastic support. Kreisberg et al.[57] used a poly-HEMA substrate to alleviate the problem. Cells grown on this support are less adherent and shape change is more easily identified. Singhal et al.[58] and Barnett et al.[59] used a silicone rubber support and identified contraction by the resultant wrinkles in the support. Simonsen and Dunn[60] used Teflon membranes.

Mesangial cells change shape in response to ANG II, AVP, and histamine,[1,57] agents that reduce the glomerular ultrafiltration coefficient, K_f, in vivo. It is proposed that the reduction in K_f observed with these and other agents is secondary to contraction of the mesangium in vivo, resulting in a decrease in filtration surface area. This mechanistic association remains controversial, however, Fugiwara et al.[61] found that glomerular ^{14}C-inulin space was decreased with ANG II and suggested that this was due to a decrease in glomerular intracapillary volume that could be associated with decreased glomerular capillary surface area. Haley et al.,[62] in morphological studies, demonstrated that ANG II reduced glomerular tuft volume and parenchyma but did not alter filtration surface area. Savin[63] measured no change with ANG II in fluid uptake into glomeruli suspended in a hypooncotic media. She suggested that the ANG II-mediated reduction in the K_f in vivo was due to shunting of blood flow away from some of the capillaries.

One difficulty with many of the studies conducted on contractility is that only a fraction of the cells are found to change shape. This complicates the evaluation of the mechanisms of contraction. There are many possible explanations for this heterogeneity of response. Phospholipase C activation may be hetergeneous from cell to cell. The increase in $[Ca^{2+}]_f$ and protein kinase C activity (see below) may differ greatly from cell to cell. The cellular response may depend upon the phase of the cell cycle it is in. There may be autocoid factors, such as PGE_2, which are produced to varying degrees in different cells, and feedback to prevent contraction. PGE_2 is produced by mesangial cells in response to various "contractile stimuli." There is a good deal of evidence that PGE_2 inhibits contraction,[64] and cyclooxygenase inhibitors have been found to enhance contraction.[65–67]

The evidence suggests, therefore, that mesangial cells are contractile and that glomerular contraction in vivo is related to mesangial cell contraction, and this, in turn, may represent an important regulatory influence on K_f. The mechanisms coupling mesangial cell contraction to changes in K_f are, however, not established.

The cellular mechanisms of mesangial cell contractility are incompletely defined. A number of agents other than those mentioned above, including leukotrienes, PAF, PDGF, calcium ionophores, and isoproterenol, have been shown to induce contraction of mesangial cells in culture. Many, but not all, of these agonists also increase $[Ca^{2+}]_f$. Meyer-Lehnert and Schrier have found that pretreatment of cells with cyclosporin A, which has no effect on basal $[Ca^{2+}]_f$, enhances the AVP-induced increase in $[Ca^{2+}]_f$ and also increases the percentage of cells changing shape in response to AVP. Kreisberg has reported that insulin is required for contraction in response to ANG II.[69]

Given the central role that is played by calcium in the contractile process in both cardiac and vascular smooth muscle, it is reasonable to assume that this divalent cation plays a central role in mesangial cell contraction also. Angiotensin II, AVP, PDGF, PAF, and endothelin, agents that induce contraction, increase $[Ca^{2+}]_f$. One question of importance is whether the calcium involved in contraction is derived primarily from intracellular or extracellular sources. In cardiac muscle, for example,[70] depolarization of the cell membrane leads to the opening of voltage-dependent Ca^{2+} channels. The resultant influx of Ca^{2+} contributes to both the membrane depolarization and the Ca^{2+} supply to the contractile filaments. By contrast, in vertebrate skeletal muscle contraction is observed in the absence of extracellular Ca^{2+}.[71] As in nerve axons, the Ca^{2+} necessary for cell contraction is derived from intracellular stores subsequent to cell activation mediated by voltage-dependent Na^+ and K^+ channels.[72] There are Ca^{2+} channels in skeletal muscle, but their physiological role in muscle contraction is not well established.[73]

It has been reported that the contractile response to AVP is dependent on the presence of extracellular Ca^{2+}.[74] It is, however, the "rounding up" of the cells that is extracellular Ca^{2+}-dependent and not isometric contraction. In cells exposed to AVP in media from which Ca^{2+} has been removed, isometric tension development can be clearly observed (personal communication, J. I. Kreisberg). Furthermore Okuda et al.[75] demonstrated that mesangial cells contract in response to AVP or ANG II in a Ca^{2+}-free medium containing 0.5 mM EGTA.

Singhal et al. found that the Ca^{2+} ionophore, A23187, resulted in wrinkling of the support upon which the mesangial cells were growing. This effect was also seen in some cells when they were treated with ionophore in nominally Ca^{2+}-free buffer. However, the extracellular Ca^{2+} concentration was not measured in these studies, and it therefore remains unclear to what extent release of Ca^{2+} from intracellular stores vs. entry of Ca^{2+} from the media contributed to the shape change. It is also not clear to what extent shape change reflects a contractile force.

Protein kinase C is also likely to play an important role in mesangial cell contractility. Protein kinase C phosphorylates myosin light chain kinase. In muscle cells myosin light chain kinase phosphorylates myosin light chain, which then interacts with actin to establish tension. It has been suggested by Rasmussen et al.[76] that protein kinase C activation may be responsible for the prolonged tonic contraction observed with many agonists in vascular smooth muscle. Troyer et al[77] found that phorbol esters and l-oleoyl acetylglycerol stimulated contraction of the mesangial cell in a manner synergistic with A23187. Thus Ca^{2+}, perhaps acting through calmodulin, together with protein kinase C activity, plays an important role in the contractile response of the mesangial cell.

The cAMP messenger system is also likely involved in the modulation of contractility along with Ca^{2+} and protein kinase C. Isoproterenol and PGI_2, two agents that increase cAMP levels, block shape change induced by AVP.[57] These agents, as well as dibutyryl-cAMP, decrease mesangial cell adherence and the number of focal contacts to the cell support. These effects result in a shape change, which is manifest when these cAMP elevating agents are exposed to cells in the absence of other vasoactive agents. These effects are independent of extracellular Ca^{2+}.[57] Myosin light chain phosphorylation is increased with AVP and decreased[4] with agents that enhance cAMP. We have demonstrated that dibutyryl-cAMP has no effect on $[Ca^{2+}]_f$ and does not alter the AVP-induced increase in $[Ca^{2+}]_f$. Troyer et al[78] have shown that cAMP has no effect on polyphosphoinositide metabolism.

Meyer-Lehnert et al.[16] found that atriopeptin III resulted in fewer cells changing shape in response to AVP. Since guanosine 3', 5'-cyclic monophosphate (cGMP) is believed to mediate some of the effects of atriopeptins, these investigators examined the effects of 8-bromo cGMP on AVP-induced changes in $[Ca^{2+}]_f$ and on the percent of cells changing shape with AVP. When either functional response to AVP was studied, 8-bromo cGMP was found to be inhibitory.

Ca^{2+}-Activated Cl-Channels

Few electrophysiological studies have been performed on the mesangial cell.[75,79] Okuda et al.[75] determined the resting membrane potential to be -53 ± 7 mV and Nobiling and Buhrle[79] found it to be -52 ± 29 mV. Okuda et al. found that ANG II depolarized the cells by 24 mV. The reversal potential of the depolarization response to ANG II and AVP was -29 ± 3 and -25 ± 7 mV, respectively. The reversal potential was dependent upon extracellular $[Cl^-]$, leading to a conclusion that the depolarizing effects of ANG II and AVP were due to changes in chloride conductance. The reversal potential of the depolarization response to A23187 was almost identical to that of ANG II and AVP, and was dependent upon extracellular $[Cl^-]$. Thus, the depolarization effects were likely mediated by a Ca^{2+} dependent Cl^- conductance pathway. This depolarization response was observed with ANG II or AVP, even in a Ca^{2+}-free medium containing 0.5 mM EGTA, indicating that Ca^{2+} release from intracellular storage sites mediated the enhancement of Cl^- conductance. The authors proposed that this change in permeability to Cl^- may be important to the tubuloglomerular feedback system in vivo.

Proliferation

The role of calcium in the proliferation of mesangial cells is not well established. In fact, the role of calcium in growth stimulation in general is not well characterized. Many agonists that stimulate growth of mesangial cells, such as PDGF, AVP, and endothelin, produce an increase in $[Ca^{2+}]_f$. These agents, however, also increase diacylglycerol levels and presumably increase protein kinase C activation. In addition, agonists such as epidermal growth factor, which does not increase $[Ca^{2+}]_f$, and PDGF enhance the activity of kinases that phosphorylate proteins on tyrosine residues. This tyrosine kinase activity has been proposed to be critical to mitogenesis in a number of cell systems.

Extracellular calcium concentrations can affect the ability of many other cells to proliferate.[80,81] Inhibition of lectin- or interleukin 2-stimulated DNA synthesis in lymphocytes by Ca^{2+} antagonists has led to the speculation that Ca^{2+} entry from the external milieu of the cell is necessary for initial activation of lymphocyte proliferation.[82,83] Furthermore, it has been demonstrated in other cells that levels of calmodulin, an intracellular Ca^{2+} binding protein, increase during the cell cycle, reaching maximal levels in late G1 and early S.[84] Drugs that act by inhibiting calmodulin delay the progression of cells from G1 to S.

Increasing $[Ca^{2+}]_f$ with calcium ionophores has been found to increase the expression of proto-oncogenes such as c-fos and c-myc[85-87] in a number of different cell types. We have found[88] in mesangial cells that increasing $[Ca^{2+}]_f$ results in enhanced expression of an early growth response gene, Egr-1, which has recently been cloned by Sukhatme and colleagues.[89,90] This gene is the first early-growth-related gene coding for a protein with a "zinc finger motif," similar to the motif seen in many transcription factors.[91,92] There remain some questions, however, as to what degree, if any, the effects of the Ca^{2+} ionophores are mediated by activation of protein kinase C rather than an action of Ca^{2+} per se.

If Ca^{2+} is a potentiator of mesangial cell proliferation, then agents that decrease $[Ca^{2+}]_f$ might be expected to be antiproliferative. Johnson and colleagues[18] reported that atriopeptin 28 and atriopeptin 24 decreased thymidine incorporation in mesangial cells. They also found that atriopeptin 28 decreased resting levels of $[Ca^{2+}]_f$ and attenuated the maximal levels of $[Ca^{2+}]_f$ achieved with serum. By contrast Ganz et al.[19] found no effect of atriopeptin 28 on mesangial cell proliferation in response to AVP, in spite of the fact the atriopeptin 28 decreased basal levels of $[Ca^{2+}]_f$ and peak levels of $[Ca^{2+}]_f$ achieved in the AVP.

Dibutyryl-cAMP and forskolin, an activator of adenylate cyclase, also have antimitogenic effects.[93] We did not find any modulation of the $[Ca^{2+}]_f$ response to vasopressin in the presence of dibutyryl-cAMP.[4] Thus, the antiproliferative effect of cAMP may be mediated by an effect on the cell that does not depend upon a modulation of the $[Ca^{2+}]_f$ signal.

Ganz et al.[19] evaluated the determinants of the mitogenic effect of AVP and sought to determine relationships between the ability of this agent to cause proliferation and its ability to increase $[Ca^{2+}]_f$. They found that the level to which $[Ca^{2+}]_f$ increased with AVP was decreased with atriopeptin 28 or 2,3,4-trimethoxybenzoic acid 8-(diethyl-amino) octyl ester hydrochloride (TMB-8), an inhibitor of intracellular Ca^{2+} release. Neither agent, however, inhibited mitogenesis. On the other hand preincubation of the cells with 600 nM phorbol ester for 48 hrs, designed to down-regulate protein kinase C, resulted in inhibition of proliferation while inhibiting the AVP-induced elevation of $[Ca^{2+}]_f$. These authors concluded that protein kinase C was necessary for proliferation, whereas proliferation did not depend upon a maximal, initial rise in $[Ca^{2+}]_f$.

Calcium Antagonists

Ichikawa and colleagues[94] reported that verapamil and manganese, an organic and inorganic Ca^{2+} transport inhibitor, respectively, inhibited the ANG II-induced changes in K_f in vivo. It was suggested that these effects on K_f were due to inhibition of mesangial cell contractility due to inhibition of ANG II-induced Ca^{2+} uptake involved in excitation-contraction coupling. There are other potential explanations, however. Verapamil and manganese may inhibit local production of glomerular prostaglandins, which, if produced, would contribute to contractility. Verapamil and manganese may decrease the ANG II-induced generation of an agent such as thromboxane A_2, which would otherwise contribute to the angiotensin-induced decrease in K_f.

Hassid et al.[7] found no effect of incubating mesangial cells in a high K^+ bath (50 mM) and suggested that the cells have no voltage-dependent Ca^{2+} channels. Verapamil or nifedipine did not alter the initial levels of $[Ca^{2+}]_f$, nor the relative stimulation observed in the presence of ANG II, but did prevent a secondary increase in $[Ca^{2+}]_f$ that these authors observed with ANG II. Takeda et al.[12] found inhibition of the AVP and ANG II-induced early $[Ca^{2+}]_f$ transients when mesangial cells were pre-incubated with verapamil. Verapamil inhibited ANG II-induced $^{45}Ca^{2+}$ influx. In addition the time course of return to basal $[Ca^{2+}]_f$ was significantly different in the presence of verapamil. These investigators did not observe any inhibition of contraction with verapamil. de Arriba et al.,[95] by contrast, reported that verapamil inhibited ANG II-induced contraction, although the effect of TMB-8, which blocks Ca^{2+} release from intracellular stores, was greater than that of verapamil.

Loutzenhiser et al.[96] examined the effect of diltiazem upon the reduction in volume of isolated glomeruli that was observed with U-44069, a stable prostaglandin H_2 analog. These authors found that the effect of U-44069 was neither prevented nor reversed by diltiazem.

Pfeilschifter et al.[97] reported that verapamil abolished the norepinephrine, ANG II and PAF-induced enhancement of prostaglandin E_2 synthesis in the mesangial cell. Verapamil had no effect on PGE_2 synthesis induced by addition of exogenous arachidonic acid, indicating that the action of this agent was not to inhibit the cyclooxygenase enzyme. The authors also found that verapamil inhibited basal $^{45}Ca^{2+}$ uptake and prevented any increase in $^{45}Ca^{2+}$ uptake with either norepinephrine, ANG II or PAF.

Conclusion

There is a large amount of evidence to implicate Ca^{2+} as a critical intracellular mediator of many functional and dysfunctional responses of the mesangial cell. The precise manner in which Ca^{2+} regulates processes such as contraction, proliferation, and eicosanoid production remains unclear, however. Enhanced insight into the cellular mechanisms of Ca^{2+} modulation will potentially lead to a better understanding of the pathophysiological responses of the mesangial cell in disease states, in vivo. With better understanding, greater insight into fundamental issues of cell biology will result. Furthermore, it may be possible to engineer therapeutic interventions in a such way as to interrupt the Ca^{2+}-mediated pathophysiological response.

Acknowledgments. The work discussed in this chapter was supported by National Institutes of Health grants DK 39773 and DK 38452. The author is an Established Investigator of the American Heart Association.

References

1. Ausiello DA, Kreisberg JI, Roy C, Karnovsky MJ: Contraction of cultured rat glomerular cells of apparent mesangial origin after stimulation with angiotensin II and arginine vasopressin. J Clin Invest 65:754–760, 1980.

2. Scharschmidt LA, Dunn MJ: Prostaglandin synthesis by rat glomerular mesangial cells in culture. J Clin Invest 71:1756–1764, 1983.

3. Jim K, Hassid A, Sun F, Dunn MJ: Lipoxygenase activity in rat kidney glomeruli, glomerular epithelial cells, and cortical tubules. J Biol Chem 257:10294–10299, 1982.

4. Bonventre JV, Skorecki KL, Kreisberg JI, Cheung JY: Vasopressin increases cytosolic free calcium concentration in glomerular mesangial cells. Am J Physiol 251(Renal Fluid Electrolyte Physiol 20):F94–F102, 1986.

5. Kremer S, Harper P, Hegele R, Skorecki K: Bradykinin stimulates a rise in cytosolic calcium in renal glomerular mesangial cells via a pertussis toxin insensitive pathway. Can J Physiol Pharm 66:43–48, 1988.

6. Mene P, Dubyak GR, Scarpa A, Dunn MJ: Stimulation of cytosolic free calcium and inositol phosphates by prostaglandins in cultured rat mesangial cells. Biochem Biophys Res Comm 142:579–586, 1987.

7. Hassid A, Pidikiti N, Gammero D: Effects of vasoactive peptides on cytosolic calcium in cultured mesangial cells. Am J Physiol 251(Renal Fluid Electrolyte Physiol 20):F1018–F1028, 1986.

8. Badr KF, Murray JJ, Brezer MD, et al: Mesangial cell, glomerular and renal vascular responses to endothelin in the rat kidney. Elucidation of signal transduction pathways. J Clin Invest 83:336–342, 1989.

9. Bonventre JV, Weber PC, Gronich JH: PAF and PDGF increase cytosolic [Ca^{2+}] and phospholipase activity in mesangial cells. Am J Physiol 254(Renal Fluid Electrolyte Physiol 23):F87–F94, 1988.

10. Cheung JY, Constantine JM, Bonventre JV: Regulation of cytosolic free calcium in cultured renal epithelial cells. Am J Physiol 251(Renal Fluid Electrolyte Physiol 20):F690–F701, 1986.

11. Volpe P, Krause K-H, Hashimito S, et al: "Calciosome," a cytoplasmic organelle: The inositol 1,4,5-trisphosphate-sensitive Ca^{2+} store of nonmuscle cells? Proc Natl Acad Sci (USA) 85:1091–1095, 1988.

12. Takeda K, Meyer-Lehnert H, Kim JK, Schrier RW: Effect of angiotensin II on Ca^{2+} kinetics and contraction in cultured rat glomerular mesangial cells. Am J Physiol 254(Renal Fluid Electrolyte Physiol 23):F254–F266, 1988.

13. Simonson MS, Wann S, Mene P, et al: Endothelin stimulates phospholipase C, Na$^+$/H$^+$ exchange, c-fos expression, and mitogenesis in rat mesangial cells. J Clin Invest 83:708–712, 1989.

14. Mene P, Abboud HE, Dubyak GR, et al: Effects of PDGF on inositol phosphates, Ca^{2+}, and contraction of mesangial cells. Am J Physiol 253(Renal Fluid Electrolyte Physiol 22):F458–F463, 1987.

15. Kester M, Mene P, Dubyak GR, Dunn MJ: Elevation of cytosolic free calcium by platelet-activating factor in cultured rat mesangial cells. FASEB J 1:215–219, 1987.

16. Meyer-Lehnert H, Tsai P, Caramelo C, Schrier RW: ANF inhibits vasopressin-induced Ca^{2+} mobilization and contraction in glomerular mesangial cells. Am J Physiol 255(Renal Fluid Electrolyte Physiol 24):F771–F780, 1988.

17. Hassid A: Atriopeptins decrease resting and hormone-elevated cytosolic Ca in cultured mesangial cells. Am J Physiol 253(Renal Fluid Electrolyte Physiol 22):F1077–F1082, 1987.

18. Johnson A, Lermioglu F, Garg UC, et al: A novel biological effect of atrial natriuretic hormone: inhibition of mesangial cell mitogenesis. Biochem Biophys Res Commun 152:893–897, 1988.

19. Ganz MB, Pekar SK, Perfetto MC, Skerzel RB: Arginine vasopressin promotes growth of rat glomerular mesangial cells in culture. Am J Physiol 255(Renal Fluid Electrolyte Physiol 24):F898–F906, 1988.

20. Appel RG, Dubyak GR, Dunn MJ: Effect of atrial natriuretic factor on cytosolic free calcium in rat glomerular mesangial cells. FEBS Lett 224:396–400, 1987.

21. Exton JH: Mechanisms of action of calcium-mobilizing agonists: Some variations on a young theme. FASEB J 2:2670–2676, 1988.

22. Troyer DA, Kreisberg JI, Schwertz DW, Venkatachalam MA: Effects of vasopressin on phosphoinositides and prostaglandin production in cultured mesangial cells. Am J Physiol 249(Renal Fluid Electrolyte Physiol 18):F139–F147, 1985.

23. Bonventre JV, Swidler: Calcium dependency of prostaglandin E_2 production in rat glomerular mesangial cells. Evidence that protein kinase C modulates the Ca^{2+} -dependent activation of phospholipase A_2. J Clin Invest 82:168–176, 1988.

24. Pfeilschifter J, Bauer C: Pertussis toxin abolishes angiotensin II-induced phosphoinositide hydrolysis and prostaglandin synthesis in rat renal mesangial cells. Biochem J 236:289–294, 1986.

25. Schlondorf D, Satriano JA, DeCandido S: Different concentrations of pertussis toxin have opposite effects on agonist-induced PGE_2 formation in mesangial cells. Biochem Biophys Res Comm 141:39–45, 1986.

26. Orita Y, Fujiwara Y, Ochi S, Tanaka Y, Kamada T: Calcium-activated, phospholipid-dependent protein kinase in cultured rat mesangial cells. FEBS Lett 192:155–158, 1985.

27. Pfeilschifter J: Protein kinase C from rat mesangial cells: its role in homologous desensitization of angiotensin II-/! induced polyphosphoinositide hydrolysis. Biochem Biophys Acta 969:263–270, 1988.

28. Pfeilschifter J: Tumour promotor 12-0-tetradecanoylphorbol 13-acetate inhibits angiotensin II-induced inositol phosphate production and cytosolic Ca^{2+} rise in rat renal mesangial cells. FEBS Lett 203:262–266, 1986.

29. Pfeilschifter J, Bauer C: Different effects of phorbol ester on angiotensin II- and stable GTP analogue-induced activation of polyphosphoinositide phosphodiesterase in membranes isolated from rat renal mesangial cells. Biochem J 248:209–215, 1987.

30. Scharschmidt LA, Dunn MJ: Prostaglandin synthesis by rat glomerular mesangial cells in culture. Effects of angiotensin II and arginine vasopressin. J Clin Invest 71:1756–1764, 1983.

31. Ardaillou N, Nivez MP, Striker G, Ardaillou R: Prostaglandin synthesis by human glomerular cells in culture. Prostaglandins 26:773–784, 1983.

32. Schlondorff D, Satriano JA, Hagege J, et al: Effect of platelet-activating factor and serum-treated zymosan on prostaglandin E_2 synthesis, arachidonic acid release, and contraction of cultured rat mesangial cells. J Clin Invest 73:1227–1231, 1984.

33. Sraer J, Siess W, Moulonguet-Doleris L, et al: In vitro prostaglandin synthesis by various rat renal preparation. Biochem Biophys Acta 710:45–52, 1982.

34. Jim K, Hassid A, Sun F, Dunn MJ: Lipoxygenase activity in rat kidney glomeruli, glomerular epithelial cells, and cortical tubules. J Biol Chem 257:10294–10299, 1982.

35. Schlondorf D, DeCandido S, Satriano JA: Angiotensin II stimulates phospholipase C and A_2. Am J Physiol 253:C113– C120, 1987.

36. Derksen A, Cohen P: Patterns of fatty acid release from endogenous substrates by human platelet homogenates and membranes. J Biol Chem 250:9342–9347, 1975.

37. Frei E, Zahler P: Phospholipase A_2 from sheep erythrocyte membranes. Ca^{2+} dependence and localization. Biochem Biophys Acta 550:450–463, 1979.

38. Brugge JS: The p35/p36 substrates of protein-tyrosine kinases as inhibitors of phospholipase A_2. Cell 46:149–150, 1986.

39. Clark MA, Conway TM, Shorr RGL, Cooke ST: Identification and isolation of a mammalian protein which is antigenically and functionally related to the phospholipase A_2 stimulating peptide mellitin. J Biol Chem 262:4402–4406, 1987.

40. Bonventre JV: Prostaglandin E_2 synthesis by renal mesangial cells is enhanced by protein kinase C activation. A possible role for lipocortins. Proc Xth Int Cong Nephrol 225, 1987.

41. Pepinsky RB, Sinclair LK, Browning JL, et al: Purification and partial sequence analysis of a 37-kDa protein that inhibits phospholipase A_2 activity from rat peritoneal exudates. J Biol Chem 261:4239–4246, 1986.

42. Davidson FF, Dennis EA, Powell M, Glenney JR Jr: Inhibition of phospholipase A_2 by "lipocortins" and calpactins. J Biol Chem 262:1698–1705, 1987.

43. Gronich JH, Bonventre JV, Nemenoff RA: Identification and characterization of a hormonally-regulated form of phospholipase A_2 in rat renal mesangial cells. J Biol Chem 263:16645-16651, 1988.

44. Thuren T, Tulkki A-P, Virtanen JA, Kinnunen PKJ: Triggering of the activity of phospholipase A_2 by an electric field. Biochemistry 26:4907–4910, 1987.

45. Sweatt JD, Blair IA, Cragoe EJ, Linbird LE: Inhibitors of Na^+/H^+ exchange block epinephrine- and ADP- induced stimulation of human platelet phospholipase C by blockade of arachidonic acid release at a prior step. J Biol Chem 261:8660–8666, 1986.

46. Burch RM, Luini A, Axelrod J: Phospholipase A_2 and phospholipase C are activated by distinct GTP-binding proteins in response to α_1-adrenergic stimulation in FRTL5 thyroid cells. Proc Natl Acad Sci (USA) 83:7201–7205, 1986.

47. Jelsema CL: Light activation of phospholipase A_2 in rod outer segments of bovine retina and its modulation by GTP-binding proteins. J Biol Chem 262:163–168, 1987.

48. Lianos EA, Zanglis A: Biosynthesis and metabolism of 1-0-alkyl-2-acetyl-sn-glycerol-3-phosphocholine in rat glomerular mesangial cells. J Biol Chem 262: 8990–8993, 1987.

49. Elias H, Hossman A, Barth IB, Solmor A: Blood flow in the renal glomerulus. J Urol 83:790–798, 1960.

50. Richards AN, Schmidt CF: A description of the glomerular circulation in the frog's kidney and observations concerning the action of adrenaline and various other substances. Am J Physiol 7:178–208, 1924.

51. Bernik MB: Contractility of human glomeruli in culture. Nephron 6:1–10, 1969.

52. Latta H: Ultrastructure of the glomerular and juxtaglomerular apparatus. In Orloff J, Berliner RW (eds): Handbook of Physiology. Renal Physiology. Washington, DC, Am Physiol Soc, 1973, p 1.

53. Becker CG: Demonstration of actomyosin in cells of the renal glomerulus. Am J Pathol 66:97–110, 1972.

54. Mahieu PR, Foidart JB, Dubors CH, et al: Tissue culture of normal rat glomeruli: Contractile activity of the cultured mesangial cells. Invest Cell Pathol 3:121–128, 1980.

55. Foidart J, Sraer J, Delarue F, Mahieu P, Ardaillou R: Evidence for mesangial cell glomerular receptors for angiotensin II linked to mesangial cell contractility. FEBS Lett 121:333–339, 1980.

56. Mahieu PR, Foidart JB, Bubois CH, et al: Tissue culture of normal rat glomeruli: Contractile activity of the cultured mesangial cells. Invest Cell Pathol 3:121–138, 1980.

57. Kreisberg JI, Venkatachalam M, Troyer D: Contractile properties of cultured glomerular mesangial cells. Am J Physiol 249(Renal Fluid Electrolyte Physiol. 18):F457–F463, 1985.

58. Singhal PC, Scharschmidt LA, Gibbons N, Hays RM: Contraction and relaxation of cultured mesangial cells on a silicone rubber surface. Kidney Int 30:862–873, 1986.

59. Barnett R, Goldwasser P, Scharschmidt LA, Schlondorff D: Effects of leukotrienes on isolated rat glomeruli and cultured mesangial cells. Am J Physiol 250(Renal Fluid Electrolyte Physiol 19): F838–F844, 1986.

60. Simonson MS, Dunn MJ: Leukotriene C_4 and D_4 contract rat glomerular mesangial cells. Kidney Int 30:524–531, 1986.

61. Fujiwara Y, Kikkawa R, Kitamura E, et al: Angiotensin II effects upon glomerular intracapillary volume in the rat. Renal Physiol 7:344–348, 1984.

62. Haley DP, Sarrafian M, Bulger RE, et al: Structural and functional correlates of effects of angiotensin-induced changes in the rat glomerulus. Am J Physiol 253(Renal Fluid Electrolyte Physiol 22):F111–F119, 1987.

63. Savin VJ: In vitro effects of angiotensin II on glomerular function. Am J Physiol 251(Renal Fluid Electrolyte Physiol 20): F627–F634, 1986.

64. Mene P, Dunn MJ. Eicosanoids and control of mesangial cell contraction. Cicr Res 62:916–925, 1988.

65. Schlondorff D, Satriano JA, Hagege J, et al: Effect of platelet activating factor and serum-treated zymosan on PGE_2 synthesis, arachidonic acid release, and contraction of cultured rat mesangial cells. J Clin Invest 73:1227–1231, 1984.

66. Scharschmidt LA, Simonson M, Dunn MJ: Glomerular prostaglandins, angiotensin II, and nonsteroidal antiinflammatory drugs. Am J Med 81(suppl 2B): 30–42, 1986.

67. Ardaillou N, Hagege J, Nivez MP, et al: Vasoconstrictor-evoked prostaglandin synthesis in cultured human mesangial cells. Am J Physiol 248(Renal Fluid Electrolyte Physiol 17): F240–F246, 1985.

68. Meyer-Lehnert H, Schrier RW: Cyclosporine A enhances vasopressin-induced Ca^{2+} mobilization and contraction in mesangial cells. Kidney Int 34:89–97, 1988.

69. Kreisberg JI: Insulin requirement for contraction of cultured rat glomerular mesangial cells to angiotensin II. Possible role for insulin in modulating glomerular hemodynamics. Proc Natl Acad Sci (USA) 79:4190–4192, 1982.

70. Beeler, GW Jr, Reuter H: Membrane calcium current in ventricular myocardial fibers. J Physiol (Lond) 207:191–209, 1970.

71. Armstrong CM, Bezanilla FM, Horowicz P: Twitches in the presence of ethylene glycol bis(B-aminoethyl ether)-N,N'-tetraacetic acid. Biochem Biophys Acta 267:605–608, 1972.

72. Pappone PA: Voltage-clamp experiments in normal and denervated mammalian skeletal muscle fibers. J Physiol (Lond) 306:377–410, 1980.

73. Almers W, McCleskey EW, Palade PT: Calcium channels in vertebrate skeletal muscle. In Rubin RP, Weiss GB, Putney JW Jr (eds): Calcium in Biological Systems. New York, Plenum Press, 1985, pp 321–330.

74. Venkatachalam MA, Kreisberg JI: Agonist-induced isotonic contraction of cultured mesangial cells after multiple passage. Am J Physiol 249(Cell Physiol 18):C48–C55, 1985.

75. Okuda T, Yamashita N, Kurokawa K: Angiotensin II and vasopressin stimulate calcium-activated chloride conductance in rat mesangial cells. J Clin Invest 78:1443–1448, 1986.

76. Rasmussen H, Takuwa Y, Park S: Protein kinase C in the regulation of smooth muscle contraction. FASEB J 1:177–185, 1987.

77. Troyer DA, Gonzalez OF, Venkatachalam MA, Kreisberg JI: Elevation of cAMP in cultured mesangial cells diminishes vasopressin-stimulated increases of phosphate uptake and ^{32}p-specific activity in ATP but has no effect on phosphoinositide metabolism. J Biol Chem 262:1614–1617, 1987.

78. Troyer DA, Gonzalez OF, Douglas JG, Kreisberg JI: Phorbol ester inhibits arginine vasopressin activation of phospholipase C and promotes contraction of, and prostaglandin production by, cultured mesangial cells. Biochem J 251:907–912, 1988.

79. Nobiling R, Buhrle CP: The mesangial cell culture: A tool for the study of the electrophysiological and pharmacological properties of the glomerular mesangial cell. Differentiation 36:47–56, 1987.

80. Balk SD: Calcium as a regulator of the proliferation of normal but not of transformed chicken fibroblasts in plasma-containing medium. Proc Natl Acad Sci 68:271–275, 1971.

81. Hazelton B, Mitchell B, Tupper J: Calcium, magnesium and growth control in the WI-38 human fibroblast cell. J Cell Biol 83:487–498, 1979.

82. Birx DL, Berger M, Fleisher TA: The interference of T cell activation by calcium channel blocking agents. J Immunol 133:2904–2909, 1984.

83. Grier CE, Mastro AM: Mitogen and co-mitogen stimulation of lymphocytes inhibited by three Ca^{2+} antagonists. J Cell Physiol 124:131–136, 1985.

84. Chafouleas JG, Bolton WE, Hidaka H, et al: Calmodulin and the cell cycle:involvement in regulation of cell cycle progression. Cell 28:41–50, 1982.

85. Bravo R, Burckhardt J, Curran T, Muller R: Stimulation and inhibition of growth by EGF in different A431 cell clones is accompanied by the rapid induction of a c-fos and c-myc proto-oncogenes. EMBO J 4:1193–1198, 1985.

86. Tsuda T, Kaibuchi K, West B, Takai Y: Involvement of Ca^{2+} in platelet-derived growth factor-induced expression of c-myconcogene in Swiss 3T3 fibroblasts. FEBS Lett 187:43–46, 1985.

87. Reed JC, Nowell PC, Hoover RG: Regulation of c-myc mRNA levels in normal human lymphocytes by modulators of cell proliferation. Proc Natl Acad Sci 82:4221–4224, 1985.

88. Bonventre JV, Sullivan S, Sukhatme V, Ouellette AJ: Vasopressin increases the expression of the early growth response gene, *Egr-1*, in cultured mesangial cells. Kidney Int 24:169, 1989.

89. Sukhatme VP, Kartha S, Toback EG, et al: A novel early growth response gene rapidly induced by fibroblast, epithelial cell and lymphocyte mitrogens. Oncogene Res 1:343–355, 1987.

90. Sukhatme VP, Cao X, Chang LC, et al: A zinc finger- encoding gene coregulated with c-fos during growth and differentiation, and after cellular depolarization. Cell 53:37– 43, 1988.

91. Brown RS, Sander C, Argos P: The primary structure of transcription factor TF111A has 12 consecutive repeats. FEBS Lett 186:271–274, 1985.

92. Rhodes D, Klug A: An underlying repeat in some transcriptional control sequences corresponding to half a double helical turn of DNA. Cell 46:123–132, 1986.

93. Abboud HE, Throckmorton D, Weinshell E, Jaffer F: Differential modulation of mesangial cell proliferation by peptide growth factors and cyclic adenosine monophosphate (cAMP). FASEB J 2:A627, 1988.

94. Ichikawa I, Miele JF, Brenner BM: Reversal of renal cortical actions of angiotensin II by verapamil and manganese. Kidney Int 16:137–147, 1979.

95. deArriba G, Barrio V, Olivera A, Rodriguez-Puyol D, Lopez-Novoa JM: Atrial natriuretic peptide inhibits angiotensin II-induced contraction of isolated glomeruli and cultured glomerular mesangial cells of rats: The role of calcium. J Lab Clin Med 111:466–474, 1988.

96. Loutzenhiser R, Epstein M, Horton C, Sonke P: Reversal of renal and smooth muscle actions of the thromboxane mimetic U-44069 by diltiazen. Am J Physiol 250(Renal Fluid Electrolyte Physiol 19):F619–F626, 1986.

97. Pfeilschifter J, Kurtz A, Bauer C: Role of phospholipase C and protein kinase C in vasoconstriction-induced prostaglandin synthesis in cultured rat renal mesangial cells. Biochem J 234:125–130, 1986.

P. Darwin Bell, Ph.D
Martha Franco, M.D

6

Regulation of Renal Epithelial Cell Function and Tubuloglomerular Feedback by Cytosolic Calcium

Within the last few years there has been an increasing awareness that intracellular calcium subserves an important role in the control and regulation of many intrarenal events. This applies not only to the calcium-mediated excitation-contraction-coupling of the renal microvasculature, but also to the control of many renal tubular epithelium processes. At this later site, cytosolic calcium and other intracellular messenger systems may serve in the regulation of transepithelial transport and in the responsiveness of the renal epithelium to hormonal regulation. Since the nephron is composed of a number of distinct morphological and functional segments, this provides for an interesting diversity in the way that intracellular calcium participates in epithelial function. However, this diversity does prevent the development of a "unified view" concerning the role of intracellular calcium in nephron function. The purpose of this review is to exemplify some of the roles that calcium may play in the control and regulation of epithelial cell function. Because of the breadth of this subject, this review will not be comprehensive and will not consider each individual nephron segment. Specifically, we will address the following issues: (1) regulation of cytosolic calcium concentration by renal epithelia; (2) cytosolic calcium regulation of transepithelial transport; (3) the effects of adenosine receptor activation on transport and cytosolic calcium concentration in the cortical thick ascending limb (cTAL), and (4) mediation of tubuloglomerular feedback signal transmission by cytosolic calcium.

Control of Cytosolic Calcium in Renal Epithelium

In recent years, efforts have been made to measure the level of cytosolic calcium in renal epithelial cells. Most measurements have been obtained in vitro using either isolated nephron segments or cultured cells derived from renal tissue. The proximal tubule has received considerable attention; however, studies have also been performed in other segments such as the cortical collecting tubule. Measurements of cytosolic calcium concentration have been performed using a variety of techniques, including Ca^{2+} microelectrodes,[1] aequorin,[2] arsenazo III,[3] the null-point method,[4] and the recently developed fluorescent indicators Quin 2 and the newer generation Fura 2.[3,5-8] Each technique has potential problems and technical limitations, but each method can provide at least an estimate of cytosolic calcium levels. In general, proximal cell cytosolic calcium concentration, whether derived from freshly dissected tubules or from cell culture, is in the range of 75 to 200 nM. As shown in Figure 1, studies from our laboratory on the cortical thick ascending limb (cTAL) indicate that under control conditions, cytosolic calcium concentration in this nephron segment is similar, averaging approximately 100 nM. In addition, Figure 1 shows that in this segment cytosolic calcium concentration is sensitive to alterations in external calcium concentration. Removal of bath calcium, which lowers external calcium concentration from 1.5 mM to approximately 100 μM, decreased cytosolic calcium from 125 nM to 50 nM. Accordingly, most values obtained under control conditions from nonstimulated renal epithelial cells indicate that calcium concentration is within the low nanomolar range. This fact should not be surprising since it agrees with values obtained in nearly all living cells. In fact, maintenance of the gradient, 10^{-3} M extracellular versus 10^{-7} M cytosol, for calcium is probably one important criteria for determining cell life.[10] Maintenance of this gradient is dependent upon calcium transport mechanisms located at both plasma membrane and intracellular organelles.

Studies of cell membrane transport mechanisms that help maintain and regulate cytosolic calcium concentration in renal cells are complex due, in part, to epithelial cell polarization resulting in different transport properties for apical and basolateral surfaces. Another complicating feature is that certain tubular segments, such as the proximal tubule and thick ascending limb, exhibit net transepithelial transport of calcium. These cells must contend not only with forces that work against the maintenance of low intracellular cytosolic calcium concentration but also must be capable of adapting to conditions that alter transcellular calcium transport.

Evidence from studies in the proximal tubules indicates that the major route for calcium movement across the basolateral membrane is through the Ca^{2+} ATPase transporter.[11,12] It has also been argued that this transporter is primarily responsible for the control and regulation of cytosolic calcium concentration. Calcium transport through this pathway is markedly stimulated in the presence of the calcium-binding protein, calmodulin. Kinetic studies indicate during activation of Ca^{2+} ATPase by calmodulin that this transporter has a large capacity for calcium transport and an affinity for calcium that is within the physiological range of resting or stimulated cytosolic calcium concentrations (100 to 600 nM).[13] The structure, function, and calcium affinity of the renal Ca^{2+} ATPase appears to be very similar to the Ca^{2+} ATPase found in other tissues.[14] Thus, under conditions in which there are increases in cytosolic calcium concentration, calcium binding to calmodulin would activate Ca^{2+} ATPase and result in increased calcium efflux from the cell. Potentially Ca^{2+} ATPase could return cytosolic calcium concentration back to control levels. Other transport mechanisms exist, and it cannot be concluded with certainty that the Ca^{2+} ATPase is entirely responsible for the final regulation of cytosolic calcium levels. For instance, one such transporter that is thought to participate in renal epithelial calcium transport is the Na^+/Ca^{2+} exchanger.

Within the kidney the Na^+/Ca^{2+} exchanger is present at the basolateral membrane of at least the proximal tubule and cortical collecting tubule. The physiological role of this transporter has, however, remained controversial. Studies in basolateral vesicles have found that under conditions of zero external sodium and preloading

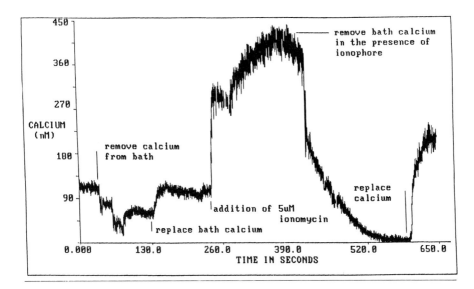

FIGURE 1. Rabbit cortical thick ascending limbs were dissected in an isotonic dissecting media containing 5 μM Fura-2 AM for 1 hour. Tubules were transferred to a chamber mounted on an inverted microscope, cannulated, and perfused with isotonic perfusates. Fura-2 fluorescence was measured using a spectrophotometer with excitation monchrometers set at 340 nm and 380 nm. Emission wavelength was set at 515 nm. Fluorescence intensity was quantitated using a variable diaphragm and a photometer-based system. Calibration procedures and cytosolic calcium concentration was calculated using standard techniques. Initial cytosolic calcium concentration $[Ca^{++}]$ was 95 nM and decreased to about 50 nM upon removal of extracellular Ca^{++}. $[Ca^{++}]$ returned to 95 nM after readdition of normal Ca^{++}. Ionomycin (5 μM) increased $[Ca^{++}]$ to over 400 nM. $[Ca^{++}]$ was reduced to near zero with the addition of a bathing solution containing no Ca^{++} and 5 μM EGTA.

with calcium, addition of sodium to the epithelial membrane results in calcium efflux and sodium influx. The converse experiment is also true. Under conditions of high intravesicular sodium and no external calcium, addition of calcium results in sodium efflux and calcium influx.[11] In the intact cell, assessing the direction and rate of calcium transport is complex, since it requires knowledge of the affinity of the exchanger for both calcium and sodium, intracellular and extracellular calcium and sodium activities, and membrane electrical potential. Kinetic analysis indicates that the affinity of the exchanger for Ca^{2+} is considerably higher than the affinity of Ca^{2+} ATPase for calcium.[15] In fact, there is the possibility that this exchanger may not participate, in a meaningful way, in calcium extrusion from the cell, although this point is controversial. At the present time, it is not known whether, under normal in vivo conditions, the Na^+/Ca^{2+} exchanger produces Ca^{2+} influx or efflux, or if the exchanger is at thermodynamic equilibrium with little flux of sodium of calcium through this transporter. However, as shown in studies by Yang, Lee and Windhager,[1] under most circumstances where there are experimentally induced decreases in the electrochemical gradient for sodium, there are measured increases in cytosolic calcium concentration. For instance, these investigators found that maneuvers such as removal of bath potassium, or administration of either ouabain or gramicidin, resulted in increases in intracellular sodium concentration and increases in cytosolic calcium concentration. Likewise reductions in the sodium concentration of the bathing solution to 10 mM reduced the electrochemical driving force for sodium across the basolateral membrane and increased cytosolic calcium concentration from about 82 nM to 585 nM. Thus, it appears from these studies that intracellular calcium concentration is, under at least some conditions, influenced by changes in sodium electrochemical potential across the basolateral membrane.

Much less is known concerning transport by the apical or luminal membrane. Calcium entry occurs through a specific transport pathway, however, little is known concerning the kinetics and regulation of this pathway.

Regulation of cytosolic calcium concentration also involves calcium fluxes between intracellular calcium binding sites, mitochondria, and endoplasmic reticulum. As in other cell types, renal proximal tubular cell mitochondria and endoplasmic reticulum can sequester and release calcium. The mitochondria has a large capacity to store calcium but can only reduce free calcium levels to approximately 500 nM.[16] The endoplasmic reticulum has a lower calcium storage capacity but can reduce free calcium concentration down to physiological levels.[17] In addition, the endoplasmic reticulum contains an inositol 1,4,5-trisphosphate(IP$_3$) sensitive calcium pool that can be released during intracellular calcium mobilization.[17] Finally, a great deal of intracellular calcium is bound to cell membranes and intracellular proteins. Regulation of these calcium pools is not well understood.

Regulation of Transepithelial Transport by Cytosolic Calcium

The modification of tubular fluid that occurs along the length of the nephron is a consequence of the transport of water, electrolytes, and solutes across the renal epithelium. There are numerous mechanisms, both intrinsic and extrinsic, that serve to regulate transport processes within each nephron segment. Both extrinsic (e.g., hormones, nerves)[18] and intrinsic (see below) mechanisms influence nephron function through the activation of intracellular messenger systems; cytosolic calcium contributes importantly to the regulation of transepithelial transport.[19,20] Studies in the proximal tubule and collecting duct have shown that experimental manipulations that increase cytosolic calcium concentration result in diminished sodium and water transport.[19−21] Addition of the calcium ionophore A23187, which markedly increases cytosolic calcium concentration, inhibits volume reabsorption. Similarly, inhibition of transport was found during administration of quinidine, an agent that has been reported to mobilize intracellular calcium.[22] In isolated perfused proximal tubule experiments, reductions in extracellular calcium concentration resulted in enhanced proximal tubular reabsorption.[21] As indicated previously, alterations in extracellular calcium concentration can influence cytosolic calcium concentration. Thus, these studies indicate that increases in cytosolic calcium concentration, at least in the proximal tubule and cortical collecting tubule, are associated with decreases in transepithelial transport, whereas decreases in cytosolic calcium concentration are associated with increases in transport.

The mechanism by which increases in cytosolic calcium concentration inhibit transepithelial sodium transport is not known with certainty. Studies by Yang, Lee and Windhager[1] indicate that, in the proximal tubule, elevations of intracellular calcium with either ionomycin or quinidine result in decreases in intracellular sodium concentration. This argues for calcium inhibition of sodium transport at the apical membrane and not at the basolateral membrane. In other studies, using patch clamp techniques,[23,24] increased calcium levels inhibited apical sodium channel activity; however, this effect occurred only with cell-attached patches, and no inhibition occurred in excised patches. Inhibition of the channel may be due to some secondary event, since reductions in sodium current with increased cytosolic calcium were relatively slow (minutes). Taken together, these studies indicate that elevations in intracellular calcium concentration decrease transport, probably through an inhibition of sodium entry across the apical membrane, although the mechanism for this inhibition remains to be determined.

A number of studies have examined the regulation of transepithelial sodium transport by cytosolic calcium via basolateral Na^+/Ca^{2+} exchange.[20,21,25] As shown in Figure 2, under conditions of enhanced sodium entry across the apical membrane, intracellular sodium concentration would rise, thereby decreasing the electrochemical gradient for sodium across the basolateral membrane. A decrease in the electrochemical gradient for sodium might stimulate calcium influx through the Na^+/Ca^{2+} exchanger and increase cytosolic calcium concentration. The increase in intracellular calcium would result in an inhibition of sodium entry across the apical membrane, leading to a fall in intracellular sodium concentration. This intrinsic mechanism would serve in the control of sodium reabsorption, providing a means of coupling the apical sodium entry with the exit of sodium across the basolateral membrane.

Other pathways for calcium regulation across the basolateral membrane may exist in renal epithelial cells. Administration of calcium antagonists induces diuresis and natriuresis that appear to be independent of alterations in blood flow and glomerular filtration rate. It has been suggested that the effects of calcium antagonists may be the result of inhibition of the neurogenic regulation of renal transport.[25a] Alternatively it has been suggested that calcium antagonists directly inhibit transepithelial transport, perhaps at some distal nephron site. However, voltage-sensitive

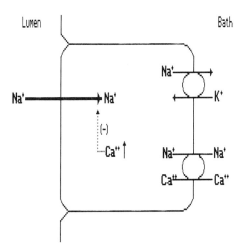

FIGURE 2.   Model representing the regulation of transepithelial sodium transport by cytosolic Ca^{++} via $Na^+/Ca++$ exchange. See text for explanations

calcium channels have not, as yet, been identified within renal epithelia. Thus, the mechanism by which calcium antagonists induce salt and water excretion by the kidney remains to be determined.

In recent studies, [9] we have examined the possibility that intracellular calcium may participate in the regulation of Na^+Cl^- transport in the cortical thick ascending limb (cTAL). Numerous studies[26-29] have indicated that the entry step for Na^+Cl^- across the apical membrane is through the furosemide sensitive $Na^+:2Cl^-:K^+$ triporter. Reabsorption of Na^+Cl^- by the water impermeant cTAL results in the dilution of tubular fluid; at the end of the cTAL, Na^+ Cl^- values can reach 20 to 25 mM. At the basolateral membrane, there is an abundance of Na^+K^+ ATPase as well as a chloride conductive pathway. Na^+Cl^- transport by the cTAL results in the generation of a transepithelial potential that is lumen-positive with respect to the bath. As shown by Greger and coworkers,[27] the positive luminal potential can be used as an index of Na^+Cl^- transport by this segment. The electrical potential difference is sensitive to luminal administration of furosemide or other "loop diuretics," which reduce the potential difference to near zero.

In order to determine the effects of increased cytosolic calcium concentration on cTAL transport, we measured the effects of luminal administration of the calcium ionophore, ionomycin, on transepithelial potential difference. Administration of the calcium ionophore resulted in a substantial decrease in transepithelial potential difference towards zero. In fact, ionomycin was just as effective as furosemide in reducing the transepithelial potential difference and therefore in inhibiting Na^+Cl^- transport in this segment. As indicated earlier, in the proximal tubule and collecting duct increases in cytosolic calcium concentration inhibit transport by blocking the apical entry step. It is not known at what site calcium inhibits transport in the TAL; however, possible sites of action include the $Na^+:2Cl^-:K^+$ triporter or a K^+ conductance that recycles potassium across the apical membrane.

Since cytosolic calcium may participate in the regulation of transepithelial transport in the cTAL, it was of interest to determine if the same model for the regulation of transport via Na^+/Ca^{2+} exchange was also applicable to this epithelium. To accomplish this goal, we tested the effects of alterations in bathing solution sodium concentration on cytosolic calcium concentration.[30] Studies were performed in the nonperfused collapsed tubule in order to mitigate the complication of simultaneous transport occurring across the apical membrane. Figure 3 shows a schematic of the experimental design and Figure 4 is an example of an experiment testing the effects of changes in external sodium concentration on cytosolic calcium concentration. The cTALs were dissected and bathed in a solution containing 2 or 6 mM sodium. The experimental period consisted of rapidly switching to a bathing solution that contained normal amounts of sodium (Na^+ = 140 mM). If Na^+/Ca^{2+} exchange was present in this nephron segment, then two predictions obtain. First, under conditions of reduced extracellular sodium concentration, TAL cytosolic calcium concentration should be increased as found in proximal and collecting duct tubules. [1,21,31] Second, reintroduction of sodium should initially result in an increase in the electrochemical driving force for sodium across the basolateral membrane and a decrease in cytosolic calcium concentration.

As shown in Figure 4, the control Fura 2 fluorescent ratio yields a calculated value for cytosolic calcium concentration control of 133 nM in the absence of extracellular sodium. This value is within the normal range of cytosolic calcium concen-

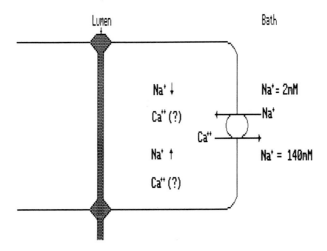

FIGURE 3. Schematic of experiment testing the effects of reduced bathing solution sodium concentration of cTAL cytosolic calcium concentration. These experiments were performed in nonperfused tubules in order to negate the effects of transport across the luminal membrane. Under control conditions, the bath contained 2 or 6 mM sodium. The experimental period consisted of increasing bath sodium concentration to 140 mM.

trations measured in cTALs bathed with a complete Ringer's solution. With the reintroduction of sodium, cytosolic calcium concentration increased to 253 nM and did not decrease as expected. Thus, these results are not consistent with the presence of a Na^+/Ca^{2+} exchange mechanism located on the basolateral membrane of the cTAL. However, these results suggest that changes in intracellular sodium can alter cTAL cytosolic calcium concentration. Low extracellular sodium would presumably decrease intracellular sodium concentration while reintroduction of extracellular sodium would result in the movement of sodium into the cell and transiently increase intracellular sodium concentration. It is possible that increases in intracellular sodium concentration may either directly or indirectly result in increased cytosolic calcium concentration.

It was also of interest to determine if elevations in cytosolic calcium concentration during increased extracellular sodium was due to calcium entry across the basolateral membrane or calcium mobilization from internal stores. The previous studies were repeated, except that all calcium was removed and 5 mM EGTA was added to the bathing solution immediately prior to sodium reintroduction. Although removal of extracellular calcium resulted in a decline of basal cytosolic calcium concentration, addition of sodium resulted in a large transient increase in cytosolic calcium concentration. In other studies, addition of TMB-8, an intracellular calcium antagonist that binds to bound or sequestered calcium[32,33] and prevents calcium release, completely abolished the rise in cytosolic calcium concentration during sodium reintroduction, suggesting that the increase in cytosolic calcium concentration during addition of sodium was due to calcium mobilization.

These studies indicate that in the cTAL cytosolic calcium participates in the regulation of transepithelial transport. Increases in intracellular calcium appear to

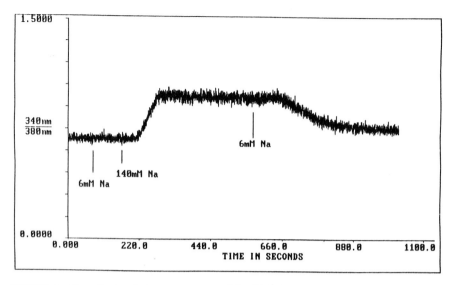

FIGURE 4. The effects of changes in extracellular [Na$^+$] on ratio of Fura 2 fluorescence in cortical thick ascending limb. The initial ratio represents a [Ca^{++}] of 133 nM, which is within the normal range. With the introduction of a bathing solution containing 140 mM Na$^+$, the ratio increased and calculated cytosolic [Ca^{++}] rose to 253 nM. This increase was reversible with reintroduction of the 6 mM Na$^+$ containing bathing solution.

have a "furosemide-like effect," and it is possible that calcium inhibits an apical transport event. Unlike the proximal tubule or collecting duct, the cTAL does not appear to possess a basolateral Na$^+$/Ca^{2+} exchanger; however, these studies suggest the intriguing possibility that changes in intracellular sodium may directly result in calcium mobilization.

Hormonal Regulation of Transport in the cTAL

It is generally accepted that autocoids and humoral substances play an important role in the control of renal epithelial transport.[18] It is also clear that each nephron segment contains specific receptors that are linked to intracellular messenger systems. Although a great deal of information is now known regarding the mechanisms responsible for transepithelial transport in the cTAL,[26] little is known concerning the effects of autocoids or hormones on the regulation of transport in this segment. Based on certain considerations, we felt it likely that adenosine might play a role in the regulation of cTAL transport. Adenosine is produced by metabolic breakdown of ATP and is transported out of cells and into extracellular fluid.[34,35] It is also found in urine, so that at least some of the adenosine that is produced by renal cells enters tubular fluid. Presently, there is evidence for two adenosine receptors (A1 and A2) located on the external surface of cells. The A2 receptor stimulates the formation of cAMP, whereas the A1 receptor inhibits cAMP generation and may in some cells result in increased cytosolic calcium concentration.[36,37]

It is possible that adenosine or activation of adenosine receptors influences transport at some site(s) within the kidney.[34,38,39] Systemic administration of adenosine induces
natriuresis, which may be unrelated to the affects of these agents on hemodynamics and glomerular filtration rate.[40] In addition, adenosine receptors have been identified within the kidney.[41] These studies have not provided specific location of the receptors, i.e., which cell type and whether or not there is a preferential location of the receptors to one specific area of the cell.

In recent studies in shark rectal gland, Kelly and coworkers[42] found that adenosine may serve as a negative modulator of chloride secretion. In this epithelium, chloride secretion proceeds via a furosemide-sensitive pathway. Numerous secretagogues can activate chloride secretion, and it was found that stimulation of chloride secretion resulted in increased adenosine production. In fact there was a close correlation between the level of chloride secretion and the amount of adenosine produced by the gland. In addition, inhibition of adenosine A1 receptors resulted in enhanced chloride secretion. Thus, in this system enhanced chloride secretion produced increased adenosine production, resulting in a feedback inhibition of chloride secretion. These results indicate that adenosine may be an important local regulator of transepithelial transport.

In recent studies we have evaluated the effects of adenosine receptor agonists and antagonists on cTAL transport. We chose to examine the effects of the A1 receptor agonist CPA,[43] since A1 agonists have been shown by Arend et al.[44] to increase cytosolic calcium concentration in cultured cortical-collecting tubule cells. In previous tubuloglomerular feedback studies, the receptor agonist produced responses when added to the lumen, and this provided the impetus to first examine the effects of these agents when added to the luminal perfusate. Addition of the adenosine A1 receptor agonist was found to decrease the transepithelial potential difference by some 40%. This indicates that the adenosine A1 receptor was effective in reducing the rate of transepithelial transport in the cTAL. In other studies, we examined the effects the A1 receptor agonist on cTAL cytosolic calcium concentration using Fura 2. As shown in Figure 5, addition of the agonist resulted in an increase in cytosolic calcium concentration. Maximal concentrations of the agonist produced approximately a twofold increase in cytosolic calcium concentration. This increase was blocked by coinfusion of the receptor blocker. Interestingly, the increase in cytosolic calcium concentration with the A1 receptor agonist was found only when the agonist was administered into the lumen; no change in cytosolic calcium concentration was observed when the agonist was added to the bathing solution. These results suggest that, like the shark rectal gland, adenosine may participate in the regulation of transport in the cTAL. In addition adenosine may act not from the basolateral side but rather by activation of receptors located on the apical membranes of cTAL. Figure 6 outlines our current working hypothesis regarding the role of cytosolic calcium and adenosine receptors in the control of cTAL transport.

Calcium Mediation of Macula Densa Tubuloglomerular Feedback Signals

As discussed in the preceding section, reabsorption of Na^+ Cl^- by the water impermeant cTAL results in a diminution of luminal Na^+ Cl^- concentration along the

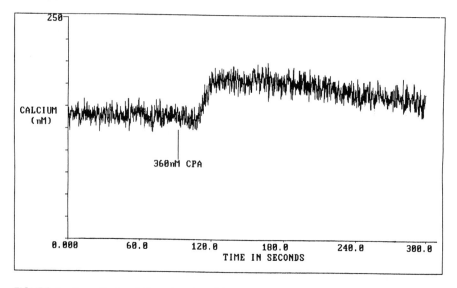

FIGURE 5 The effects of the adenosine A1 receptor agonists (CPA) on cytosolic calcium concentration in the cortical thick ascending limb. See Figure 1 legend for details of methodology.

length of the cTAL. Na^+ Cl^- reabsorption is, however, flow-dependent and varies directly with the initial flow rate into the cTAL. At low flow rates, Na^+ Cl^- at the end of the cTAL is reduced to low concentrations (15 to 30 mM) but can increase up to isotonic values at high luminal flow rates. Near the end of the cTAL, there is an area of contact between the cTAL and its own glomerulus. At the site of contact between glomerulus and tubule, the tubular cells facing the glomerulus are specialized and are referred to as macula densa cells. These cells rest on layers of diffuse intermingling extraglomerular mesangial cells; the extraglomerular mesangial cells are contiguous with the intraglomerular mesangial cells as well as the smooth muscle cells of the arterioles. Specialized gap junctions are clearly evident throughout this area, except between macula densa cells and extraglomerular mesangial cells. [45,46]

As discussed in several recent reviews,[46-49] the macula densa cells are involved in a unique intrarenal mechanism that participates in the regulation of glomerular filtration rate. The macula densa cells appear to detect changes in luminal fluid composition and transmit signals to the afferent arteriole and perhaps other contractile elements within the glomerulus. Under conditions where luminal Na^+ Cl^- concentration and osmolality increase, macula densa cells transmit vasoconstrictor signals, resulting in decreases in glomerular filtration rate. On the other hand, reductions in luminal Na^+ Cl^- concentration and osmolality produce vasodilation and increases in glomerular filtration rate. This intranephron signaling process is termed tubuloglomerular feedback and is considered to be an important regulator of renal hemodynamics.

Most of the information that is available concerning the tubuloglomerular feedback mechanism has been obtained using in vivo micropuncture and microperfusion techniques. Using this methodology, it has been possible to characterize the tubuloglomerular feedback responses in several species including dog and rat.

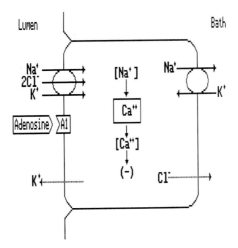

FIGURE 6. Proposed model for the regulation of transport by cortical thick ascending limb (cTAL). According to this model, enhanced transport into the cTAL increases intracellular sodium concentration, which then leads directly or indirectly to calcium mobilization. Increased cytosolic calcium concentration decreases transport in this segment. Another means of regulating transport is through activation of adenosine A1 receptors. Activation of these receptors increases cytosolic calcium concentration and decreases transport in the cTAL.

As shown in Figure 7, increases in flow rate into the late proximal tubule results in elevations in distal tubule fluid osmolality and sodium chloride concentration. This elevation in distal tubular fluid composition results in decreases in single-nephron glomerular filtration rate and stop-flow pressure, an index of glomerular capillary pressure. A number of studies have attempted to define the specific compositional change that is detected by the macula densa cells. These studies have involved measuring feedback responses during microperfusion with solutions containing different osmolalities and different sodium chloride concentrations. This issue has remained controversial, and it is not entirely clear whether these cells detect changes in osmolality or specific changes in sodium or chloride concentration. Indeed the macula densa cells may respond to several different physico-chemical-humoral components of tubular fluid. However, the relative importance of these initial "activators" in the feedback transmission process is not well understood.

It has recently been possible to study the macula densa cells directly using an isolated perfused thick ascending limb–macula densa preparation. This technique has provided the opportunity to directly examine the effects of changes in luminal fluid composition on macula densa cells. With this approach studies[50] have examined the effects of changes in luminal fluid osmolality on the morphology of macula densa cells. With the use of differential-interference contrast optics, changes in the width of the lateral intercellular spaces between macula densa cells have been examined in response to alterations in luminal fluid osmolality. When luminal fluid osmolality was reduced from isotonic to hypotonic values, the spaces between the macula densa cells dilated and the height of the macula densa cells increased, suggesting that the macula densa plaque is permeable to water. In recent work, Ribadeniera and Barfuss[51] directly measured macula densa water permeability using the concentration

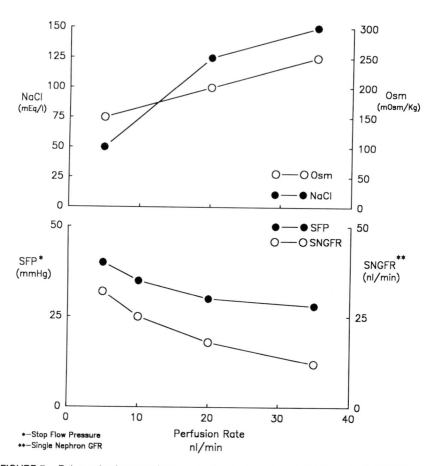

FIGURE 7. Relationship between late proximal perfusion rate and distal tubular fluid NaCl concentration and osmolality (top panel) and stop flow pressure (SFP) and single nephron glomerular filtration rate (SNGFR) (bottom panel) obtained in rat micropuncture experiments. Increases in perfusion rate results in elevations in osmolality and NaCl concentration at the macula densa and feedback mediated decreases in SFP and SNGFR.

of a volume marker added to the luminal fluid. They found that the macula densa cells exhibit a very high degree of water permeability, which was in fact higher than the water permeability calculated for the proximal tubule. The macula densa cells therefore appear to be a highly water permeable plaque of cells surrounded by epithelium that is, for all practical purposes, impermeable to water. Thus, changes in cell volume or water flow across macula densa cells may be one means by which these cells detect changes in luminal fluid composition.

Recent studies have also shown that macula densa cells respond to specific alterations in luminal Na^+ Cl^-. Using microelectrodes,[52] it has been possible to impale macula densa cells and to measure basolateral membrane potentials (Vbl). The Vbl of macula densa cells in the presence of 10 mM luminal Na^+ Cl^- averaged -56 mV.

As luminal Na^+ Cl^- was increased to 150 mM, macula densa Vbl depolarized by over 30 mV. In some experiments Vbl was decreased to near zero in the presence of 150 mM Na^+ Cl^-. On the average, macula densa Vbl decreased to -26 mV in the presence of 150mM luminal Na^+Cl^-. The Vbl responses to alterations in luminal Na^+ Cl^- represented steady state changes and were not transient events. In addition, Vbl was most sensitive to alterations in luminal fluid Na^+ Cl^- between 10 and 45 mM, and this is similar to the range of Na^+ Cl^- at which the tubuloglomerular feedback mechanism is most responsive.[47] Thus, the macula densa cells exhibit a remarkable electrical responsiveness to alterations in luminal Na^+ Cl^-, and it is possible that these changes in macula densa Vbl could participate in the transmission of feedback signals.

It is also possible that the macula densa cells may be responsive to or activated by humoral agents. We have been particularly interested in the role of adenosine in the transmission of feedback signals. It is clear that the renal microvasculature contains both adenosine A1 and A2 receptors. Studies by Churchill[53,54] in the isolated perfused kidney have shown that administration of an A1 receptor agonist into the renal artery produces vasoconstriction, whereas infusion of the A2 receptor agonist produces vasodilation. In other studies,[55] it has been demonstrated that systemic infusions of putative adenosine receptor blockers (methylxanthines) inhibit tubuloglomerular feedback responses. These results might suggest that adenosine A1 receptors located on smooth muscle cells could be involved in the transmission of feedback signals. However, in recent studies from our laboratory[56], we tested the effects of a newer and more specific adenosine receptor blocker on the transmission of feedback responses. In these studies, the adenosine receptor blocker PSPX was infused systemically and tubuloglomerular feedback responses were assessed using micropuncture techniques. Systemic administration of this receptor blocker did not inhibit tubuloglomerular feedback responses, suggesting that the previous inhibition of feedback responses obtained with the less specific methylxanthines may be due to other effects of these agents, such as inhibition of phosphodiesterase activity and elevations in cAMP. Since vascular adenosine A1 receptors did not appear to be involved in the transmission of feedback signals, further studies were performed in which the A1 receptor agonist was infused into the tubular lumen in order to directly test the effects of A1 receptor activation on feedback responses. As shown in Figure 8, administration of the adenosine A1 agonist, CPA, produced significant feedback responses that could be blocked with coinfusion of the receptor antagonist. Similar results have also been obtained by Schnermann and coworkers.[57] These results indicate that, besides the vascular adenosine receptors, there may be other adenosine receptors involved in the transmission of feedback signals that are located at an extravascular site. Indeed, as suggested for the cTAL, it is possible that these receptors may be located on the luminal membrane of macula densa cells. Presumably adenosine, which is generated by macula densa, cTAL, or prior nephron segments, could enter the lumen and activate macula densa cells, thereby resulting in the transmission of vasoconstrictor signals. Thus, under conditions where tubular flow rate was elevated, enhanced tubular transport would lead to the generation of adenosine. In the cTAL, adenosine would serve to down-regulate transport and presumably protect the cTAL from the increased Na^+ Cl^- load, whereas in the macula densa, adenosine would activate the transmission of feedback signals, thereby decreasing glomerular filtration rate and reducing Na^+ Cl^- delivery.

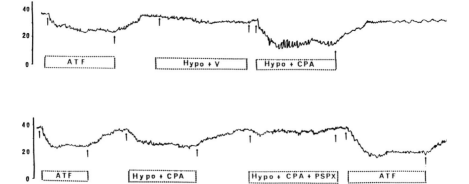

FIGURE 8. The effects of the adenosine A1 receptor agonist CPA, on retrograde tubuloglomerular feedback responses assessed by stop flow pressure (SFP) feedback responses. Decreases in SFP indicate vasoconstriction. ATF is a complete perfusate containing 150 mM NaCl. Hypo is the same solution but with NaCl reduced to 20mM. V is the vehicle (DMSO) used to dissolve CPA. PSPX is the adenosine receptor blocker. ATF produced feedback mediated decreases in SFP of about 12mmHg. Perfusion into the distal tubule with the hypo solution did not elicit a response. However, addition of the adenosine A1 receptor agonist to the Hypo solution resulted in markedly enhanced feedback responses. This enhanced response could be blocked by the receptor blocker.

Thus, when delivery into the cTAL and to the macula densa cells is increased, elevations in tubular fluid osmolality would alter water flow across the macula densa; increased luminal Na^+ Cl^- would depolarize Vbl; and generation of adenosine could bind to adenosine A1 receptors. Each of these events may participate in the activation of macula densa cells, leading to the transmission of tubuloglomerular feedback signals and decreases in glomerular filtration rate.

Over the last few years, we have examined the notion that the macula densa cells may respond to changes in luminal fluid composition and transmit signals to the vasculature through a cytosolic calcium system. These studies have involved both in vivo micropuncture techniques, as well as the isolated perfused thick ascending limb–macula densa preparation.[57–60] Using micropuncture methodology, we examined the effects of maneuvers that would presumably alter macula densa cytosolic calcium concentration on transmission of tubuloglomerular feedback signals. We found that the calcium ionophore A23187, when perfused into the tubular lumen in the presence of a hypotonic solution that alone does not cause feedback responses, resulted in the marked enhancement of feedback responses. This effect was calcium-specific, since removal of luminal calcium blunted the increased feedback responses obtained with the ionophore. These results suggested that an increase in cytosolic calcium concentration, presumably in the macula densa cells, resulted in the transmission of vasoconstrictor feedback signals.

Presumably under normal conditions, an increase in luminal-fluid sodium chloride concentration or osmolality would increase macula densa cytosolic calcium concentration. If so then the source of the elevated calcium could be due to calcium mobilization and/or calcium entry. A role for calcium entry across the luminal membrane was tested by removal of luminal calcium and addition of a calcium chelator.

In the presence of an isotonic solution, deletion of luminal calcium did not influence feedback responses, eliminating a role for calcium entry across the luminal membrane and into the macula densa cells. In other studies, the intracellular calcium antagonist TMB-8 was introduced into the lumen in the presence of an isotonic solution. This agent, which has been shown to prevent calcium mobilization, resulted in a substantial reduction in the magnitude of feedback responses. This inhibition was also specific for calcium, since the inhibition by TMB-8 could be overcome by the simultaneous addition of the calcium ionophore. These results suggest that, in the macula densa, a rise in cytosolic calcium concentration occurring as a consequence of calcium mobilization serves as an important part of the feedback signal transmission process.

This conclusion has been recently confirmed in the in vitro perfused thick ascending limb–macula densa preparation. As shown in Figure 9, increases in luminal fluid Na^+ Cl^- from 45 mM to 150 mM resulted in a substantial increase in macula densa cytosolic calcium concentration as assessed by Fura 2 fluorescence. These studies directly support the notion that changes in luminal fluid composition directly alter macula densa cytosolic calcium concentration and further substantiate the hypothesis that macula densa cytosolic calcium serves in the transmission of tubuloglomerular feedback signals. The mechanism by which changes in luminal fluid composition alters cytosolic calcium concentration is not known. Figure 10 offers some possibilities. Presumably alterations in water flow across the macula densa cells could directly alter cell volume and change calcium concentration. Likewise activation of adenosine A1 receptors could increase cytosolic calcium concentration similar to what was found for the cTAL. Finally, it is interesting to speculate that increases in luminal fluid Na^+ Cl^- concentration may alter macula densa cytosolic calcium concentration through an effect on the basolateral membrane potential (Vbl). Although previous studies indicate

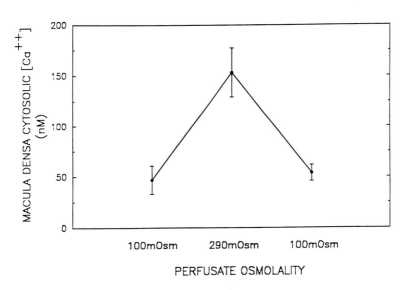

FIGURE 9. The effects of changes in luminal fluid osmolality (by varying NaCl concentration) on macula densa cytosolic calcium concentration. Details of the Fura 2 fluorescence methodology are given in Figure 1.

that calcium mobilization occurs during transmission of feedback signals, in most cell types sustained activation of a cytosolic calcium system requires both calcium mobilization as well as calcium entry. Although calcium entry across the apical membrane does not appear to participate in feedback signal transmission, this does not rule out a role for calcium entry across the basolateral membrane. It is intriguing to speculate that the large depolarization of Vbl in the presence of high luminal Na^+ Cl^- concentrations could serve to promote calcium entry across this membrane. In this regard it will be interesting to examine whether calcium antagonists can block the effects of increases in cytosolic calcium concentration induced by elevations in luminal Na^+ Cl^- concentration.

The transmission process from macula densa cells to the glomerular vasculature is not well understood; however, it is known that the final step in feedback signal transmission involves calcium-mediated excitation-contraction coupling in smooth muscle cells of the afferent arteriole. This final step in the transmission of feedback signals is highly sensitive to calcium antagonists. In previous micropuncture studies, Muller-Suur et al.[61] found that systemic administration of verapamil blocked stop-flow pressure feedback responses. In a more recent study, Mitchell[62] examined the effects of infusions of nifedipine into surrounding peritubular capillaries during simultaneous measurements of tubuloglomerular feedback responses. In the presence of nifedipine, both stop-flow pressure and single nephron glomerular filtration rate feedback responses were almost completely inhibited. These results suggest that the tubuloglomerular feedback mechanism elicits vasoconstriction through the activation of voltage-dependent calcium channels that are sensitive to calcium channel blockers such as nifedipine.

In summary, cytosolic calcium is an important regulator in renal epithelial cells. In the cTAl, as in the proximal tubule and collecting duct, cytosolic calcium serves in the regulation of transepithelial transport. In each of these segments, increases

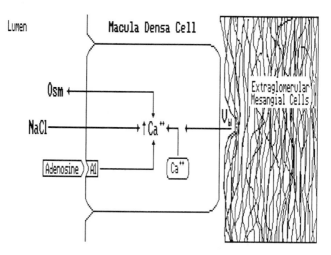

FIGURE 10. Model of the possible ways that changes in the composition of tubular fluid could alter macula densa cytosolic calcium concentration. See text for details.

in transepithelial transport results in elevations in cytosolic calcium concentration, which, in turn, down-regulates transport. In contrast to the proximal tubule and collecting duct, alterations in cytosolic calcium concentration in the cTAL during variations in transepithelial transport does not involve coupling to a basolateral Na^+/Ca^{2+} exchanger, but rather elevations in cytosolic sodium concentration may directly mobilize calcium. In the cTAL, recent evidence indicates that adenosine A1 receptors may be located on the apical membranes of these cells and that activation of these receptors increases cTAL cytosolic calcium concentration and decreases transepithelial transport. Cytosolic calcium also appears to be important in the macula densa–tubuloglomerular feedback mechanism. Increases in luminal fluid osmolality, Na^+Cl^- and adenosine may all increase macula densa cytosolic calcium concentration. Transmission of feedback signals to the glomerular vasculature results in calcium-mediated excitation-contraction coupling. This feedback-mediated event is dependent upon voltage-dependent calcium channels and can be inhibited by calcium channel blockers.

Acknowledgments. The author's work was supported by grants from NIH (AM32032 and HL18426) and the American Heart Association (831122). We thank Michael Higdon and Martha Yeager for their help in preparing this manuscript and express our thanks to previous collaborators. P.D. Bell is an Established Investigator of the American Heart Association. M. Franco is a visiting scientist the Instituto Nacional de Cardiologia I. Chavez, Mexico City, Mexico.

References

1. Yang JM, Lee CO, Windhager EE: Regulation of cytosolic free calcium in isolated perfused proximal tubules of necturus. Am J Physiol (Renal Fluid Electrolyte Physiol 24):F787-799, 1988.

2. Snowdowne KW, Borle AB: Measurement of cytosolic free calcium in mammalian cells with aequorin. Am J Physiol 247:C396–C408, 1984.

3. Bonventre JV, Cheung TY: Cytosolic free calcium concentration in cultured renal epithelial cells. Am J Physiol 250:F329–F338, 1986.

4. Murphy E, Mandel LJ: Cytosolic free calcium levels in rabbit proximal kidney tubules. Am J Physiol 242(Cell Physiol 11):C124–C128, 1982.

5. Grynkiewicz G, Poenie M, Tsien RY: A new generation of Ca^{2+} indicators with greatly improved fluorescence properties. J Biol Chem 260:3440–3450, 1985.

6. Tsien, RY, Rink TJ, Poenie M: Measurement of cytosolic free Ca^{2+} in individual small cells using fluorescence microscopy with dual excitation wavelengths. Cell Calcium 6:145-158, 1985.

7. Goligorsky M, Hruska K, Loftus D, Elson E: Alpha 1- adrenergic stimulation and cytoplasmic free calcium concentration in cultured renal proximal tubular cells: evidence for compartmentalization of quin-2 and fura-2. J Cell Physiol 128:466–475, 1986.

8. Goligorsky M, Loftus D, Hruska K: Cytoplasmic Ca^{2+} in individual proximal tubular cells in culture: effects of PTH. Am J Physiol 251:F938–944, 1986.

9. Bell PD, Franco M, Higdon M: The effects of adenosine A1 agonist on transepithelial potential difference and cytosolic calcium concentration in the cortical thick ascending limb: Kidney Int 35:1–309, 1989.

10. Rasmussen H, Barrett PQ: Calcium messenger system: An integrated view: Physiol Rev 64 (3): 1984.

11. Gmaj P, Murer H, Calcium transport mechanisms in epithelial cell membranes: Miner Electrolyte Metab 14:22–28, 1988.

12. Ghijsen WEJM, DeJong MD, van Os CH: ATP-dependent calcium transport and its correlation with Ca^{2+} ATPase activity in basolateral plasma membranes of rat duodenum. Biochim Biophys Acta 689:327–336, 1982.

13. Gmaj P, Murer H, Carafoli E: Localization and properties of a high-affinity (Ca^{2+} + Mg^{2+})-ATPase in isolated kidney cortex plasma membranes. FEBS Lett 144:226–230, 1982.

14. Carafoli E: Membrane Transport of Calcium. New York, Academic Press, 1982, p 266.

15. Scoble JE, Mills S, Hruska KA: Calcium transport in canine renal basolateral membrane vesicles. Effects of parathyroid hormone. J Clin Invest 75:1096–1105, 1985.

16. Becker GL, Fiskum G, Lehninger A: Regulation of free Ca^{2+} by liver mitochondria and endoplasmic reticulum. J Biol Chem 255:909–914, 1980.

17. Thevenod F, Streb H, Ullrich KJ, Schultz I: Inositol 1,4,5-trisphosphate releases Ca^{2+} from a nonmitochondrial store site in permeabilized rat cortical kidney cells. Kidney Int 29:695–702, 1986.

18. Rasmussen H, Kojima I, Apfeldorf W, Barrett P: Cellular mechanism of hormone action in the kidney: Messenger function of calcium and cyclic AMP. Kidney Int 29:90–97, 1986.

19. Chase HS Jr: Does calcium couple the apical and basolateral membrane permeabilities in epithelia? Am J Physiol 247(Renal Fluid Electrolyte Physiol 16):F869–876, 1984.

20. Frindt G, Lee CO, Yang JM, Windhager EE: Potential role of cytoplasmic calcium ions in the regulation of sodium transport in renal tubules. Miner Electrolyte Metab 14:40–47, 1988.

21. Friedman PA, Figueiredo JF, Maack T, Windhager EE: Sodium-calcium interactions in the renal proximal convoluted tubule of the rabbit. Am J Physiol 240:F558–F568, 1981.

22. Lorenzen M, Lee CO, Windhager EE: Cytosolic Ca^{2+} and Na^+ activities in perfused proximal tubules of Necturus kidney. Am J Physiol 247:F93–F102, 1984.

23. Palmer LG, Frindt G: Amiloride-sensitive Na channels from the apical membrane of the rat cortical collecting tubule. Proc Nat Acad Sci USA 83:2767–2770, 1986.

24. Palmer LG, Frindt G: Epithelial Na channels: characterization using the patch lamp technique. Fed Proc 45:2708-2712, 1986.

25. Taylor A, Windhager EE: Possible role of cytosolic calcium and Na–Ca exchange in regulation of transepithelial sodium transport. Am J Physiol 236:F505–F512, 1979 or Am J Physiol:Renal Fluid Electrolyte Physiol 5:F505–512, 1979.

25a. Johns EJ, Manitius J: The renal actions of nitrendipine and its influence on the neural regulation of calcium and sodium reabsorption in the rat.J Cardiovasc Pharmacol 9(Suppl 1):S49–S56, 1987.

26. Greger R: Ion transport mechanisms in thick ascending limb of Henle's Loop of mammalian nephron. Physiol Rev 65 (3): 1985.

27. Greger RE, Schlatter E, Lang F: Evidence for electroneutral sodium chloride cotransport in the cortical thick ascending limb of Henle's loop of rabbit kidney. Pflugers Arch 396:308–314, 1983.

28. Greger R, Schlatter E: Properties of the basolateral membrane of the cortical thick ascending limb of Henle's loop of rabbit kidney. Pflugers Arch 396:325–334, 1983.

29. Wright FS, Briggs JP: Feedback control of glomerular blood flow pressure and filtration rate. Physiol Rev 59:958–1006, 1979.

30. Bell PD, Higdon M: Participation of cytosolic calcium in cortical thick ascending limb (cTAL) transport. FASEB J (submitted).

31. Snowdowne KW, Borle AB: Effects of low extracellular sodium on cytosolic ionized calcium. J Biol Chem 260: 14998–15007, 1985.

32. Chiou CY, Malagodi MH: Studies on the mechanism of action of a new Ca^{2+} antagonist, 8-N(N,N-diethylamino)-octyl-3,4,5-trimethoxybenzoate hydrochloride in smooth and skeletal muscle. Br J Pharmacol 53:279–285, 1975.

33. Bell PD, Reddington M: Intracellular calcium in the transmission of tubuloglomerular feedback signals. Am J Physiol 245(Renal Fluid Electrolyte Physiol 14):F295–F302, 1983.

34. Spielman WS, Thompson CI: A proposed role for adenosine in the regulation of renal hemodynamics and renin release. Am J Physiol 242(Renal Fluid Electrolyte Physiol 11):F423–435, 1982.

35. Trimble ME, Coulson R: Adenosine transport in perfused rat kidney and cortical membrane vesicles. Am J Physiol 246(Renal Fluid Electrolyte Physiol 15):F794–F803, 1984.

36. Daly JW: Adenosine receptors: Target for future drugs. J Med Chem 25:197–207, 1982.

37. Fredholm BB: Adenosine receptors. Med Biol 60:289-293, 1982.

38. Osswald H: The role of adenosine in the regulation of glomerular filtration rate and renin secretion. Trends in Pharmacol Sci 5:94–97, 1984.

39. Lear S, Silva P, Epstein M: Adenosine and PGE$_2$ modulate transport by isolated thick ascending limb. Clin Res 33:586, 1985.

40. Osswald H: Adenosine and renal function. In Bernes R, Rall TW, Rubio R (eds): Regulatory Function of Adenosine, Boston, Martinus nijoff 1983, pp 399–415.

41. Brines ML, Forrest JN Jr: Autoradiographic localization of A1 adenosine receptors to tubules in the red medulla and papilla of the rat kidney. Kidney Int 33:109, 1987.

42. Kelley GG, Barron H, Andreoni K, et al: A1 adenosine receptors inhibit chloride transport in the shark rectal gland by N$_1$-coupled cyclic AMP dependent and cyclic AMP independent mechanisms. Kidney Int 31:274, 1987.

43. Bell PD, Franco M, Higdon M: Adenosine A1 agonist increases cytosolic calcium concentration in the isolated perfused cortical thick ascending limb. Fed Proc 72:3681, 1988.

44. Arend LJ, Sonnenburg WK, Smith WL, Spielman WS: A1 and A2 adenosine receptors in the rabbit cortical collecting tubule cells. Modulation of hormone-stimulated cAMP. Clin Invest 79:710-714, 1982.

45. Barajas L. The juxtaglomerular apparatus: Anatomical considerations in the feedback control of glomerular filtration rate. Fed Proc 40:78–86, 1981.

46. Bell PD, Navar LG. Macula densa feedback control of glomerular filtration: Role of cytosolic calcium. Miner Electrolyte Metab 8:61–77, 1982.

47. Bell PD, Franco M, Navar LG. Calcium as a mediator of tubuloglomerular feedback. Ann Rev Physiol 49:275–293, 1987.

48. Bell PD: Calcium antagonists and intrarenal regulation of glomerular filtration rate. Am J Nephrol 7(suppl 1): 24–31, 1987.

49. Briggs JP, Schnermann J: The tubuloglomerular glomerular feedback mechanism: Functional and biochemical aspects. Ann Rev Physiol 49:251–273, 1987.

50. Kirk KL, Bell PD, Barfuss DW, Ribadenerira M: Direct visualization of the isolated and perfused macula densa. Am J Physiol 248(Renal Fluid Electrolyte Physiol 17):F890–894, 1985.

51. Ribadeniera M, Barfuss DW: Hydraulic conductivity of the isolated perfused macula densa. J Am Soc Neph 1:352A, 1988.

52. Bell P, LaPoint JY, Cardinal J: Direct measurement of basolateral membrane potentials from cells of the macula densa. Am J Physiol (submitted).

53. Churchill PC, Bidani A: Renal effects of selective adenosine receptor agonists in anesthetized rats. Am J Physiol 252(Renal Fluid Electrolyte Physiol):F299–F303, 1987.

54. Rossi NF, Churchill PC, Jacobsond KA, Leahy AE: Further characterization of the renovascular effects of N6-cyclohexyladenosine in the isolated perfused rat kidney. J Pharmacol Exp Ther 240:911–915, 1987.

55. Schnermann J, Osswald H, Hermle M: Inhibitory effect of methylxanthines on feedback control of glomerular filtration rate in the rat kidney. Plugers Arch 369:39–48, 1977.

56. Franco M, Bell PD, Navar LG: Effect of adenosine A1 analog on tubuloglomerular feedback mechanism. Am J Physiol (submitted).

57. Schnermann J: Effect of adenosine analogues on tubuloglomerular feedback responses. Am J Physiol 255(Renal Fluid Electrolyte Physiol 24):F33–F42, 1988.

58. Bell PD, Navar LG: Cytoplasmic calcium in the mediation of macula densa tubuloglomerular feedback responses. Science 215:670–673, 1982.

59. Bell PD: Cyclic AMP-calcium interaction in the transmission of tubuloglomerular feedback signals. Kidney Int 28:728–732, 1985.

60. Bell PD, Krause A, Franco M: Macula densa cytosolic calcium concentration during changes in luminal fluid osmolality. Kidney Int 33:150, 1988.

61. Muller-Suur R, Gutsche HU, Schurek HJ. Acute and reversible inhibition of tubuloglomerular feedback mediated afferent vasoconstriction by the calcium antagonist verapamil. Curr Probl Clin Biochem 6:291–298, 1976.

62. Mitchell KD, Navar LG. Inhibition of tubuloglomerular feedback responses during peritubular capillary infusions of calcium channel blockers (submitted).

Paul C. Churchill, Ph.D.

7

Calcium, Calcium Antagonists, and Renin Secretion

The renin-angiotensin system plays a central role in salt and water balance and in the regulation of arterial blood pressure. The level of activity of this system is determined primarily by the rate at which the granulated juxtaglomerular cells (JG cells) in the kidney secrete renin into the blood. Physiologically, the renin secretory rate is controlled by a number of first messengers: afferent arteriolar transmural pressure or some function of pressure, such as stretch (baroreceptor mechanism); solute transport in the macula densa segment of the tubule (the macula densa mechanism); catecholamines released from the renal nerves and from the adrenal medulla (the β adrenergic mechanism); extracellular concentrations of many organic and inorganic substances, including angiotensin II, vasopressin, potassium, and magnesium.[29,47,87] In addition to these physiological first messengers, a number of pharmacological agents affect renin secretion.[47] This chapter concerns the effects of calcium (Ca) channel blockers on renin secretion.

It is an accepted principle of cellular biology that first messengers act by affecting the intracellular concentrations of only a few second messengers. There is evidence to suggest that cyclic AMP, cyclic GMP, and free ionic calcium (Ca^{2+}) are second messengers in renin secretion. The evidence Ca^{2+} is an inhibitory second messenger, i.e., that JG cell Ca^{2+} is inversely related to secretory activity, has been discussed at length elsewhere[13,36-38] and only those details relevant to understanding the effects of Ca channel blockers are discussed in the following chapter. An inverse relationship between renin secretion and JG cell Ca^{2+} might suggest that Ca channel blockers should stimulate renin secretion, by antagonizing Ca^{2+} influx and thereby decreasing intracellular Ca^{2+} (Ca_i^{2+}). How can this prediction be reconciled with the array of experimental observations? Calcium channel blockers can increase,[1,2,4,26,44,45,55-57,59,60,79,90] have no effect on,[28,31,44,94] or actually decrease[7,79] renin secretory rate and/or plasma renin. Review articles have been cited almost exclusively, and these can be consulted for further detail. Space considerations alone preclude citing the original research articles.

Regulation of Cell Calcium

Extracellular and Intracellular Calcium

Recently, Kurtz et al.[49] used the quin-2 fluorescence method to measure JG cell Ca^{2+}, and the results of one experiment indicate a concentration of about 3×10^{-7} M. A priori, despite the paucity of direct measurements, JG cell Ca_i^{2+} must be about 10^{-7} M in the steady state,[13] since JG cells contain mitochondria and since Ca_i^{2+} must be about 10^{-7}M in order for oxidative phosphorylation to occur.[9] Moreover, Ca_i^{2+} in other cells ranges between 5×10^{-8} and 3.5×10^{-7} M in the non-Ca–activated state to about 1.5×10^{-6} M in the Ca-activated state, a concentration range that is consistent with the Ca-binding constants of Ca-modulated proteins such as calmodulin.[77,78] If JG cell Ca^{2+} is approximately 10^{-7} M, an enormous electrochemical gradient for Ca^{2+} influx exists, since extracellular Ca^{2+} (Ca_e^{2+}) is approximately 10^{-3} M, and since JG cell membranes are electrically polarized, intracellular fluid about 60–70 mV negative with respect to extracellular fluid.[8,32]

How can the JG cell maintain such a low Ca_i^{2+} in the face of such a large electrochemical gradient for Ca^{2+} influx (Fig. 1)? Perhaps the JG cell membrane is relatively impermeable to Ca^{2+}, and perhaps JG cells, like other cells, buffer Ca_i^{2+} by mitochondrial uptake, by Ca^{2+} binding to intracellular molecules such as calmodulin, and by Ca^{2+} sequestration in organelles such as the endoplasmic reticulum.[3,9,76–78,80,86] However, in the final analysis, JG cells must possess specific Ca^{2+} extrusion mechanisms, since cell membranes are not completely impermeable to Ca^{2+} and since no buffering mechanism has infinite capacity. Only two mechanisms for cellular Ca^{2+} extrusion are known to exist[3,5,77,80,86]: Na-Ca exchange, which is ultimately dependent on the active transport of Na^+ and K^+ (Fig. 2), and primary active, ATP-

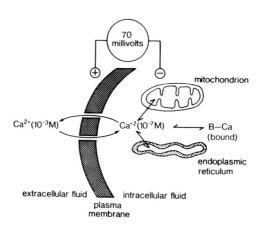

FIGURE 1. A hypothetical JG cell. The large electrochemical gradient favoring Ca^{2+} influx suggests that efflux pathways must exist, even if intracellular Ca^{2+} can be buffered by mitochondrial uptake, by sequestration in endoplasmic reticulum, and by Ca-binding molecules such as proteins and nucleotides. Reproduced with permission from Churchill.[13]

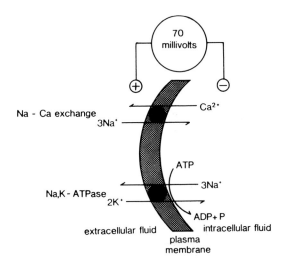

FIGURE 2. A hypothetical JG cell plasma membrane. The Na-Ca exchange carrier binds Na^+ and Ca^{2+} in a 3:1 ratio. In the presence of a normal transmembrane electrochemical gradient for Na^+, Na^+ influx down its gradient is coupled with Ca^{2+} efflux against its gradient. Decreases in the Na + electrochemical gradient, due to membrane depolarization or increased intracellular or decreased extracellular Na^+, decrease the rate of Ca^{2+} efflux (and conversely). Transmembrane Na^+ and K^+ concentration gradients, and ultimately the transmembrane potential, are maintained by primary active transport of Na^+ and K^+ (Na,K-ATPase). Reproduced with permission from Churchill.[13]

dependent, Ca transport (Fig. 3). It seems reasonable to infer that one or both of these mechanisms must contribute to regulating JG cell Ca_i^{2+}. The pharmacological evidence that supports this inference is presented in the following section on "Calcium Efflux and Sequestration."

It should be stressed that an inverse relationship between Ca_i^{2+} and renin

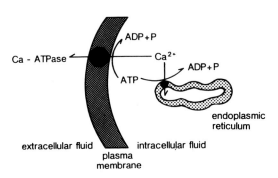

FIGURE 3. ATP-dependent Ca^{2+} transport in a hypothetical JG cell. Ca-activated ATPase activity, associated with the plasma membrane and with the membranes of organelles such as endoplasmic reticulum, is the biochemical correlate of primary active Ca^{2+} efflux and nonmitochondrial Ca^{2+} sequestration. Reproduced with permission from Churchill.[13]

secretion (Ca^{2+} acting as a second messenger) does not imply an inverse relationship between Ca_e^{2+} and renin secretion (Ca^{2+} acting as a first messenger). The implicit assumption, that changes in Ca_e^{2+} induce parallel or proportionate changes in Ca_i^{2+}, is incorrect. Indeed, Ca_i^{2+} can change in opposite directions to changes in Ca_e^{2+}, due to the membrane-stabilizing property of Ca_e^{2+}. Increasing Ca_e^{2+} decreases cell membrane Ca^{2+} permeability,[76,78,80,86,91] and can actually decrease Ca^{2+} influx as exemplified by the observations that increased Ca_e^{2+} antagonizes vascular smooth muscle contractility[91] and pancreatic β-cell secretory activity,[34] yet increased Ca_i^{2+} triggers increased vascular smooth muscle contractility and increased insulin secretion. Conversely, decreasing Ca_e^{2+} destabilizes and depolarizes cell membranes, and depending upon the transmembrane concentration gradient, Ca^{2+} influx and Ca_i^{2+} can increase as Ca_e^{2+} decreases.[76] For this reason, one must be cautious in interpreting the results of in vitro experiments in which cells were exposed to nominally "Ca-free" physiological saline solution. A gradient of indeterminant magnitude for Ca^{2+} influx still exists in this situation since Ca_i^{2+} is submicromolar and since "Ca-free" solutions without chelators invariably contain 1–10 μM Ca^{2+}, depending upon the quality of the water, the quality of the reagents, and the amount of Ca^{2+} leached from glass.[76] It is not surprising, therefore, that "Ca-free" extracellular fluid has been observed to inhibit, to stimulate, and to have no effect on in vitro renin release.[13] Similarly, increased plasma Ca^{2+} has been observed to inhibit, to stimulate, and to have no effect on renin secretion or on plasma renin in intact animals.[47] Since the effects of Ca_e^{2+} on Ca_i^{2+} are unpredictable, except when the transmembrane concentration gradient is actually reversed (by adding a Ca chelator to "Ca-free" solutions) or the cell membrane Ca^{2+} permeability is increased (by ionophores), these observations cannot be taken as evidence for or against a second messenger role of Ca_i^{2+}.

Adding a Ca-binding substance to a nominally Ca-free physiological saline solution reverses the normal transmembrane Ca^{2+} concentration gradient, which favors Ca^{2+} influx, and EDTA and/or EGTA have been shown to stimulate renin release in several in vitro preparations, including rat glomeruli, rat renal cortical slices, pig renal cortical slices, and isolated perfused rat kidneys.[13,35–38,53,70,72,73,89] Moreover, chelator-stimulated renin release cannot be attributed to the leakage of renin across permeabilized cell membranes, since EGTA-stimulated renin release is unrelated to the release of lactate dehydrogenase,[10,58] another intracellular protein. Therefore, the observation that reversal of the transmembrane Ca^{2+} concentration gradient, which cannot fail to decrease JG cell Ca_i^{2+}, stimulates renin secretion can be taken as one piece of evidence that Ca_i^{2+} is an inhibitory second messenger.

The renin secretory effects of La^{3+}, Mg^{2+}, and Ca ionophores strengthen this evidence. La^{3+} blocks transmembrane Ca^{2+} fluxes,[78,80] and La^{3+} blocks the stimulatory effect of chelators on renin secretion.[13] Mg^{2+} acts as a membrane stabilizer, reducing cell membrane Ca^{2+} permeability.[76,78,80] In the presence of a normal Ca_e^{2+}, increased extracellular Mg^{2+} stimulates renin secretion in vivo, in isolated perfused rat kidneys, and in rat renal cortical cell suspensions.[13,37,38] Ca ionophores facilitate passive Ca^{2+} fluxes in either direction across cell membranes. In general, Ca ionophores appear either to inhibit or stimulate renin secretion in vitro, depending upon whether the Ca^{2+} concentration gradient favors influx or efflux, respectively.[13,37,38]

Calcium Efflux and Sequestration

The Sodium-Calcium Exchange Mechanism

According to the Na-Ca exchange model shown in Figure 2, Na,K-ATPase inhibitors should inhibit renin secretion (increased Na_i^+, decreased Na^+ gradient, decreased Ca^{2+} efflux, and increased Ca_i^{2+}), and Ca chelators should block the inhibitory effect by promoting Ca^{2+} efflux. Conversely, Na,K-ATPase stimulators should stimulate renin secretion (decreased Na_i^+, increased Na^+ gradient, increased Ca^{2+} efflux, and decreased Ca_i^{2+}) and agents that increase Ca_i^{2+} should block the stimulatory effect. A number of experimental observations are consistent with these predictions.

Na,K-ATPase Inhibitors. Ouabain, vanadate, and K-free extracellular fluid inhibit Na,K-ATPase activity, and all three have inhibitory effects on renin secretion.[10,13,17,23,25,27,28,36–38,47,55,58,69,70] The inhibitory effects are mediated by increased Ca_i^{2+}, since they can be blocked by reversing the transmembrane Ca^{2+} gradient.

Na,K-ATPase Stimulators. Na,K-ATPase is activated by increasing K_e^+ from 0 to approximately 2 mM, and can be stimulated further by phenytoin and by β-adrenergic agonists, via cyclic AMP.[74,81] Increasing K_e^+ from 0 to 2 mM stimulates renin secretion,[13,16,21] and both phenytoin[13] and β-adrenergic agonists[13,29,35–38,41,47,72] stimulate renin secretion. Moreover, ouabain blocks the stimulatory effects on renin secretion of increasing K_e^+, of phenytoin, of isoproterenol, and of dibutyryl cyclic AMP.[13]

Primary Active Calcium Transport

Primary active Ca^{2+} transport is depicted in Figure 3 as Ca-activated ATPase activity associated with the plasma membrane and the membranes of organelles such as the endoplasmic reticulum. According to this model, Ca-ATPase inhibitors and stimulators should increase and decrease Ca_i^{2+}, respectively, thereby inhibiting and stimulating renin secretion.

Vanadate inhibits Na,K-ATPase activity, but it also inhibits Ca-ATPase activity; either action would produce an increase in Ca_i^{2+} that could be blocked by Ca chelators. Therefore, its inhibitory effect on renin secretion and the blockade of this effect by Ca chelation can be taken as evidence that Ca^{2+} is an inhibitory second messenger, but it cannot be taken as evidence of a specific mechanism of action. Similarly, although there is agreement that β-adrenergic agonists, via cyclic AMP, promote Ca^{2+} efflux from many cells[5,74,77,86] there is controversy concerning the mechanism: cyclic AMP-stimulated Na,K-ATPase activity, which would increase Ca^{2+} efflux via Na-Ca exchange, versus cyclic AMP-stimulated Ca-ATPase activity, which would increase active Ca^{2+} efflux and sequestration. Whichever mechanism is involved, Ca_i^{2+} decreases, and two pieces of evidence indicate that this cyclic AMP-dependent increase in Ca^{2+} efflux mediates the stimulatory effect on renin secretion. First, La^{3+} blocks Ca^{2+} efflux[78,80] and La^{3+} blocks the stimulatory effect of isoproterenol on renin secretion.[54] Second, several manipulations and substances antagonize and/or block isoproterenol-stimulated (and dibutyryl cyclic AMP-stimulated) renin secretion, and the only known effect they have in common is to increase Ca_i^{2+} : α-adrenergic agonists, angiotensin II, vasopressin, ouabain, vanadate, K-free extracellular fluid, and K-depolarization.[13,16,17,35–38,41,53,54,67,71]

Variations in the rates of intracellular Ca^{2+} sequestration and mobilization can affect Ca_i^{2+}, and therefore potentially affect renin secretion. Consistently, TMB-8 (8-(N,N-diethylamino) octyl 3,4,5-trimethoxy-benzoate) antagonizes Ca^{2+} mobilization from intracellular sequestration sites, and this compound stimulates renin secretion in in vitro preparations.[38]

In summary, all the above observations indicate that Ca^{2+} is an inhibitory second messenger in renin secretion, and further, that JG cell Ca^{2+} can be affected by the rates of two Ca^{2+} efflux mechanisms (Na-Ca exchange; primary active Ca^{2+} transport) and the rates of intracellular Ca^{2+} sequestration and mobilization. Potentially, then, first messengers (and the second messenger—cyclic AMP) could affect renin secretion by affecting any or all of these processes, and theoretically these renin secretory affects would be immune to antagonism by Ca channel blockers.

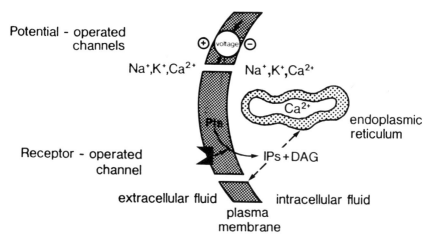

FIGURE 4. A hypothetical JG cell membrane with potential-operated and receptor-operated channels. Potential operated channels for Na^+, K^+, and Ca^{2+} have been characterized in many cells. Potential operated Ca channels are opened by membrane depolarization and by channel agonists (BAY K 8644); Ca channel blockers (nifedipine, verapamil) antagonize depolarization-induced Ca^{2+} influx. Similarly, potential-operated Na^+ channels are opened by membrane depolarization and by channel agonists (veratridine), and Na^+ channel blockers (tetrodotoxin) antagonize depolarization-induced Na^+ influx. In contrast, receptor-operated channels are activated when an agonist occupies its receptor on the cell membrane; this usually leads to stimulation of phospholipase activity, hydrolysis of phosphoinositides (PIs) associated with the membrane, and the production of inositol phosphates (IPs) that increase Ca^{2+} influx and/or mobilize sequestered Ca_i^{2+} and diacylglycerol (DAG). Receptor antagonists block agonist-induced changes in ion permeability, but in general, agonist-induced ion fluxes are resistant to the effects of channel blockers (e.g., tetrodotoxin, nifedipine). Probably angiotensin II and vasopressin, and possibly A_1-adenosine receptor agonists and α-adrenergic agonists, activate JG cell receptor-operated ion channels.

Calcium Influx and Mobilization

Receptor Operated Ca Channels

Phenomenologically, receptor-operated ion channels are local increases in ion permeability that result from the interaction of an agonist with its specific receptor on the cell membrane[6,65,76-78,80] (Fig. 4). Agonist-induced increases in ion permeability are not initiated by membrane depolarization, but they can produce either depolarization or hyperpolarization, depending upon the ion selectivity (e.g., neurotransmitter-induced excitatory and inhibitory postsynaptic potentials). Receptor operated Ca channels, specifically, are agonist-induced increases in Ca_i^{2+} that are attributable to phosphoinositide hydrolysis and the production of inositol phosphates, which increase Ca^{2+} influx and/or mobilize Ca^{2+} from intracellular sites of sequestration, and of diacylglycerol, which, together with the increased Ca_i^{2+}, activates protein kinase C.[65] Since receptor-mediated increases in Ca_i^{2+} are not dependent upon membrane depolarization, they are resistant to the effects of Ca channel blockers.[6,33,78]

The observation that secretory and smooth muscle cells have receptor operated Ca Channels,[6,65,76-78,80,86] taken together with the observation that the renin-secreting JG cells are derived from smooth muscle, suggests that JG cell Ca^{2+} might be increased by activation of receptor operated Ca channels like those of vascular smooth muscle. Indeed, Peart[72] pointed out many years ago that substances that increase vascular smooth muscle contractility, presumably by receptor-mediated increases in Ca_i^{2+}, tend to inhibit renin secretion. Four examples of this are considered below: angiotensin II, vasopressin, A_1-adenosine receptor agonists, and α-adrenergic agonists.

Angiotensin II and Vasopressin. Both of these vasoconstrictors inhibit renin secretion, and it is very likely that the inhibitory effects are mediated by increased phospholipid turnover[51] and an increase in Ca_i^{2+} that is attributable, at least in part, to mobilization from intracellular sites of sequestration.[13] Although chelation of Ca_e^{2+} blocks the inhibitory effects on renin secretion of both angiotensin II and vasopressin,[11-13,89] the blockade is not instantaneous, which is consistent with the concept that mobilization of Ca_i^{2+}, rather than influx of Ca_e^{2+}, is involved. Furthermore, although both angiotensin II and vasopressin reportedly depolarize JG cells[8] and increase JG cell membrane Ca^{2+} permeability,[50,51] their inhibitory effects on renin secretion have been shown to be completely independent of membrane potential[11-13,24] (Fig. 5).

A_1 Adenosine Receptor Agonists. Adenosine and adenosine analogs that act as adenosine receptor agonists affect both renal vascular smooth muscle contractility and renin secretion.[13,15,21,29,41,47,59,62,63,68,83,85] It has been shown, using selective agonists, that A_1 adenosine receptor occupation leads to increased contractility and decreased renin secretion; in contrast, A_2 adenosine receptor occupation leads to decreased contractility and increased renin secretion[13,15,21,62,63]; (Figs. 6 and 7). Increased Ca_i^{2+} has been shown to mediate both of the A_1 responses—the increased contractility and the decreased rate of renin secretion—but the mechanism leading to increased Ca_i^{2+} in vascular smooth muscle cells apparently is not the same as that in JG cells. EGTA blocks the renin secretory effect,[21] demonstrating mediation

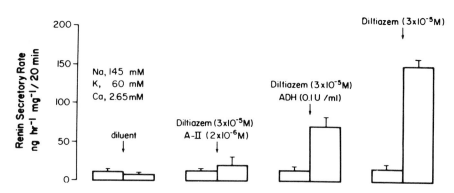

FIGURE 5. Renin secretory rates of rat renal cortical slices; each pair of columns represents secretory rates during two consecutive incubation periods in a given experiment. K-depolarization reduces secretory rate to a very low level (left pair of columns), and adding diltiazem completely blocks the inhibitory effect (right pair of columns). However, this concentration of diltiazem fails to block the inhibitory effect of angiotensin II (AII; compare with the right pair of columns) or the inhibitory effect of antidiuretic hormone (ADH; compare with the right pair of columns). Since both angiotensin II and antidiuretic hormone produced inhibitory effects when the cells were already completely depolarized with 60 mM K$^+$, the inhibitory effects are independent of cell membrane potential. Reproduced with permission from Churchill, et al.[24]

by increased Ca$_i^{2+}$, but Ca channel blockers do not block,[21,59] demonstrating that a depolarization-induced Ca^{2+} influx does not account for the increased Ca$_i^{2+}$. In contrast, Ca channel blockers abolish adenosine-induced renal vasoconstriction,[59] demonstrating that the effect is mediated by increased Ca$_i^{2+}$ resulting from depolarization-induced Ca^{2+} influx.

α-**Adrenergic Agonists.** It is well known that α-adrenergic agonists increase vascular smooth muscle contractility, and that they inhibit basal and/or antagonize stimulated renin secretion, particularly in in vitro preparations.[47,50,51,53,67,72] Several observations indicate that the inhibitory effect is mediated by activation of α$_1$-adrenergic receptors followed by increased Ca$_i^{2+}$. Norepinephrine activates both α- and β-adrenergic receptors, and both verapamil and Mn^{2+} (an inorganic Ca channel blocker,[78,80]) enhance norepinephrine-stimulated renin secretion in isolated perfused rat kidneys.[53] Presumably, by blocking the Ca-dependent inhibitory effect of α-receptor activation on renin secretion, the stimulatory effect of β-adrenergic receptor occupation is unmasked. In accord with this interpretation, it has been shown that phenylephrine antagonizes isoproterenol-stimulated renin secretion in isolated perfused rabbit kidneys, and that either methoxyverapamil or EGTA blocks the antagonistic effect.[67] Collectively, the effects of EGTA and the inorganic and organic Ca channel blockers suggest that either α-agonists activate potential operated Ca channels directly (like BAY K 8644, vide infra), or they activate a receptor-operated ion channel that induces depolarization, and depolarization in turn activates potential operated Ca channels. The recent findings that norepinephrine depolarizes JG cells[8] and increases the Ca permeability of their plasma membranes[51] are consistent with either possibility. In summary, renal vascular smooth muscle contractility is increased and renin secre-

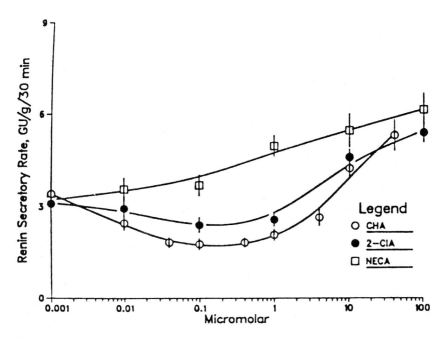

FIGURE 6. Renin secretory rate of rat renal cortical slices versus the logarithm of the concentrations of three adenosine receptor agonists: CHA (N^6-cyclohexyladenosine), 2-ClA (2-chloroadenosine), and NECA (N-ethylcarboxamide adenosine). Means ± S.E.M.s; n = 12–30 separate observations for each point. The basal secretory rate, not shown, averaged 3.9 GH/g/30 (different units from Figure 5). The order of potency for inhibition, in comparison with this basal rate, was CHA › 2-ClA ›› NECA; this order, and the concentration range, demonstrate that A_1-adenosine receptors inhibit renin secretion. The order of potency for stimulation of secretion was NECA ›› 2-ClA › CHA; this order, and the concentration range, demonstrate that A_2-adenosine receptors stimulate renin secretion. Reproduced with permission from Churchill and Churchill.[21]

tion is decreased by agonists of four distinct receptors: angiotensin II, vasopressin, A_1-adenosine, and α-adrenergic. Both cellular responses are mediated by increased Ca_i^{2+}. Angiotensin II, vasopressin, and α-adrenergic agonists may increase Ca_i^{2+} by identical mechanisms in both vascular smooth muscle and JG cells, but adenosine does not. The inhibitory effect of α-adrenergic agonists on renin secretion may be dependent upon a depolarization-induced influx of Ca^{2+}, but the inhibitory effects of angiotensin II, vasopressin, and A_1 adenosine receptor agonists are independent of membrane potential.

Potential Operated Ca Channels

Potential operated, or voltage dependent, channels for Na^+, K^+, and Ca^{2+} have been described and characterized in many secretory and contractile cells.[6,33,40,76,77,80,86] This observation, taken together with the observation that the renin-secreting JG cells are derived from smooth muscle, suggests that depolarization of the JG cell might activate potential operated Ca channels and increase Ca^{2+} influx (Fig. 4). Although few electrophysiological data are available, the membrane potential of JG

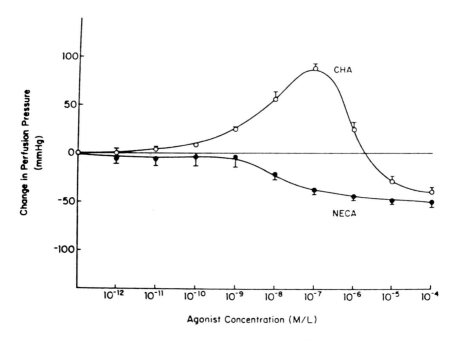

FIGURE 7. The effects of adenosine receptor agonists (CHA, N^6-cyclohexyladenosine; NECA, N-ethylcarboxamide adenosine) on perfusion pressure of isolated rat kidneys perfused at constant flow. Increases and decreases in pressure reflect increases and decreases in renovascular resistance, respectively. The order of potency for increased resistance (CHA › NECA) implies that A_1-adenosine receptors induce vasoconstriction; the order of potency for decreased resistance (NECA ›› CHA) implies that A_2-adenosine receptors induce vasodilation (reproduced from Murray and Churchill[63]). Compare Figures 6 and 7. CHA produces vasoconstriction (increases Ca_i^{2+}) over the same range of submicromolar concentrations that it inhibits renin secretion; at 0.1 μM, there are inflection points in both dose response curves, and CHA begins to vasodilate and to stimulate renin. At and above 10 μM, CHA stimulates renin secretion above baseline and vasodilates below baseline (decreases Ca_i^{2+}). NECA only stimulates renin secretion and vasodilates the kidney.

cells approximates a K-diffusion potential[8,32] and increasing K_e^+ causes a progressive depolarization.[32] K-depolarization (50 - 60 mM K_e^+) has been shown to inhibit renin secretion in isolated perfused rat kidneys and in pig, dog, rabbit, and rat renal cortical slices.[11–14,16–18,21,24,25,35–38,69–71] Several observations demonstrate that the inhibitory effect is mediated by increased Ca^{2+} influx through potential operated Ca channels, resulting in increased Ca_i^{2+}. Chelation of Ca_e^{2+} reverses the transmembrane Ca^{2+} gradient and abolishes the inhibitory effect.[18,70] Furthermore, the inhibitory effect is antagonized in a concentration-dependent manner by four organic Ca channel blockers: nifedipine,[22] methoxyverapamil[11,18] (Fig. 8), verapamil[18] (Fig. 9), and diltiazem[24] (Fig. 10). The estimated IC_{50}'s are 5 x 10^{-8}, 10^{-7}, 5 x 10^{-7}, and 2 x 10^{-6} M, respectively. The same order of potency and similar IC_{50}'s have been reported for antagonizing potential-operated Ca channels that have been characterized electrophysiologically. Lowering Ca_e^{2+} potentiates the ability of Ca channel

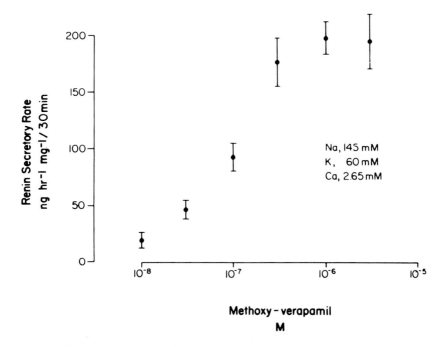

FIGURE 8. The effect of methoxyverapamil (D-600) on the renin secretory rate of K-depolarized rat renal cortical slices. Incubation of slices in 60 mM KCl nearly abolishes renin secretion (in the presence of 4 mM KCl, secretory rate is approximately 200, in the same units), and methoxyverapamil antagonizes this inhibitory effect in a concentration-dependent manner. The IC_{50} is approximately 0.1 μM, and 0.5 μM restores secretory rate to the level observed in nondepolarized cells. Reproduced with permission from Churchill and Churchill.[18]

blockers to antagonize the effect of K-depolarization[18,24] (Fig. 11), which is consistent with competitive action between Ca_e^{2+} and channel blockers at potential-operated Ca channels. Finally, BAY K 8644, a Ca channel agonist, inhibits renin secretion and the inhibitory effect is antagonized by Ca channel blockers.[22,61] Collectively, even in the absence of electrophysiological data, these observations provide unequivocal pharmacological evidence that JG cells have potential-operated Ca channels, that depolarization-induced Ca influx inhibits renin secretion, and that Ca^{2+} is an inhibitory second messenger in renin secretion.

Theoretically, then, first messengers could affect JG cell Ca^{2+} and therefore renin secretion by altering the membrane potential—inhibitory first messengers by depolarizing and increasing Ca^{2+} influx, stimulatory first messengers by hyperpolarizing and decreasing Ca^{2+} influx. Indeed, the hypothesis that JG cell membrane potential controlled renin secretion was originally advanced by Fishman[32] more than a decade ago, and Fray and Park [35–38,69–71] subsequently hypothesized that Ca^{2+} influx is the link between membrane potential and renin secretion. As attractive as this unifying hypothesis is, and despite the recent evidence that can be marshalled in its support,[8] it ignores other mechanisms of altering JG cell Ca^{2+}: changes in Ca^{2+} efflux via Na-Ca exchange, changes in Ca^{2+} efflux and sequestration via Ca-ATPase,

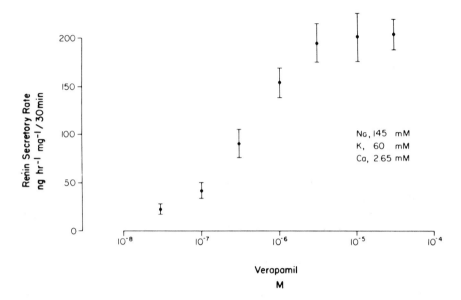

FIGURE 9.   The effect of verapamil on the renin secretory rate of K-depolarized rat renal cortical slices. Incubation of slices in 60 mM KCl nearly abolishes renin secretion (in the presence of 4 mM KCl, secretory rate is approximately 200 in the same units), and verapamil antagonizes this inhibitory effect in a concentration-dependent manner. The IC_{50} is approximately 0.5 μM, and 1 μM restores secretory rate to the level observed in nondepolarized cells. Reproduced with permission from Churchill and Churchill.[18]

and receptor-mediated mobilization of sequestered Ca^{2+}. Moreover, there is evidence that the stimulatory effects of β-adrenergic agonists[16] (Fig. 12) and the inhibitory effects of angiotensin II and vasopressin[11,12,24] (Fig. 5) are completely independent of membrane potential.

Although increased plasma K^+ inhibits renin secretion in vivo, it is very unlikely that this effect is mediated by K-depolarization of the JG cells. Increasing plasma K^+ by as little as 0.5 mM inhibits renin secretion in vivo,[88] and increases in K_e^+ of this magnitude have no appreciable effect on JG cell membrane potential.[32] More definitively, although K-depolarization of JG cells would occur independently of glomerular filtration, the inhibitory effect of increased plasma K^+ is observed in filtering kidneys but not in nonfiltering kidneys.[82] This finding suggests that the inhibitory effect of increased plasma K^+ is mediated by a tubular mechanism, e.g., by a K^+-induced increase in macula densa NaCl load.

In summary, JG cells appear to have potential-operated Ca channels, and Ca^{2+} influx through these channels leads to inhibition of renin secretion. The effects of both agonists (BAY K 8644) and antagonists (nifedipine, methoxyverapamil, verapamil, diltiazem) are consistent. However, several stimulatory and inhibitory first messengers apparently act independently of JG cell membrane potential, even if they act by changing JG cell Ca^{2+}. What first messenger does act by changing JG cell membrane potential? A reasonable possibility is discussed in the section on "Physiological Regulation of Renin Secretion" below.

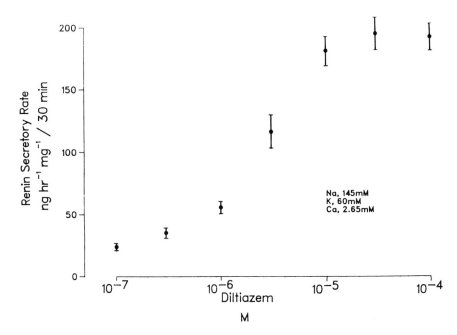

FIGURE 10. The effect of diltiazem on the renin secretory rate of K-depolarized rat renal cortical slices. Incubation of slices in 60 mM KCl nearly abolishes renin secretion (in the presence of 4 mM KCl, secretory rate is approximately 200 in the same units), and diltiazem antagonizes this inhibitory effect in a concentration-dependent manner. The IC_{50} is approximately 5 μM, and 30μM restores secretory rate to the level observed in nondepolarized cells. Reproduced with permission from Churchill et al.[24]

Calcium as an Inhibitory Second Messenger

Collectively, the above observations provide strong evidence that Ca^{2+} is an inhibitory second messenger in renin secretion. This appears to be one of only a very few exceptions to the rule that Ca is a stimulatory second messenger.[3,5,6,33,40,65,76–78,80,86] It is completely obvious that some step must be reversed in the process leading from a change in Ca_i^{2+} to changes in the secretory activities of JG cells versus adrenal medullary chromaffin cells, for example. If both JG and chromaffin cells release their stored secretory products by a process that involves exocytosis, then increased Ca_i^{2+} must change the concentration/effect of some unknown intermediate (a phosphorylated protein?) in precisely the opposite directions in JG and chromaffin cells. So far, the intermediate remains elusive.

Regardless of whether Ca^{2+} is an inhibitory or a stimulatory second messenger in cells, some intracellular entity must act as a "Ca receptor" and calmodulin is a likely candidate. Further, if Ca^{2+} is an inhibitory second messenger and if calmodulin is the receptor, then antagonists of Ca-calmodulin activity should stimulate renin secretion. Ca-calmodulin antagonists have been shown to stimulate basal renin secretion and antagonize the effects of several inhibitors of renin secretion[13,19,38,41,50,71] (Fig. 13). However, these observations cannot be taken as evidence of Ca-calmodulin involve-

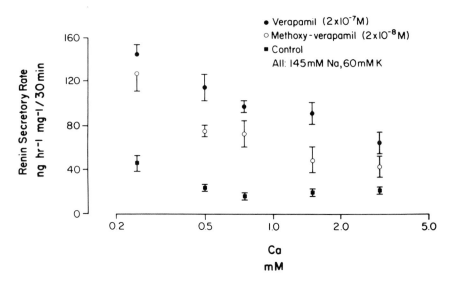

FIGURE 11. The effects of extracellular calcium, in the absence and the presence of low concentrations of verapamil and methoxyverapamil, on renin secretory rate of K-depolarized rat kidney slices. K-depolarization nearly abolishes renin secretion (in the presence of 4 mM KCl, secretory rate is approximately 200 in the same units), and reducing calcium from normal to one-tenth normal has little effect. The low concentrations of Ca antagonists have little effect at normal Ca^{2+} concentration, but as Ca^{2+} is lowered, their antagonism of the inhibitory effect of K-depolarization is potentiated. Reproduced with permission from Churchill and Churchill.[18]

ment, since several Ca-calmodulin antagonists including trifluoperazine, calmidazolium, and chlorpromazine have repeatedly been shown to block Ca^{2+} influx, especially depolarization-induced Ca^{2+} influx.[48] This effect could account for their stimulatory effects on basal secretion and their antagonism of the effects of some inhibitors, especially the inhibitory effect of K-depolarization (Fig. 13). In other words, the renin secretory effects of Ca-calmodulin antagonists can be explained equally well by either their putative intracellular effect of binding to and antagonizing the Ca-calmodulin complex, or their effect on the cell membrane of antagonizing Ca^{2+} influx independently of any direct interaction with Ca-calmodulin. Indeed, although they do not interpret their results in this manner, Kurtz et al.[50] have shown that trifluoperazine is as effective as verapamil in blocking ^{45}Ca influx in cultured JG cells. Therefore, calmodulin could be the intracellular receptor which mediates the effects of Ca_i^{2+} on renin secretion, but there is no strong evidence that it is.

The Ca-activated phospholipid-dependent protein kinase C is also an intracellular Ca^{2+} receptor, and activation of this enzyme is believed to be involved in the secretory process in some cells.[65] Tumor-promoting phorbol esters, such as 12-O-tetradecanoylphorbol 13-acetate (TPA) activate protein kinase C in two ways, by substituting for diacylglycerol and by increasing the Ca^{2+} affinity such that ambient Ca_i^{2+} is sufficient. If the inhibitory effect of increased Ca_i^{2+} on renin secretion is mediated by Ca-activation of protein kinase C, then TPA should inhibit renin secretion. TPA has been shown to inhibit renin secretion in in vitro preparations.[20,51] These results are consistent with, but do not validate, the hypothesis that activation of protein kinase C leads to inhibition of renin secretion.

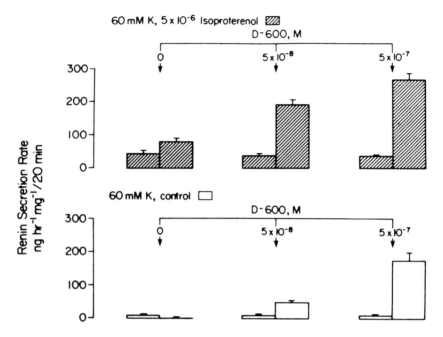

FIGURE 12. The effects on basal and isoproterenol-stimulated renin secretion (in rat kidney slices) of adding methoxyverapamil (D-600) to K-depolarizing media. Each pair of columns represents renin secretory rate in two consecutive periods in a given experiment. It can be seen, in the lower panel, that K-depolarization nearly abolishes renin secretion, and that adding methoxyverapamil produces a concentration-dependent antagonism of this inhibitory effect. Isoproterenol was present in the experiments of the upper panel; it can be seen that isoproterenol stimulates renin secretion despite K-depolarization. Therefore, its stimulatory effect cannot be attributed to hyperpolarization. Reproduced with permission from Churchill and Churchill.[16]

In summary, the detailed mechanisms by which increases and decreases in Ca_i^{2+} lead to decreases and increases in renin secretion, respectively, remain to be fully elucidated.

Other Second Messengers

Cyclic AMP as a Stimulatory Second Messenger

Sutherland's criteria[92] for establishing cyclic AMP as a stimulatory second messenger are: (1) Is there a hormone-sensitive adenylate cyclase activity associated with the cell membrane? (2) Does the hormone produce a change in intracellular cyclic AMP that precedes or coincides with the cellular response? (3) Does exogenous cyclic AMP, or a cyclic AMP analog, mimic the effect of the hormone? (4) Do methylxanthines (via phosphodiesterase inhibition) mimic or potentiate the hormone effect? With respect to the role of cyclic AMP in renin secretion, most of these criteria are impossible to satisfy, primarily because there are no techniques for obtaining a pure population of JG cells large enough to do the biochemical studies. However, there is strong indirect evidence that cyclic AMP is a stimulatory second messenger.

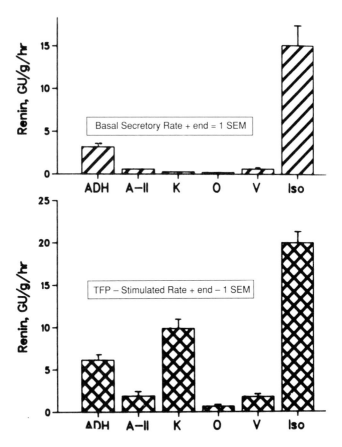

FIGURE 13. Upper panel: renin secretory rates of rat kidney slices incubated in media containing antidiuretic hormone (ADH), angiotensin II (A-II), high extracellular K^+ (K), ouabain (O), vanadate (V), and isoproterenol (Iso). The horizontal rectangle represents the mean $\pm$ S.E.M. of the basal renin secretory rate; in comparison, ADH, A-II, K, O, and V inhibited whereas Iso stimulated. Lower panel: renin secretory rates of rat kidney slices incubated in media containing trifluoperazine (TFP) plus the same inhibitors and stimulator; the horizontal rectangle represents the mean $\pm$ S.E.M. of the secretory rate of slices incubated in the presence of TFP alone. It can be seen that TFP stimulates renin secretion above the basal level, and that in the presence of TFP, ADH, A-II, K, O, and V still inhibited secretion and that Iso still stimulated. However, trifluoperazine was <u>most</u> effective in antagonizing the inhibitory effect of K-depolarization. Reproduced with permission from Churchill and Churchill.[19]

Stimulation and Inhibition of Adenylate Cyclase. β-Adrenergic agonists stimulate renin secretion, the stimulatory effect is receptor-mediated since it can be blocked by receptor antagonists, and the receptors are on JG cells since the renin stimulatory effects can be elicited in dispersed isolated cells.[47] There are no known instances of β-adrenergic receptor occupation which do not lead to activation of adenylate cyclase followed by an increase in cyclic AMP. Therefore, by strong inference,[75] cyclic AMP is a stimulatory second messenger in renin secretion. Furthermore, renin secretion is stimulated by several substances known to activate adenylate cyclase in some cells (dopamine, glucagon, histamine, A_2 adenosine receptor agonists, prostaglandins E_2 and I_2, forskolin), and renin secretion is inhibited by several substances known to inhibit adenylate cyclase in some cells (α-adrenergic and A_1 adenosine receptor agonists).[13,17,21,29,38,39,41,43,47,62,63] However the correlation between stimulators/inhibitors of adenylate cyclase and stimulation/inhibition of renin secretion is not perfect. For example, angiotensin II and vasopressin stimulate adenylate cyclase in some cells, yet both peptides inhibit renin secretion. Moreover, even if α-adrenergic and A_1 adenosine receptor agonists inhibit adenylate cyclase in some cells, it cannot be assumed that their inhibitory effects on renin secretion are mediated by decreased cyclic AMP; in fact, their inhibitory effects appear to be mediated by increased Ca_i^{2+} (vide supra).

Exogenous cyclic AMP and analogs. Sutherland's criterion that exogenous cyclic AMP should mimic the hormone effect (i.e., β-adrenergic) has come under criticism[92] since cell membranes are relatively impermeable to intact nucleotides and since extracellular cyclic AMP is extensively metabolized and some of the products have very potent effects, e.g., adenosine. This is not a trivial possibility, since although cyclic AMP should stimulate renin secretion, adenosine can either stimulate or inhibit (Fig. 6). In any case, several investigators have studied the renin secretory effects of exogenous cyclic AMP and cyclic AMP analogs, and as might be expected with the benefit of hindsight, cyclic AMP has been observed to inhibit (due to conversion to adenosine?), to have no effect on, and to stimulate renin secretion.[47]

Phosphodiesterase Inhibitors. Sutherland's criterion that phosphodiesterase inhibitors should mimic or potentiate the hormone effect has come under criticism also,[92] because nearly mM concentrations of, for example, theophylline are required to block phosphodiesterase activity,[93] yet plasma concentrations more than an order of magnitude lower produce toxic effects that are frequently lethal. Therefore, the effects of theophylline in intact animals simply cannot be attributed to phosphodiesterase inhibition; another mechanism of action must prevail. Antagonism of the effects of endogenously released adenosine is a very likely possibility, since theophylline and other alkyxanthines act, at μM concentrations, as competitive antagonists of adenosine receptors. Theophylline occasionally has been found to stimulate renin secretion in intact animals,[47] and antagonism of the inhibitory effect of endogenously released adenosine could be the mechanism of this action. In in vitro studies, alkylxanthines can be used in concentrations sufficient to inhibit phosphodiesterase activity, and there are several reports that high concentrations of alkylxanthines stimulate renin secretion.[13,17,29,38,41,47,68]

In conclusion, the best available proof that cyclic AMP is a stimulatory second messenger in renin secretion is by strong inference: renin secretion is stimulated by a β-adrenergic mechanism, and all known β-adrenergic receptors are coupled to adenylate cyclase in a stimulatory manner.

Ca_i^{2+} and Cyclic AMP Interactions. There are three possible ways that Ca_i^{2+} and cyclic AMP could act or interact as second messengers in renin secretion (Fig. 14). First, cyclic AMP could be the ultimate, or the final, "second" messenger and Ca-induced changes in renin secretion could be mediated by changes in cyclic AMP. That is, a substance that affects renin secretion but that has no direct effects on either adenylate cyclase or phosphodiesterase, such as ouabain (Na,K-ATPase is the only known molecule that is directly affected by ouabain[76]), could affect renin secretion by the following sequence of events: Na,K-ATPase inhibition, followed by increased Ca_i^{2+} due to the Na-Ca exchange mechanism, followed either by inhibition of adenylate cyclase or stimulation of phosphodiesterase (since both of these enzymes are Ca-calmodulin-dependent[77]), followed by decreased cyclic AMP, followed in turn by inhibition of renin secretion. Some observations seemingly rule out this possibility: dibutyryl cyclic AMP stimulates renin secretion (adenylate cyclase is not involved in the response, and dibutyryl cyclic AMP is resistant to hydrolysis), and the stimulatory effect is blocked by several agents that increase Ca_i^{2+}.[17] Second, Ca_i^{2+} could be the ultimate, or the final, "second" messenger, and cyclic AMP-induced changes in renin secretion could be mediated by changes in Ca_i^{2+}. That cyclic AMP can induce opposite changes in Ca_i^{2+} by affecting Ca^{2+} efflux and sequestration mechanisms has been discussed above. Therefore, a substance that affects renin secretion but that has no direct effects on Ca_i^{2+}, such as isoproterenol, could act by the following sequence of events: stimulation of adenylate cyclase, followed by increased cyclic AMP, followed by decreased Ca^{2+}. The results of the experiment just described[17] are consistent with such a sequence of events, but they do not rule out the third possibility, namely, that some step in the secretory process subsequent to both Ca_i^{2+} and cyclic AMP, presumably protein phosphorylation, is affected in opposite directions by Ca_i^{2+} and cyclic AMP acting independently. To date, no definitive experiments have been done

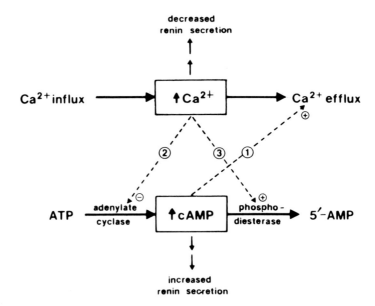

FIGURE 14. Possible interactions between Ca_i^{2+} and cyclic AMP second messenger systems in renin secretion. Experimental observations indicate that Ca_i^{2+} is inhibitory (top) and that cyclic AMP is stimulatory (bottom). Increased cyclic AMP could decrease Ca_i^{2+} by stimulating Ca^{2+} efflux and/or sequestration (pathway 1), since there is evidence that cyclic AMP stimulates both primary active Ca^{2+} efflux and sequestration (Ca-ATPase) and Na-Ca exchange (via stimulation of Na,K-ATPase). Conversely, increased Ca_i^{2+} could decrease cyclic AMP by inhibiting its synthesis (adenylate cyclase; pathway 2) and/or by stimulating its destruction (phosphodiesterase; pathway 3).

to distinguish between these two possibilities, although the observation that La^{3+} blocks the stimulatory effect of isoproterenol on renin secretion,[54] coupled with the observation that La^{3+} blocks Ca^{2+} efflux,[76,78,80] certainly favors the possibility that cyclic AMP stimulates renin secretion only by virtue of producing a decrease in Ca_i^{2+}.

Cyclic GMP as an Inhibitory Second Messenger

The recent results of Kurtz et al.[49] demonstrate that cyclic GMP mediates the inhibitory effects of atriopeptin and of nitroprusside on renin secretion. The inhibitory effect of nitroprusside on renin secretion in isolated cells[49] contrasts with the stimulatory effect of nitroprusside on renin secretion in intact animals.[47] However, this stimulatory effect is believed to be produced by nitroprusside-induced hypotension, followed by reflex activation of the renal sympathetic nerves, rather than by direct action on JG cells to increase their cyclic GMP levels.

Prostaglandins

Based on the observations that exogenous arachidonic acid and several prostaglandins (PGs) stimulate renin secretion, and that cyclooxygenase inhibitors often decrease basal and antagonize stimulated renin secretion, it has been hypothesized that PG synthesis "mediates" renin secretion, or that PGs act as second messengers.[39,43,47] Despite the validity of the experimental observations, the hypothesis itself is questionable, because the first step in PG synthesis—release of arachidonic acid from membrane phospholipids—is stimulated by increased Ca_i^{2+}. Therefore, if it is accepted that Ca_i^{2+} is an inhibitory second messenger in renin secretion, then increased JG cell Ca_i^{2+} would simultaneously stimulate PG synthesis and inhibit renin secretion. In fact, several stimulators of PG synthesis do inhibit renin secretion, and conversely some inhibitors of PG synthesis stimulate renin secretion.[23,25]

Collectively, the above observations are very difficult to reconcile with the hypothesis that renin secretion is causally related to the synthesis, by the JG cell, of any PG derived from arachidonate. However, all the experimental observations are consistent with the hypothesis that PGs synthesized by non-JG cells (e.g., endothelial cells, macula densa cells, etc.) act on JG cells as first messengers, thereby altering the concentrations of one or more second messengers, and thereby altering renin secretion. In fact, those PGs that stimulate renin secretion are the same as those which tend to vasodilate (suggestive of a decrease in JG cell Ca_i^{2+}), whereas those that inhibit renin secretion are the same as those that tend to vasoconstrict (suggestive of an increase in JG cell Ca_i^{2+}).

Physiological Regulation of Renin Secretion

Intrarenal Mechanisms

Baroreceptor Mechanism. It is well established that renin secretion is physiologically controlled, at least in part, by an intrarenal baroreceptor mechanism. The secretory activity of JG cells, which are found primarily in the media of the afferent arteriole, is influenced by physical changes in the afferent arteriole. Most experimental observations are consistent with the hypothesis that renin secretion is inversely related to transmural pressure or to stretch of the afferent arteriole: increased renal perfusion pressure increases stretch and inhibits renin secretion, whereas decreased renal perfusion pressure (or increased interstitial pressure) decreases stretch and stimulates renin secretion.[29,35,36,47,87]

Fray and co-workers[35-38] have marshalled evidence to support the hypothesis that voltage-dependent changes in Ca^{2+} influx underlie the baroreceptor mechanism for controlling renin secretion: increased stretch leads to depolarization, followed by increased Ca^{2+} influx, which then leads to increased JG cell Ca_i^{2+} and inhibited renin secretion. Conversely, decreased stretch leads to hyperpolarization (or to less depolarization), followed by decreased Ca^{2+} influx, leading to decreased JG cell Ca_i^{2+} and stimulated renin secretion (Fig. 15). Several experimental observations support the hypothesis. Increased stretch inhibits renin secretion of isolated JG cells,[35] mechanical distortion and stretch depolarize isolated JG cells,[32], depolarization with high K^+ inhibits renin secretion (vide supra), and Ca channel blockers antagonize the inhibitory effects of K-depolarization (vide supra) and of high perfusion pressure[35-38] on renin secretion.

JG cells are not unique in exhibiting stretch-induced membrane depolarization followed by increased Ca^{2+} influx. This is also exhibited by renal afferent arteriolar vascular smooth muscle cells,[42] and, in fact, this phenomenon can account for autoregulatory changes in afferent arteriolar resistance: increased stretch leads to depolarization and increased Ca^{2+} influx, followed by increased contraction and resistance, whereas decreased stretch leads to hyperpolarization (or to less depolarization) and decreased Ca^{2+} influx, followed by decreased contraction and resistance. Consistently, Ca channel blockers abolish renal autoregulation.[36,66]

Macula Densa Mechanism. It is well established that renin secretion is physiologically controlled, at least in part, by an intrarenal chemoreceptor mechanism that is sensitive to some function of tubular fluid NaCl in the macula densa segment of the nephron. Most experimental observations are consistent with Vander's original hypothesis,[87] that renin secretion is inversely related to some function of transepithelial NaCl transport: increased load of NaCl delivered to the macula densa leads to increased transport and inhibited renin secretion, whereas decreased NaCl load leads to decreased transport and stimulated renin secretion.

How the macula densa cells in the early distal tubule transmit information concerning NaCl transport to the renin-secreting JG cells is not clear. Some granulated, and therefore renin-secreting, cells are quite far away from any macula densa cells. A plausible hypothesis, originally advanced by Tagawa and Vander,[85] is that as macula densa transepithelial transport increases, ATP hydrolysis and adenosine production increase; adenosine, released from the macula densa cells, inhibits the secretory activity of nearby JG cells.

Extrarenal Mechanisms

In addition to the two completely intrarenal mechanisms, the baroreceptor and macula densa mechanisms, a whole host of extrarenal mechanisms is involved in the physiological control of renin secretion.[29,47,87] Among the most important, as

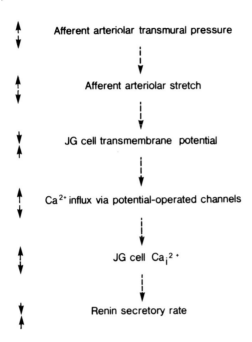

FIGURE 15. The putative mode of operation of the "intrarenal baroreceptor mechanism" for controlling renin secretion. Increased renal perfusion pressure stretches the afferent arterioles, thereby depolarizing the JG cells which are located therein, and a depolarization-induced influx of Ca^{2+} leads to inhibition of renin secretion (and conversely). Ca channel blockers antagonize the inhibitory effects on renin secretion of increased renal perfusion pressure, increased stretch, and K-depolarization (see text).

assessed by the renin secretory effects of their blockade, are: the β-adrenergic stimulation of renin secretion by increased activity of the renal nerves and increased plasma concentrations of catecholamines (β-blockers almost invariably inhibit renin secretion), and the negative-feedback inhibition of renin secretion by plasma angiotensin II (blockers of the renin-angiotensin system almost invariably stimulate renin secretion).

Renin Secretory Effects of Calcium Channel Antagonists in Vivo

Ca channel blockers are not an exception to the rule that the specificity of a drug is inversely related to the time that has elapsed since it was discovered. Although Ca channel blockers may have a number of nonspecific effects, when they act specifically, they block Ca^{2+} influx through potential operated Ca channels, channels which are gated or opened by membrane depolarization.[33,40,78] Receptor operated Ca channels are relatively resistant to the effects of Ca channel blockers,[6] as evidenced by the fact that the IC_{50}'s for antagonizing vascular smooth muscle contractions produced by K-depolarization versus α-adrenergic agonists and angiotensin II generally differ by several orders of magnitude.[78] Moreover, Ca channel blockers are not thought to affect the two Ca^{2+} efflux and sequestration mechanisms: Na-Ca exchange and Ca-ATPase. It follows that Ca channel blockers antagonize "specifically" the effects of only those first messengers that act by cell membrane depolarization.

There is strong pharmacological evidence for the existence of JG cell potential-operated channels (vide supra), but there is very little evidence that these channels play a significant role in the physiological regulation of renin secretions. If they did, then Ca channel blockers would invariably stimulate renin secretory rate and increase plasma renin concentration, and they do not[14]; stimulatory effects,[1,2,4,26,45,55−57,59,79] no effects,[27,31,44,94] and even inhibitory effects[7,79] have been documented. To illustrate this point more forcefully, if angiotensin's effect on renin secretion were mediated by a depolarization-induced Ca^{2+} influx, as has been concluded by some,[8,50,69] then Ca channel blockers would interrupt the negative feedback loop and stimulate renin secretion as effectively as converting enzyme inhibitors.

A hypothetical explanation of the diverse effects of Ca channel blockers on renin secretion can be advanced. In vivo, the secretory activity of JG cells is simultaneously affected by numerous signals—afferent arteriolar transmural pressure or stretch, NaCl load or flux in the macula densa segment, the activity of the renal sympathetic nerves, and the plasma concentrations of both inhibitors (angiotensin II, vasopressin) and stimulators (catecholamines). There is evidence that baroreceptor-mediated changes in renin secretion are produced by depolarization-induced Ca^{2+} influx (vide supra), but perhaps the baroreceptor mechanism is the only controlling mechanism operative in vivo that is susceptible to Ca channel blockade. If so, one would predict that Ca channel blockers should stimulate renin secretion (by blocking the inhibitory effect of the prevailing renal perfusion pressure) but only if Ca channel blockers don't produce some other effect that counteracts the stimulation. In fact, Ca channel blockers have at least two effects which could mask this putative stimulatory effect. First, Ca channel blockers antagonize neurotransmitter release and catecholamine release from the adrenal medulla.[80] Such actions could inhibit renin secretion by reducing any stimulatory input to the JG cells from the renal adrenergic nerves and from circulating catecholamines. Second, Ca channel blockers frequently induce natriuresis,[1,2,7,30,31,45,46,60,64,79,94] at least acutely. Therefore, they could increase NaCl load in the macula densa segment, and thereby increase the intensity of inhibitory input to the JG cells from the macula densa cells. In this context, adenosine is the putative chemical signal between macula densa and JG cells, and Ca channel blockers do not antagonize its inhibitory effect on renin secretion (vide supra). The results of one study support this interpretation: verapamil induced a natriuresis and inhibited renin secretion in filtering dog kidneys, but stimulated renin secretion in nonfiltering dog kidneys, in which macula densa influences on renin secretion are either excluded or unchanging.[79]

Summary and Conclusions

The renin-angiotensin-aldosterone system plays a central role in salt and water balance and in the regulation of arterial blood pressure. The level of activity of this system is determined primarily by the rate at which the granulated JG cells secrete renin into the blood. Although the first messengers that affect renin secretion in vivo are many and diverse, they undoubtedly affect the activity of the renin-secreting JG cell by altering its intracellular concentrations of only a few second messengers. Ca_i^{2+} is an important second messenger in all cells. However, in contrast to its stimulatory roles in most cells, Ca_i^{2+} appears to play an inhibitory second messenger role in renin secretion. The evidence that renin secretory rate is inversely related to JG cell Ca_i^{2+}, as shown in Figure 16, was reviewed in this chapter.

It can be seen in Figure 16 that since Ca_i^{2+} is affected by Ca^{2+} influx, mobilization, efflux, and sequestration pathways, first messengers can alter JG cell Ca_i^{2+} and thereby alter renin secretion by a variety of mechanisms. Ca^{2+} influx through potential operated channels has an inhibitory effect on renin secretion. These channels are activated or opened by Ca channel agonists (BAY K 8644) and by K-depolarization. There is evidence that α-adrenergic agonists produce membrane depolarization and inhibit renin secretion, and that the baroreceptor mechanism for controlling renin secretion operates via changes in membrane potential (increased perfusion pressure leads to increased stretch and to membrane depolarization, and conversely). Consistently, Ca channel blockers antagonize the inhibitory effects of Ca channel agonists, K-depolarization, α-adrenergic agonists, and increased perfusion pressure. Ca channel blockers frequently stimulate renin secretion in vivo, presumably by blocking the inhibitory effect of the prevailing perfusion pressure. However, no effects or even inhibitory effects are also found, which suggests that other effects of these drugs (e.g., natriuretic effects) must mask or counteract the stimulatory effect.

In contrast to α-adrenergic agonists, other vasoconstrictors (e.g., angiotensin II, vasopressin, and possibly A_1 adenosine agonists) inhibit renin secretion by Ca-dependent mechanisms that are independent of membrane potential and resistant to the effects of Ca channel blockers. It is likely that these agonists activate receptor-operated Ca channels (increase phospholipid metabolism and the production of inositol phosphates) and mobilize sequestered Ca_i^{2+}.

JG cell Ca_i^{2+} is also affected by two mechanisms of efflux/sequestration: Na-Ca exchange across the plasma membrane and the primary active Ca transport (Ca-

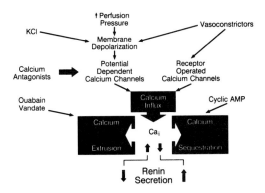

FIGURE 16. Intracellular Ca^{2+} is controlled by two mechanisms of Ca^{2+} influx and/or mobilization (potential-operated and receptor-operated channels) and two mechanisms of Ca^{2+} efflux and/or sequestration (Na-Ca exchange and primary active Ca_i^{2+} transport). There is evidence to suggest that first messengers affect Ca_i^{2+} by affecting these efflux, sequestration, influx, and mobilization pathways, and that renin secretion is inversely related to JG cell Ca_i^{2+} (see text).

ATPAse) across both the plasma membrane and the membranes of intracellular organelles. Specific inhibitors of Na,K-ATPase, such as ouabain, inhibit renin secretion presumably by increasing Na_i^+, thereby decreasing Ca^{2+} efflux via Na-Ca exchange. Vanadate's inhibitory effect on renin secretion could be produced by an increase in Ca_i^{2+} brought about by inhibition of either Na,K-ATPase (and consequently, Na-Ca exchange) or Ca-ATPase. Cyclic AMP is a stimulatory second messenger, and its effect could be produced by a decrease in Ca_i^{2+} brought about by stimulation of either Na,K-ATPase (and consequently, Na-Ca exchange) or Ca-ATPase.

The events leading from a change in JG cell Ca_i^{2+} to a change in renin secretion are unknown. The Ca-calmodulin complex and/or the Ca-activated phospholipid-dependent protein kinase C may be involved, but there is no definitive evidence, pro or con, for the involvement of either. The role played by Ca^{2+} in the secretory process in other cells has been studied extensively for decades, but to date no model of secretion has ever been proposed that can account for both inhibitory and stimulatory second messenger roles. How increased Ca_i^{2+} can stimulate the release of, for example, catecholamines, which are stored in chromaffin cell granules, yet inhibit the release of renin, which is stored in JG cell granules, is an interesting mystery.

Acknowledgments. I am very grateful that my work has been supported for several years by Grant HL-24880 from the National Institutes of Health.

References

1. Abe Y, Komori T, Miura K, et al: Effects of the calcium antagonist nicardipine on renal function and renin release in dogs. J Cardiovasc Pharmacol 5:254–259, 1983.

2. Abe Y, Yukimura T, Iwao H, Mori N, Okahara T, Yamamoto K: Effects of EDTA and verapamil on renin release in dogs. Jpn J Pharmacol 33:627–633, 1983.

3. Baker PF: The regulation of intracellular calcium. In Duncan CJ: Calcium in Biological Systems. Cambridge, UK, Cambridge University Press, 1976, pp 67–88.

4. Blackshear JL, Orlandi C, Williams GH, Hollenberg NK: The renal response to diltiazem and nifedipine: comparison with nitroprusside. J Cardiovasc Pharmacol 8:37–43, 1986.

5. Blaustein MP: The interrelationship between sodium and calcium fluxes across cell membrane. Rev Physiol Biochem Pharmacol 70:33–82, 1974.

6. Bolton TB: Mechanisms of action of transmitters and other substances on smooth muscle. Physiol Rev 59:606–718, 1979.

7. Brown B, Churchill P: Renal effects of methoxyverapamil in anesthetized rats. J Pharmacol Exp Ther 225:372–377, 1983.

8. Buhrle CP, Nobiling R, Taugner R: Intracellular recordings from renin-positive cells of the afferent glomerular arteriole. Am J Physiol 249:F272–F281, 1985.

9. Carafoli E, Crompton M: Calcium ions and mitochondria. In Duncan CJ: Calcium in Biological Systems. Cambridge, UK, Cambridge University Press, 1976, pp 89–116.

10. Churchill PC: Possible mechanism of the inhibitory effect of ouabain on renin secretion from rat renal cortical slices. J Physiol (London) 294:123–134, 1979.

11. Churchill PC: Effect of D-600 on inhibition of in vitro renin release in the rat by high extracellular potassium and angiotensin II. J Physiol (Lond) 304:449–458, 1980.

12. Churchill PC: Calcium dependency of the inhibitory effect of antidiuretic hormone on in vitro renin secretion in rats. J Physiol (Lond) 315:21–30, 1981.

13. Churchill PC: Second messengers in renin secretion. Am J Physiol 249:F175–F184, 1985.

14. Churchill PC: Calcium channel antagonists and renin secretion. Am J Nephrol 7(suppl 1):32–38, 1987.

15. Churchill PC, Bidani AK: Renal effects of selective adenosine receptor agonists. Am J Physiol 252:F299–F303, 1987.

16. Churchill PC, Churchill MC: Biphasic effect of extracellular [K] on isoproterenol-stimulated renin secretion from rat kidney slices. J Pharmacol Exp Ther 214:541–545, 1980.

17. Churchill PC, Churchill MC: Isoproterenol-stimulated renin secretion in the rat: second messenger roles of Ca and cyclic AMP. Life Sci 30:1313–1319, 1982.

18. Churchill PC, Churchill MC: Ca-dependence of the inhibitory effect of K-depolarization on renin secretion from rat kidney slices. Arch Int Pharmacodyn Ther 258:300–312, 1982.

19. Churchill PC, Churchill MC: Effects of trifluoperazine on renin secretion from rat kidney slices. J Pharmacol Exp Ther 224:68–72, 1983.

20. Churchill PC, Churchill MC: 12-O-tetradecanoylphorbol 13-acetate inhibits renin secretion of rat renal cortical slices. J Hypertension 2(suppl 1): 25–28, 1984.

21. Churchill PC, Churchill MC: A_1 and A_2 adenosine receptor activation inhibits and stimulates renin secretion of rat renal cortical slices. J Pharmacol Exp Ther 232:589–594, 1985.

22. Churchill PC, Churchill MC: BAY K 8644, a calcium channel agonist, inhibits renin secretion in vitro. Arch Int Pharmacodyn Ther 285:87–97, 1987.

23. Churchill PC, Churchill MC, McDonald FD: Quinacrine antagonizes the effects of Na,K-ATPase inhibitors on renal prostaglandin E_2 release, but not their effects on renin secretion. Life Sci 36:277–282, 1985.

24. Churchill PC, McDonald FD, Churchill MC: Effect of diltiazem, a calcium antagonist, on renin secretion from rat kidney slices. Life Sci 29:383–389, 1981.

25. Churchill PC, Savoy-Moore RT, Churchill MC: Lack of relationship between prostaglandin E_2 release and renin secretion in rat renal cortical slices. J Pharmacol Exp Ther 226:46–51, 1983.

26. Corea L, Miele N, Bentivoglio M, Boschetti E, Agabiti-Rosei E, Muiesan G: Acute and chronic effects of nifedipine on plasma renin activity and plasma adrenaline and noradrenaline in controls and hypertensive patients. Clin Sci 57:115S–117S, 1979.

27. Cruz-Soto MA, Benabe JE, Lopez-Novoa JM, Martinez-Maldonado M: Renal Na^+–K^+–ATPase in renin release. Am J Physiol 243:F598–F603, 1982.

28. Cruz-Soto M, Benabe JE, Lopez-Novoa JM, Martinez-Maldonado M: Na^+–K^+–ATPase inhibitors and renin release: relationship to calcium. Am J Physiol 247:F650–F655, 1984.

29. Davis JO, Freeman RH: Mechanisms regulating renin release. Physiol Rev 56:1–56, 1976.

30. DiBona GF, Sawin LL: Renal tubular site of action of felodipine. J Pharmacol Exp Ther 228:420-424, 1984.

31. Dietz JR, Davis JO, Freeman RH, Villarreal D, Echtenkamp SF: Effects of intrarenal infusion of calcium entry blockers in anesthetized dogs. Hypertension 5:482–488. 1983.

32. Fishman MC: Membrane potential of juxtaglomerular cells. Nature 260:542–544, 1976.

33. Fleckenstein A: Specific pharmacology of calcium in myocardium, cardiac pacemakers, and vascular smooth muscle. Ann Rev Pharmacol Toxicol 17:149–166, 1977.

34. Frankel BJ, Atwater I, Grodsky GM: Calcium affects insulin release and membrane potential in islet β-cells. Am J Physiol 240:C64–C72, 1981.

35. Fray JCS, Lush DJ: Stretch receptor hypothesis for renin secretion: the role of calcium. J Hypertension 2(suppl 1):19–23, 1984.

36. Fray JCS, Lush DJ, Park CS: Interrelationship of blood flow, juxtaglomerular cells, and hypertension: role of physical equilibrium and Ca. Am J Physiol 251:R643–R662, 1986.

37. Fray JCS, Lush DJ, Valentine AND: Cellular mechanisms of renin secretion. Fed Proc 42:3150–3154, 1983.

38. Fray JCS, Park CS, Valentine AND: Calcium and the control of renin secretion. Endocrine Rev 8:53–93, 1987.

39. Freeman RH, Davis JO, Villarreal D: Role of renal prostaglandins in the control of renin release. Circ Res 54:1–9, 1984.

40. Godfraind T: Mechanisms of action of calcium entry blockers. Fed Proc 40:2866–2871, 1981.

41. Hackenthal E, Schwertschlag U, Taugner R: Cellular mechanisms of renin release. Clin Exp Hypertens A5(7&8):975–993, 1983.

42. Harder DR, Gilbert R, Lombard JH: Vascular smooth muscle cell depolarization and activation in renal arteries on elevation of transmural pressure. Am J Physiol 253:F778–F781, 1987.

43. Henrich WL: Role of prostaglandins in renin secretion. Kidney Int 19:822–830, 1981.

44. Hiramatsu K, Yamagishi F, Kubota T, Yamada T: Acute effects of the calcium antagonist, nifedipine, on blood pressure, pulse rate, and the renin-angiotensin-aldosterone system in patients with essential hypertension. Am Heart J 104:1346–1350, 1982.

45. Imagawa J, Kurosawa H, Satoh S: Effects of nifedipine on renin release and renal function in anesthetized dogs. J Cardiovasc Pharmacol 8:636–640, 1986.

46. Johns EJ: The influence of diltiazem and nifedipine on renal function in the rat. Br J Pharmacol 84:707–713, 1985.

47. Keeton TK, Campbell WB: The pharmacologic alteration of renin release. Pharmacol Rev 32:81–227, 1980.

48. Klockner U, Isenberg G: Calmodulin antagonists depress calcium and potassium currents in ventricular and vascular myocytes. Am J Physiol 253:H1601–H1611, 1987.

49. Kurtz A, Bruna RD, Pfeilschifter J, Taugner R, Bauer C: Atrial natriuretic peptide inhibits renin release from juxtaglomerular cells by a cGMP-mediated process. Proc Natl Acad Sci (USA) 83:4769–4773, 1986.

50. Kurtz A, Pfeilschifter J, Bauer C: Is renin secretion governed by the calcium permeability of the juxtaglomerular cell membrane? Biochem Biophys Res Commun 124:359–366, 1984.

51. Kurtz A, Pfeilschifter J, Hutter A, et al: Role of protein kinase C in inhibition of renin release caused by vasoconstrictors. Am J Physiol 250:C563–C571, 1986.

52. Lederballe Petersen O: Calcium blockade in arterial hypertension. Hypertension 5:1174–1179, 1983.

53. Logan AG, Chatzilias A: The role of calcium in the control of renin release from the isolated rat kidney. Can J Physiol Pharmacol 58:60–66, 1980.

54. Logan AG, Tenyi I, Quesada T, Peart WS, Breathnach AS Martin BGH: Blockade on renin release by lanthanum. Clin Sci Mol Med 48:31s–32s, 1975.

55. Lopez-Novoa JM, Garcia JC, Cruz-Soto MA, Benabe JE, Martinez-Maldonado M: Effect of sodium orthovanadate on renal renin secretion in vivo. J Pharmacol Exp Ther 222:447–451, 1982.

56. Loutzenhiser R, Epstein M, Horton C, Hamburger R: Nitrendipine-induced stimulation of renin release by the isolated perfused rat kidney. Proc Soc Exp Biol Med 180:133–136, 1985.

57. Luft FC, Aronoff GR, Sloan RS, Fineberg NS, Weinberger MH: Calcium channel blockade with nitrendipine. Effects on sodium homeostasis, the renin-angiotensin system, and the sympathetic nervous system in humans. Hypertension 7:438–442, 1985.

58. Lyons HJ: Studies on the mechanism of renin release from rat kidney slices: calcium, sodium and metabolic inhibition. J Physiol (Lond) 304:99-108, 1980.

59. Macias-Nunez JF, Garcia-Iglesias C, Santos JC, Sanz E, Lopez-Novoa JM: Influence of plasma renin content, intrarenal angiotensin II, captopril, and calcium channel blockers on the vasoconstriction and renin release promoted by adenosine in the kidney. J Lab Clin Med 1065:562–567, 1985.

60. Marre M, Misumi J, Raemsch K-D, Corvol P, Menard J: Diuretic and natriuretic effects of nifedipine on isolated perfused rat kidneys. J Pharmacol Exp Ther 223:263–270, 1982.

61. Matsumura Y, Sasaki Y, Shinyama H, Morimoto S: The calcium channel agonist, BAY K 8644, inhibits renin release from rat kidney cortical slices. Eur J Pharmacol 117:369–373, 1985.

62. Murray RD, Churchill PC: The effects of adenosine receptor agonists in the isolated, perfused rat kidney. Am J Physiol 247:H343–H348, 1984.

63. Murray RD, Churchill PC: The concentration-dependency of the renal vascular and renin secretory responses to adenosine receptor agonists. J Pharmacol Exp Ther 232:189–193, 1985.

64. Narita H, Nagao T, Yabana H, Yamaguchi S: Hypotensive and diuretic actions of diltiazem in spontaneously hypertensive and Wistar Kyoto rats. J Pharmacol Exp Ther 227:472–477, 1983.

65. Nishizuka Y: Turnover of inositol phospholipids and signal transduction. Science 225:1365–1369, 1984.

66. Ono H, Kokubun H, Hashimoto K: Abolition by calcium antagonists of the autoregulation of renal blood flow. Naunyn-Schmiedeberg's Arch Pharmacol. 285:201–207, 1974.

67. Opgenorth TJ, Zehr JE: Role of calcium in the interaction of alpha and beta adrenoceptor-mediated renin release in isolated, constant pressure perfused rabbit kidneys. J Pharmacol Exp Ther 227:144-149, 1983.

68. Osswald H: The role of adenosine in the regulation of glomerular filtration rate and renin secretion. Trends Pharmacol Sci 5:94–97, 1984.

69. Park CS, Han DS, Fray JCS: Calcium in the control of renin secretion: Ca^{2+} influx as an inhibitory signal. Am J Physiol 240:F70–F74, 1981.

70. Park CS, Malvin RL: Calcium in the control of renin release. Am J Physiol 235:F22–F25, 1978.

71. Park CS, Sigmon DH, Han DS, Honeyman TW, Fray JCS: Control of renin secretion by Ca^{2+} and cyclic AMP through two parallel mechanisms. Am J Physiol 251:R531–R536, 1986.

72. Peart WS: Intra-renal factors in renin release. Contrib Nephrol 12:5–15, 1978.

73. Peart WS, Quesada T, Tenyi I: The effects of EDTA and EGTA on renin secretion. Br J Pharmacol 59:247–252, 1977.

74. Phillis JW, Wu PH: Catecholamines and the sodium pump in excitable cells. Prog Neurobiol 17:141–184, 1981.

75. Platt JR: Strong inference. Science 146:347–353, 1964.

76. Putney JW Jr, Askari A: Modification of membrane function by drugs. In Andreoli TE, Hoffman JF, Fanestil DD (eds): Physiology of Membrane Disorders. New York, Plenum, 1978, pp 417–445.

77. Rasmussen H, Barrett PQ: Calcium messenger system: an integrated view. Physiol Rev 64:938–984, 1984.

78. Rosenberger L, Triggle DJ: Calcium, calcium translocation, and specific calcium antagonists. In Weiss GB (ed): Calcium in Drug Action. New York, Plenum, 1978, pp 3–31.

79. Roy MW, Guthrie GP Jr, Holladay FP, Kotchen TA: Effects of verapamil on renin and aldosterone in the dog and rat. Am J Physiol 245:E410–E416, 1983.

80. Rubin RP: Calcium and Cellular Secretion. New York, Plenum, 1982.

81. Schwartz A, Lindenmayer GE, Allen JC: The sodium-potassium adenosine triphosphatase: pharmacological, physiological and biochemical aspects. Pharmacol Rev 27:3–134, 1975.

82. Shade RE, Davis JO, Johnson JA, Witty RT: Effects of arterial infusion of sodium and potassium on renin secretion in the dog. Circ Res 31:719–727, 1972.

83. Spielman WS, Thompson CI: A proposed role for adenosine in the regulation of renal hemodynamics and renin release. Am J Physiol 242:F423–F435, 1982.

84. Sundet WD, Wang BC, Hakumaki MOK, Goetz KL: Cardiovascular and renin responses to vanadate in the conscious dog: attenuation after calcium channel blockade. Proc Soc Exp Biol Med 175:185–190, 1984.

85. Tagawa H, Vander AJ: Effects of adenosine compounds on renal function and renin secretion in dogs. Circ Res 26:327–338, 1970.

86. VanBreemen C, Aaronson P, Loutzenhiser R: Sodium-calcium interactions in mammalian smooth muscle. Pharmacol Rev 30:167–208, 1979.

87. Vander AJ: Control of renin release. Physiol Rev 47:359–382, 1967.

88. Vander AJ: Direct effects of potassium on renin secretion and renal function. Am J Physiol 219:445–449, 1970.

89. Vandongen R, Peart WS: Calcium dependence of the inhibitory effect of angiotensin on renin secretion in the isolated perfused kidney of the rat. Br J Pharmacol 50:125–129, 1974.

90. Waeber B, Nussberger J, Brunner HR: Does renin determine the blood pressure response to calcium entry blockers? Hypertension 7:223–227, 1985.

91. Webb RC, Bohr DF: Mechanism of membrane stabilization by calcium in vascular smooth muscle. Am J Physiol 235:C227–C232, 1978.

92. Weinryb I: Cyclic AMP as an intracellular mediator of hormone action: Sutherland's criteria revisited. Perspect Biol Med 22:415–420, 1979.

93. Weinryb I, Chasin M, Free CA, et al: Effects of therapeutic agents on cyclic AMP metabolism in vitro. J Pharmaceut Sci 61:1556–1567. 1972.

94. Yokoyama S, Kaburagi T: Clinical effects of intravenous nifedipine on renal function. J Cardiovasc Pharmacol 5:67–71, 1983.

Lance D. Dworkin, M.D.
Judith A. Benstein, M.D.

8

Antihypertensive Agents, Glomerular Hemodynamics and Glomerular Injury

In patients with kidney disease, clinical experience has proven that once renal excretory function is significantly compromised, progressive decline in filtration capacity will occur. In individual patients, the loss of filtration rate is linear with time and often appears to be independent of the activity of the process by which the kidney was initially damaged.[1] Ultimately, most patients require some form of renal replacement therapy. Despite great progress in dialysis and transplantation, therapies that prevent progressive kidney damage in man have yet to be identified.

Forty years ago, Addis observed that restricting protein intake could preserve renal function in patients with chronic renal insufficiency. He suggested that this maneuver reduced the workload of the residual, functioning nephrons of the damaged kidney.[2] Although the concept of "renal work" has not stood the test of time, studies in experimental animals have identified other factors that may explain the protective effect of protein restriction. In particular, attention has been focused on the hemodynamic adaptations that follow nephron loss, and on the roles played by systemic and intrarenal hypertension. Specific interventions that alter these parameters and prevent or reverse experimental renal injury have been identified. The purpose of this paper is to review the evidence that alterations in glomerular hemodynamics contribute importantly to progressive injury and that reducing glomerular flows and/or pressures may significantly attenuate damage. In particular, the effects of a variety of antihypertensive pharmaceuticals on systemic and intrarenal pressure and renal injury in experimental animals will be discussed. Relevant data in man will be reviewed.

The Determinants of Glomerular Ultrafiltration of Water

As discussed below, much of our understanding of the relationship between alterations in glomerular perfusion and progressive kidney damage has been derived from experiments in which micropuncture techniques have been used to evaluate the

155

glomerular ultrafiltration process in experimental models of renal disease. In order to appreciate these experiments fully, an understanding of the forces that govern the filtration process is required. This topic has been extensively reviewed[3] and is considered briefly here.

As is the case in all capillary networks, the rate of ultrafiltration of water across the glomerular capillary depends upon the imbalance between the transcapillary hydraulic pressure gradient (ΔP), which favors filtration, and the colloid osmotic pressure gradient ($\Delta \pi$), which opposes it. For one entire glomerulus, this relationship can be expressed as:

$$SNGFR = K_f \ x \ \overline{P}_{UF}$$

$$= K_f \ x \ (\overline{\Delta P} - \Delta \pi)$$

$$= K_f \ x \ ((\overline{P}_{GC} - P_T) - (\pi_{GC} - \pi_T))$$

where SNGFR is the ultrafiltration rate of water for a single glomerulus, $\overline{P}_{UF}$ is the net force favoring ultrafiltration and K_f is the ultrafiltration coefficient for the glomerular capillary wall. $\overline{P}_{GC}$ and π_{GC} are the hydraulic and oncotic pressures within the glomerular capillary, respectively, while P_T and π_T are the corresponding pressures in Bowman's space. Because the protein concentration in Bowman's space is extremely small, π_T is negligible making $\Delta \pi$ essentially equal to π_{GC}.

Experimentally, the determinants of glomerular ultrafiltration have been directly measured in Munich-Wistar rats, a strain that possess glomeruli on the kidney surface. Representative values for the various pressures discussed above are shown in Figure 1. In the bottom panel of this figure, the net driving force for ultrafiltration is displayed

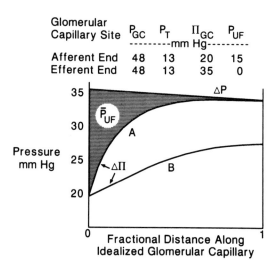

Glomerular Capillary Site	P_{GC}	P_T	Π_{GC}	P_{UF}
	---------	---------	-mm Hg-	---------
Afferent End	48	13	20	15
Efferent End	48	13	35	0

FIGURE 1. Hydraulic and colloid osmotic pressure profiles along an idealized glomerular capillary in euvolemic rats. Curves A and B represent $\Delta \pi$ profiles under conditions of normal and increased plasma flow rate, respectively. Mean net ultrafiltration pressure, P_{UF}, is equal to the shaded area between the ΔP curve and the $\Delta \pi$ curve. See text for other abbreviations. Adapted from ref. 3, with permission.

as a function of distance along the glomerular capillary network. While the hydraulic pressure gradient along the network is relatively constant (the $\overline{\Delta P}$ line), $\Delta \pi$ progressively rises, a consequence of the increasing protein concentration within the capillary as filtered plasma water passes into Bowman's space. The local net ultrafiltration pressure is determined by the difference between $\overline{\Delta P}$ and $\Delta \pi$ at any point along the network and, in normal rats, decreases from a value of ≈ 15 mmHg at the most afferent end to 0 by the efferent end of the capillary network. The net ultrafiltration pressure for the entire glomerulus is equal to the area between the ΔP and $\Delta \pi$ curves.

It should be apparent from the equation and Figure 1 that elevation in $\overline{\Delta P}$ will tend to increase $\overline{P}_{UF}$ and therefore SNGFR. Of note, in virtually all of the studies we will consider, significant alterations in ΔP result from changes in the value of $\overline{P}_{GC}$, not P_T. Conversely, elevation in plasma protein concentration, and therefore $\Delta \pi$, tend to reduce net ultrafiltration pressure and filtration rate. Declines in K_f are also predicted to cause SNGFR to decrease. What may not be clear from the preceding discussion is that increases in glomerular capillary plasma flow rate (Q_A) also cause SNGFR to rise. As plasma flow increases, the $\Delta \pi$ curve is shifted down and to the right, for example moving from curve A to curve B in Figure 1. This alteration increases the area between the $\overline{\Delta P}$ and the $\Delta \pi$ curves, and thereby increases $\overline{P}_{UF}$ and SNGFR. In the following sections, we will consider how these forces, and in particular the hydraulic pressure gradient, are modified in a variety of experimental renal diseases, and how these changes may be related to progressive kidney damage.

The Remnant Kidney Model

Surgical reduction in renal mass provides a model for the study of the response of the kidney to a decreased number of nephrons. In general, this model is produced by the combination of a unilateral total nephrectomy and the surgical removal or infarction of two-thirds to five-sixths of the remaining kidney. More than 50 years ago, Chanutin and Ferris[4] demonstrated that this procedure resulted, in the rat, in a syndrome of systemic hypertension, proteinuria and renal failure. Morphologically, end-stage remnant kidneys were characterized by extensive glomerular sclerosis, tubular atrophy and interstitial fibrosis.[2,4] Subsequent studies have examined the natural history of these lesions. Initially, after reduction in renal mass, remaining glomeruli hypertrophy. However, on sequential examination, mesangial expansion, loss of glomerular epithelial cells, and, ultimately, obliteration of capillary lumens with sclerosis are observed. Because the residual kidney tissue in this model is normal at the time of ablation, it has been suggested that the compensatory processes induced by nephrectomy were themselves responsible for the alteration in morphology.[5]

Studies of remnant kidney function reveal that surgical reduction in renal mass results in an increase in plasma flow and filtration rate in remaining nephrons of a magnitude that reflects the extent of nephron loss.[6] Advances in micropuncture techniques permitted precise characterization of the forces responsible for these adaptive changes. Following uninephrectomy (UNX), single nephron glomerular filtration rate (SNGFR) was elevated to almost twice that found in controls, an increase that was largely the result of elevation in single nephron glomerular plasma flow (Q_A).[8]

More recently, Hostetter et al. assessed the pattern of glomerular perfusion in rats subjected to more extreme degrees of renal ablation. As illustrated in Figure

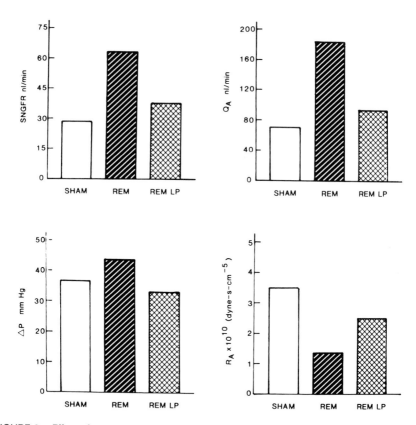

FIGURE 2. Effect of protein restriction on glomerular hemodynamics in rats subjected to subtotal renal ablation. The sham group underwent surgery without reduction in renal mass. Both experimental groups underwent $1\frac{5}{6}$ nephrectomy. The REM group was fed a diet containing 24% protein, while the REM-LP group received 6% protein in their diet. Adapted from ref. 7.

2, 1 week following $1\frac{5}{6}$ nephrectomy, SNGFR was more than twice that of sham operated controls, a consequence of significant elevation in Q_A and in $\overline{\Delta P}$, the latter resulting from an increase in $\overline{P}_{GC}$. The rise in intraglomerular pressure resulted from the combined effects of an increase in systemic blood pressure and a decline in afferent arteriolar resistance (R_A). Morphologic studies performed only 1 week following surgery in remnant kidney rats revealed early evidence of glomerular injury, including mesangial expansion and endothelial cell damage. In a group also subjected to $1\frac{5}{6}$ nephrectomy but fed a low protein diet, the rise of SNGFR was prevented, as were contributory changes in R_A, Q_A, and $\overline{\Delta P}$. Morphologic abnormalities were essentially absent in protein restricted rats and proteinuria was reduced.[8] This study provided clear evidence for a link between so-called "compensatory" hemodynamic alterations and progressive renal failure. These authors proposed that, after a loss of functioning nephrons, adaptive nephron "hyperfiltration" served initially to return the total GFR toward normal, but was, in the long run, maladaptive and responsible for the destruction of those remaining nephrons. This hypothesis, summarized in figure 3,

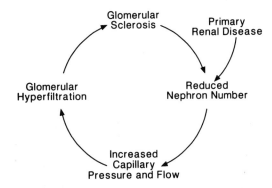

FIGURE 3. Hypothesis relating increased glomerular filtration rate to progression of renal disease. A primary renal disease results in a reduction in nephron number and filtration rate. Capillary flow and pressure increase in remnant glomeruli leading to an adaptive rise in single nephron GFR, tending to return remnant kidney GFR towards normal. Glomerular hyperfiltration contributes to progressive sclerosis of remaining glomeruli. As more nephrons are lost, flow, pressure and filtration rate increase progressively in residual glomeruli. The process is self-perpetuating and, ultimately, all nephrons are destroyed.

is attractive because it describes a final common pathway by which all human renal diseases may progress, once significant overall functional impairment has developed.

Nath et al.[9] sought to determine whether protein restriction would prevent glomerular obsolescence if imposed after the initial hemodynamic and morphologic response to ablation were present. Following $1\frac{5}{6}$ nephrectomy, rats were fed a normal protein diet for 6 weeks, and then switched to a restricted protein diet for an additional 2 weeks. Although SNGFR did not change, the period of protein restriction did result in a decline in $\overline{\Delta P}$. In a more chronic study, remnant kidney rats were fed a standard diet for 3 months. Significant proteinuria developed in these rats; however, protein restriction for an additional 3 months resulted in disappearance of proteinuria and stabilization in renal function. In this study, elevation in $\overline{\Delta P}$ was the hemodynamic abnormality most closely associated with progressive glomerular injury. Furthermore, a maneuver that reversed the glomerular hypertension was shown to be protective even when imposed after morphologic evidence of glomerular damage was present. This finding has been substantiated by work from Meyer et al.[10] In this study, a diet with only a moderately reduced protein content was imposed 8 weeks after subtotal nephrectomy. Despite sustained systemic hypertension, the low protein diet reduced $\overline{\Delta P}$, and lessened proteinuria and the prevalence of pathologic glomerular abnormalities.[10] Obviously, the ability of protein restriction to attenuate or reverse glomerular capillary hypertension and injury in animals raises the possibility that similar interventions might be used to alter the course of human renal disease.

Desoxycorticosterone-salt Hypertension

Uninephrectomy and the administration of desoxycorticosterone and 1% saline (DOC-SALT) to rats results in hypertension associated, in its early stages, with volume expansion.[11] With time, glomerular hypertrophy, vacuolar lesions and, ultimately, sclerosis supervenes.[12] In this model, efferent arteriolar dilatation is an early, prominent finding that precedes the development of overt vascular and glomerular injury. This morphologic observation led Hill and Heptinstall[12] to propose that afferent vasodilation developed early in the course of DOC-SALT hypertension. They suggested that a decline in preglomerular resistance led to an increase in glomerular pressure, and that this hemodynamic alteration, rather than ischemia, was responsible for the destruction of glomeruli.

Support for this hypothesis was provided by studies in which the pattern of glomerular perfusion was determined in rats with DOC-SALT hypertension.[13] Figure 4 summarizes these results. Two weeks after the initiation of DOC-SALT treatment and prior to the appearance of morphologic evidence of injury, arterial pressure was elevated, as were SNGFR, Q_A and $\overline{\Delta P}$. Following 4 weeks of hypertension, $\overline{\Delta P}$ was even higher, a consequence of the presence of severe systemic hypertension and the absence of a normal, autoregulatory increase in afferent arteriolar resistance.

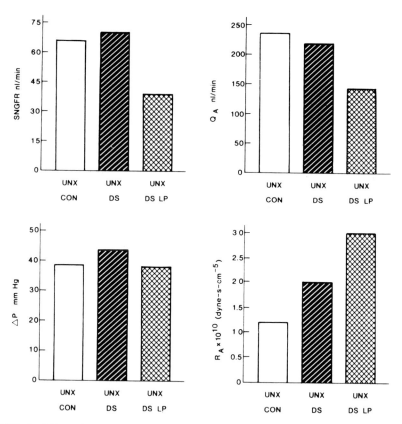

FIGURE 4. Effect of protein restriction on glomerular hemodynamics in rats after 4 weeks of mineralocorticoid and salt-induced hypertension. All three groups underwent uninephrectomy (UNX). The two experimental groups were given desoxycorticosterone acetate injections and saline to drink. The UNX DS Group was given a 24% protein diet, while the UNX DS LP group was fed a 6% protein diet. Adapted from ref. 12.

Uninephrectomized controls not given DOC and salt had similar elevations in SNGFR and Q_A, but did not develop systemic or intrarenal hypertension. Pathologic proteinuria and significant morphologic abnormalities were also absent in this group, suggesting that elevation in $\overline{\Delta P}$ is the hemodynamic alteration most closely associated with glomerular injury. When DOC-SALT rats were fed a protein restricted diet, arterial pressure was modestly reduced and afferent arteriolar resistance increased. As a result, SNGFR and Q_A declined, and the mean value for $\overline{\Delta P}$ fell to the normal level. Morphologic changes and significant proteinuria were prevented in this group, substantiating the correlation between elevations in intrarenal pressure and the development of glomerular damage.[13]

The Spontaneously Hypertensive Rat (SHR)

The SHR is a strain genetically bred to develop severe systemic hypertension. With time, proteinuria, glomerular sclerosis, and a decline in GFR are observed in these rats; however, increased protein filtration and morphologic evidence of injury involve only the juxtamedullary glomeruli.[14] Estimates of the value of SNGFR in superficial cortical nephrons of SHRs have been provided by several laboratories.[15-17] In general, despite systemic hypertension, glomerular capillary pressure is not elevated in the accessible, superficial cortical nephrons of intact SHR.[15] Thus, in this strain, the population of superficial glomeruli is protected from hypertensive damage by afferent arteriolar vasoconstriction, which prevents the transmission of an elevated perfusion pressure to the capillary level. In contrast, it has been suggested that deep nephrons of SHR may autoregulate less well and that altered hemodynamics may contribute to the development of sclerosis in these glomeruli. Due to the inaccessibility of juxtamedullary glomeruli, direct measurements of glomerular capillary pressure in these nephrons have not been made. However, compared to normotensive controls, deep cortical nephrons of SHR are characterized by elevated SNGFR,[16] an alteration which suggests that $\overline{\Delta P}$ might be abnormally high in these nephrons.

Further support for the role of glomerular capillary hypertension in the pathogenesis of glomerular injury in SHR has been provided by studies in which renal mass was surgically reduced. Uninephrectomy accelerates the development of proteinuria and glomerular sclerosis in the SHR, and results in more widespread glomerular abnormalities, so that superficial cortical as well as juxtamedullary nephrons are affected.[17] Compared to intact animals, superficial cortical nephrons of UNX SHR display elevations in Q_A, SNGFR and $\overline{\Delta P}$, which are largely a consequence of a nephrectomy-induced reduction in afferent resistance. Of note, uninephrectomized, normotensive, Wistar Kyoto (WKY) controls develop even higher mean values for plasma flow and filtration rate than UNX SHR; however, $\overline{\Delta P}$ is not significantly elevated in the WKY strain. Significant glomerular injury does not develop in UNX WKY rats, supporting the important role of glomerular capillary hypertension in the genesis of glomerular injury. Results of micropuncture studies are shown in Figure 5. When uninephrectomized SHRs were fed a diet low in protein, $\overline{\Delta P}$ and SNGFR remained within the normal range and proteinuria and histologic evidence of injury were avoided. Protection was observed even in the absence of a decline in mean arterial blood pressure, indicating that injury depends upon the extent of intrarenal, rather than systemic hypertension.[17]

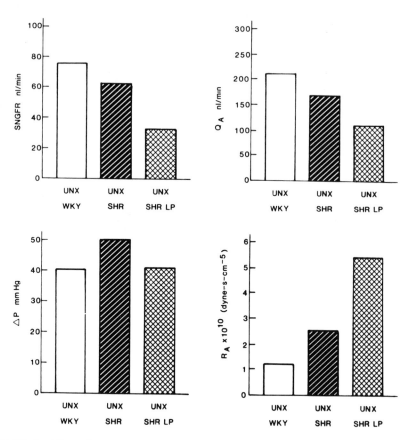

FIGURE 5. Effect of protein restriction on the glomerular hemodynamics of spontaneously hypertensive rats. Uninephrectomized Wistar-Kyoto rats (UNX WKY) served as normotensive controls. Both hypertensive groups also underwent uninephrectomy. The UNX SHR group was fed the standard 24% protein diet, while the UNX SHR LP group was given a diet containing 6% protein. Adapted from ref. 16.

Diabetes Mellitus

Disease of the renal microcirculation is the most common cause of death in patients who develop diabetes in childhood and contributes significantly to morbidity and mortality in those who become diabetic as adults.[18] Recent studies have examined the role altered renal hemodynamics play in the development of diabetic microangiopathy. Both clinically and experimentally, early diabetes is characterized by an increase in glomerular filtration rate and renal plasma flow.[19–21] In man, hyperfiltration is associated with microalbuminuria, and these two abnormalities mark those individuals destined to develop overt nephropathy.[22] In one patient with diabetes and unilateral renal artery stenosis, renal lesions were not observed in a kidney distal to the stenotic artery, where flow and pressure were probably reduced, but were seen in the contralateral kidney.[23] In rats, maneuvers that increase renal perfusion, such as nephrectomy, accelerate the pace of the disease.[24] These findings suggest that the renal vasodilation and hyperfiltration present in early diabetes contribute substantially to progressive glomerular damage and eventual real failure.[18,21]

The hemodynamic basis for hyperfiltration in diabetes has been investigated by applying micropuncture techniques to rats made diabetic by injection of streptozotocin. In this model, moderate glycemic control similar to that achieved in many clinical settings can be obtained by the daily administration of insulin. In rats, as in man, this state is associated with an increase in glomerular filtration rate. Afferent resistance is reduced and hyperfiltration results from elevations in Q_A and $\overline{\Delta P}$.[25] Thus, animals with experimental diabetes have a pattern of glomerular perfusion which resembles that observed in other nephropathies that are thought to be hemodynamically mediated.

Zatz et al.[26] examined the effect of varying protein intake on renal hemodynamics and the appearance of proteinuria and glomerular sclerosis in diabetic rats. Insulin was administered to all groups, so that the degree of metabolic control was similar in rats ingesting the different protein diets. Despite sustained hyperglycemia, protein restriction prevented hyperfiltration, hyperperfusion, and intraglomerular hypertension. After a year, no proteinuria and little pathologic evidence of injury was found in this group. In contrast, consumption of a high protein diet was associated with elevations in $\overline{\Delta P}$, Q_A, and SNGFR, and marked acceleration of the development of proteinuria and glomerular lesions. Thus, hemodynamic factors were most closely correlated with the development of diabetic nephropathy. In fact, when glomerular pressure and flow were normalized, diabetic renal disease was prevented, despite the presence of sustained hyperglycemia.

Immune-mediated Glomerular Disease

Almost 50 years ago, protein restriction was found to lessen kidney damage in animals exposed to nephrotoxic serum.[27] That finding must now be interpreted in light of our current understanding of the effects of immune injury and protein restriction on glomerular hemodynamics. Experimental models of glomerulonephritis are often characterized by heterogeneous damage, so that some glomeruli appear nearly normal whereas others are severely damaged. Nephron function is similarly heterogeneous; SNGFR is highly variable and hyperfiltering nephrons and nonfunctioning nephrons coexist.[28] Where SNGFR is elevated, $\overline{\Delta P}$ and Q_A are also increased. In a manner analogous to the residual glomeruli of the remnant kidney,[29] the population of hyperperfused, hyperfiltering nephrons within the nephritic kidney are at risk for hemodynamically-mediated damage. Accordingly, protein restriction may lessen glomerular injury in models of immune-mediated renal disease by limiting the degree of adaptive hyperperfusion that develops in those nephrons less damaged by the inflammatory process.

Recent studies have confirmed the protective effect of protein restriction in nephrotoxic serum nephritis (NSN).[29] In addition, despite persistence of high levels of autoantibodies, protein restriction attenuates renal damage in the NZB/NZW mouse, a murine model of lupus nephritis.[30] An important role for hemodynamic factors in the pathogenesis of immune-mediated renal disease was also suggested by a study in which 2-kidney, 1-clip renovascular hypertension was superimposed on NSN. Constriction of one renal artery is a maneuver that causes glomerular flows and pressures to increase in the unclipped kidney, whereas these parameters are normal or reduced on the clipped side. As predicted from these hemodynamic considerations, morphologic evidence of injury was only enhanced in the unclipped kidney.[31]

Raij et al.[32] have also examined the effect of systemic and intrarenal hypertension on immune-mediated glomerular injury. They induced ferritin/anti-ferritin immune complex disease in both SHR and DOC-SALT hypertensive rats. As discussed above, the glomerular capillaries of intact SHR are protected from elevated perfusion pressure by a high afferent resistance, whereas DOC-SALT rats have a low afferent resistance and a high $\overline{\Delta P}$. Although similar increments in systemic pressure were observed in both models, proteinuria, renal functional impairment, and glomerular sclerosis were all more prominent in DOC-SALT as compared to SHR with immune complex disease. Raij and coworkers suggested that, in the SHR, immunologic injury was not exacerbated by systemic hypertension, because afferent vasoconstriction offset the increase in perfusion pressure so that glomerular capillary pressure was not elevated. Systemic hypertension worsened immune injury only when preglomerular vasodilation rendered the glomerular capillaries vulnerable to an increase in blood pressure. Thus, even when a kidney disease is initiated by immune mechanisms, its course and outcome may be greatly influenced by hemodynamic events.

Role of Nonhemodynamic Factors in Progressive Injury

As summarized above, a considerable body of experimental evidence supports the notion that glomerular hyperperfusion is causally related to glomerular injury. However, this finding does not rule out the possibility that other, nonhemodynamic, factors participate in the complex process that culminates in glomerular destruction. In fact, evidence has been gathered which suggests that platelets, clotting factors, calcium, phosphate, lipids, ammonia and the structural changes of glomerular hypertrophy contribute to progressive renal injury. A complete discussion of the roles played by these factors is beyond the scope of this presentation; however, they are considered briefly below. For a more complete discussion of many of these factors, the reader is referred to the recent review of Klahr et al.[33]

When the endothelial cell layer that lines a blood vessel is damaged, platelets aggregate and release a number of locally acting mediators. These substances have diverse actions, including potent effects on vascular resistance, permeability, and activation of the coagulation cascade.[34] In a range of experimental models, capillary thromboses and fibrin deposition are commonly observed within glomeruli.[35] Thromboxane synthetase inhibitors, which reduce the formation of thromboxane A_2, can prevent platelet aggregation and its consequences. When these agents are administered to rats with remnant kidneys, renal plasma flow and filtration rate are preserved, proteinuria is diminished, and morphologic evidence of glomerular damage is reduced.[36] Inhibition of the clotting cascade with heparin or warfarin has also been shown to lessen renal injury in this model.[37] These findings suggest that the coagulation system may participate in the evolution of vascular injury and progressive glomerular sclerosis.

Calcium salts deposit in kidneys progressing to end-stage renal failure, suggesting that nephrocalcinosis may contribute to progressive renal damage. Hyperphosphatemia is characteristic of states in which glomerular filtration rate (GFR) is severely reduced, and phosphate feeding increases the rate of deterioration observed in rats after reduction in renal mass. Of note, the adverse effect of phosphate can be blocked by 3-phosphocitric acid, which prevents calcium phosphate crystal growth and nephrocalcinosis.[38] Diets low in phosphate slow the rate of decline in filtration function in experimental renal disease.[39] That this effect is independent of protein intake was demonstrated by a study in which a phosphate binder was administered to rats with remnant kidneys. Animals ingesting the binder had reduced tissue calcium content, less proteinuria, and a lower incidence of morphologic abnormalities of the glomeruli, tubules, and interstitium.[40] Finally, as discussed below, recent studies with the calcium-entry blocker verapamil indicate that this agent decreases renal calcium content and injury in rats with remnant kidneys.[41]

Many models in which the progressive renal disease has been studied, including the remnant kidney, DOC-SALT rat, UNX SHR, and diabetes, are characterized not only by increased glomerular pressure, but also by kidney and glomerular hypertrophy. Recently, this morphologic change has been directly associated with the development of glomerular injury. Benstein et al.[42] compared the UNX SHR fed a salt restricted diet to rats fed normal chow and to those fed normal chow but chronically given hydrochlorothiazide. Although no differences in systemic blood pressure, GFR, or its determinants were observed among the groups, proteinuria and the incidence of glomerular sclerosis were significantly less in rats on the low salt diet. Amelioration of injury was correlated with a significant reduction in kidney weight in that group. Thus, glomerular injury was found only in those rats where hypertrophy and glomerular capillary hypertension coexisted, and not when only the latter was present. Salt restriction has also been reported to retard glomerular injury in the remnant kidney model.[43]

A similar relationship between glomerular hypertrophy, hypertension and injury has been described by Yoshida et al.[44] They removed two-thirds of the left kidney, and then compared rats in which the remaining right kidney was removed to animals in which the right kidney was left in situ, but its ureter diverted to drain into the peritoneal cavity. Rats with $1\frac{2}{3}$ nephrectomy developed glomerular hyperperfusion, hyperfiltration and hypertrophy. Rats with ureteral diversion and two-third nephrectomy developed equivalent elevations in glomerular pressure, flow, and filtration rate, but no increase in glomerular size. Sclerosis was significantly more frequent in the $1\frac{2}{3}$ nephrectomized group. The mechanism by which hypertrophy contributes to glomerular injury is uncertain but may ultimately relate to hemodynamic factors (Fig. 6). According to the La Place relationship (T = P x R), wall tension (T) in a capillary is as dependent on the vessel radius (R) as it is on the transcapillary hydraulic pressure gradient (P). If capillary radius increases as glomeruli hypertrophy, as occurs following nephrectomy,[45] then at constant pressure capillary wall tension would be increased in hypertrophied kidneys. Conversely, maneuvers that prevent hypertrophy, for example salt restriction, will decrease tension.

Abnormalities in lipid metabolism are seen in a variety of renal diseases, especially those associated with the nephrotic syndrome. It has been suggested that under some circumstances, circulating lipoproteins may directly damage the glomerular basement membrane.[46] Even in the remnant kidney model, where primary abnormalities in lipid metabolism are not described, lowering of serum cholesterol with clofibrate lessens injury without preventing glomerular hypertension.[47]

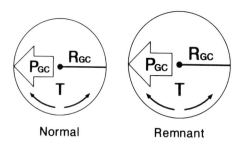

Normal   **Remnant**

FIGURE 6. Wall tension hypothesis. According to the LaPlace relationship, glomerular capillary pressure (P_{GC}) and glomerular capillary radius (R_{GC}) contribute equally to developed wall tension. In remnant kidneys, R_{GC} increases as glomeruli hypertrophy, tending to augment wall tension, and injury, on a purely morphologic basis.

Finally, increased ammonia levels in chronic renal failure may contribute to glomerular destruction. Ammonia can bind to the third component of complement and lead to activation of the entire complement system via the alternate pathway. Increased levels of this amidated form of C_3 have been observed in a model of renal failure, and complement components can be detected in glomeruli undergoing sclerosis.[48]

Therapy

As outlined above, a growing body of evidence supports the theory that intraglomerular hypertension plays a pivotal role in the progression of renal disease. It follows that systemic hypertension will affect this process only if increased pressure is transmitted to the glomerulus, an outcome dependent on the afferent and efferent arteriolar resistances. In the models described above, protein restriction was uniformly effective in reducing glomerular pressure and retarding progressive glomerular damage. This dietary manipulation reduces glomerular pressure by causing afferent arteriolar resistance to increase significantly. Unfortunately, for reasons discussed in detail elsewhere,[49] the application of dietary protein restriction to large numbers of patients with mild to moderate renal functional impairment may not be practical.

A logical alternative would seem to be the numerous antihypertensive agents currently utilized to treat patients with systemic hypertension. One might predict that pharmacologic reduction of systemic blood pressure would cause glomerular capillary pressure to decline and thereby protect the kidney from injury. However, these agents, most of which dilate resistance vessels, are unlikely to reduce glomerular capillary pressure in a manner analogous to protein restriction, which increases preglomerular resistance. Furthermore, studies in both patients and experimental animals suggest that the renal circulatory effects of various antihypertensive agents may differ significantly. Theoretically, an agent that , in addition to decreasing systemic vascular resistance, preferentially dilates the efferent arteriole, might cause $\overline{\Delta P}$ to decline and reduce the incidence of glomerular sclerosis. Alternatively, an agent that selectively dilates the preglomerular circulation might cause persistent elevation in $\overline{\Delta P}$ and little reduction in injury.[50] The hemodynamic and therapeutic effects of several agents in experimental renal disease is discussed below and summarized in Table 1.

TABLE 1. Effect of Therapy on Golmerular Hemodynamics and Injury

Therapy	Model	$\overline{\Delta}$P	Proteinuria	Morphology	Reference
HHR	Remnant	NC*	NC	NC	52
	DOC-SALT	NC	NC	NC	53
	UNX SHR	↓	↓	IMP*	59,60
	UNX NSN	↓	↓	IMP	31
Enalapril	Remnant	↓	↓	IMP	10,52
	UNX SHR	↓	↓	IMP	60
	Diabetes	↓	↓	IMP	24
Captopril	UNX SHR	↓	↓	IMP	59
Nifedipine	Remnant	?	↓	IMP	76
	DOC-SALT	NC	↓	IMP	72
Verapamil	Remnant	? ↓	NC	IMP	41,71

*NC = no change; IMP = improved; see text for other abbeviations

Older Agents

Regimens combining vasodilators and a diuretic have long been mainstays of antihypertensive therapy. The effects of the administration of hydralazine, a thiazide diuretic (hydrochlorthiazide), and reserpine (HHR) on glomerular function and injury have been examined in a number of models of hypertension and renal disease. Purkerson et al.[51] administered this regimen to rats with remnant kidneys and found that it failed to provide complete protection from glomerular damage. Using the same model, Anderson et al.[52] subsequently demonstrated that HHR, so-called "triple therapy," induced a selective decline in afferent resistance, while efferent resistance remained unchanged. This resulted in the maintenance of glomerular hypertension, even though systemic blood pressure was completely normalized. Furthermore, the HHR combination failed to prevent proteinuria and glomerular damage. It was suggested that treatment with a diuretic and vasodilator activated the renin angiotensin system, which secondarily increased efferent resistance, tending to maintain $\overline{\Delta}$P at hypertensive levels.[52]

Similar results have been described in rats with DOC-SALT hypertension, where normalization of blood pressure with hydralazine, hydrochlorthiazide, and reserpine failed to protect against injury. Glomerular hypertension persisted in these animals due to a drug-induced decline in afferent resistance.[53] The individual agent responsible for the reduction in afferent resistance was not addressed in these studies; however, former work in the SHR model[54,55] indicates that, as single agents, thiazide diuretics have little antihypertensive activity. Hydralazine, on the other hand, has been shown to increase renal blood flow and decrease renal vascular resistance.[56] Regardless of the responsible agent, these studies confirm that, if therapy causes afferent resistance to decrease selectively, then a decline in systemic blood pressure may not be associated with a beneficial effect at the glomerular level.

Somewhat different effects of HHR have been described in SHR. Early studies showed that gross evidence of renal damage could be lessened by treatment with triple therapy.[57] Subsequently, Feld et al.[58] reported that life-span was prolonged by therapy, and that evidence of renal damage was delayed, albeit not prevented. Triple therapy is also effective in uninephrectomized SHR. Reports indicate that normalization of systemic blood pressure with this regimen results in a decline in $\overline{\Delta}$P and prevents injury.[59] The explanation for the different effects of HHR in various models of hypertension and reduced renal mass is uncertain, but may result from interstudy differences in drug dose. Baseline pre- and postglomerular resistances also vary greatly among the models, being significantly greater in intact or UNX SHR[17] than in remnant[8] or DOC-SALT[13] rats.

Therapy with traditional agents has also been beneficial in immunologic models of renal disease. In a model of severe nephrotoxic serum nephritis with hypertension, proteinuria and histologic damage were reduced when blood pressure was normalized with triple therapy. Micropuncture confirmed that $\overline{\Delta P}$ was lowered by this therapy. It should be noted that, in this study, SNGFR and Q_A also declined in rats given HHR, suggesting that afferent resistance was already maximally reduced prior to drug administration. In that setting, $\overline{\Delta P}$ would be predicted to decline in proportion to the fall in systemic pressure.[31]

In SHR with Heymann nephritis, a model of membranous glomerulonephritis, proteinuria and vascular lesions were lessened by treatment with hydralazine and guanethidine.[61] While micropuncture was not done, it is reasonable to infer that, in the setting of the elevated afferent resistance of the SHR, normalization of systemic blood pressure resulted in a lowering of $\overline{\Delta P}$.

Angiotensin-converting Enzyme Inhibitors

It has been suggested [62] that the efferent arteriole is more responsive than the afferent to the vasoconstrictor effects of angiotensin II (ANG II). If so, then agents that block the conversion of ANG I to ANG II might selectively dilate the postglomerular circulation and, therefore, reduce glomerular pressure. Such an effect might depend on the level of activity of the renin-angiotensin system prior to drug therapy. For example, in the DOC-SALT model, which is characterized by volume expansion and extremely low levels for plasma renin activity,[63] converting-enzyme inhibitor (CEI) with captopril fails to reduce systemic pressure or to lessen proteinuric evidence of glomerular injury (unpublished observations).

Rats with remnant kidneys display some degree of volume expansion, and renin levels are typically not abnormally elevated.[52] Nevertheless, in the remnant model, enalapril therapy initiated soon after ablation prevented the rise in systemic and glomerular pressure usually associated with loss of renal tissue. Protein excretion failed to rise during the experimental period and glomerular sclerosis was markedly decreased in the treated group.[64] In subsequent studies, in which enalapril therapy was begun after the appearance of proteinuria and hypertension, hypertension was still controlled, proteinuria stabilized, and progressive renal damage prevented.[10]

The renal effects of CEIs have also been studied in the SHR. In intact animals, CEI is as effective as conventional therapy in preventing renal damage.[65] In the uninephrectomized SHR, both captopril and enalapril prevent systemic and glomerular hypertension and lessen injury.[59] Of note, abnormalities of vascular smooth muscle were observed in small renal cortical arteries and arterioles of SHR on CEI.[59] To date, etiology or significance of these vascular lesions has not been clarified.

Rats with experimental diabetes develop glomerular hypertension and hyperfiltration, which precede and predict the appearance of proteinuria and diabetic glomerular sclerosis, despite the absence of systemic hypertension. Zatz et al.[66] administered enalapril to diabetic rats with moderate hyperglycemia in an attempt to prevent these deleterious alterations. Therapy was begun soon after the induction of diabetes and resulted in modest reductions in systemic blood pressure in the treated group. Although hyperfiltration persisted, micropuncture studies showed that glomerular capillary hypertension was prevented. After 14 months of diabetes, heavy protein-uria and glomerular lesions were present in the untreated group, while enalapril prevented both. This study supports the importance of hemodynamic factors in the development of diabetic nephropathy and suggests that CEI, even in the absence of systemic hypertension, may reverse glomerular hypertension and prevent progressive glomerular disease.

Calcium Antagonists

Calcium antagonists lower blood pressure by interfering with calcium-mediated smooth muscle contraction.[67] In general, reduction in blood pressure does not result in activation of the renin-angiotensin system.[68] To date, there have been relatively few studies of the effects of theses agents on glomerular structure and function in models of glomerular disease. In intact normotensive rats, verapamil has little effect on systemic blood pressure or on glomerular hemodynamics. However, it antagonizes the effects of exogenously administered ANG II to increase systemic and glomerular capillary pressure.[69]

Anderson et al.[70] examined the acute effects of calcium channel blockade on glomerular hemodynamics in rats with remnant kidneys. Four weeks after subto-tal ablation, infusion of diltiazem or verapamil normalized blood pressure, lowered $\overline{\Delta P}$, and reduced SNGFR. In a long-term study, chronic administration of verapamil failed to lower systemic blood pressure or lessen proteinuria in remnant kidney rats. Nevertheless, renal function, as measured by inulin clearance, was preserved, and there was less morphologic evidence of glomerular damage.[41] In this study, the protective effect of verapamil was attributed to a reduction in cell injury resulting from a decline in the uptake of calcium by the kidney. However, because the determinants of glomerular filtration were not measured, the role of hemodynamic factors could not be assessed.

Subsequently, Pelayo et al.[71] examined the glomerular hemodynamic effects of chronic administration of a similar, subantihypertensive dose of verapamil in rats with remnant kidneys. Verapamil administration failed to alter either systemic or intrarenal vascular resistance; however, $\overline{\Delta P}$ declined secondary to a drug-associated increase in tubular pressure. The authors concluded that the protective effect of verapamil might relate to this reduction in transcapillary hydraulic pressure. However, the study is difficult to interpret for several reasons. First, the verapamil administered in this fashion was not associated with reduction in either proteinuria or morphologic evidence of glomerular injury, so that the relationship of the observed decline in $\overline{\Delta P}$ to protection was undefined. Second, the reason for the elevated tubular pressure in verapamil-treated rats was entirely unexplained and not attributable to alterations in either glomerular or tubular structure or function. Finally, it should be noted that in every instance in which reduction in $\overline{\Delta P}$ has been associated with protection from glomerular damage, $\overline{\Delta P}$ has declined secondary to a fall in glomerular capillary pressure. That a reduction in $\overline{\Delta P}$ resulting from a rise in tubular pressure may lessen glomerular damage has not been demonstrated.

In a recent preliminary report, Dworkin et al.[72] described the glomerular effects of chronic administration of nifedipine to DOC-SALT rats. The calcium antagonist was administered in a dose sufficient to normalize systemic blood pressure. Nevertheless, micropuncture studies revealed that glomerular dynamics were not different in treated and untreated rats, so that SNGFR, Q_A and $\overline{\Delta P}$ remained elevated despite nifedipine. Persistence of glomerular capillary hypertension resulted from a drug-induced reduction in afferent resistance that offset the decline in arterial pressure. Of note, selective, nifedipine-induced afferent arteriolar vasodilation has also been described in in vitro perfused kidneys,[73] and in the blood-perfused hydronephrotic kidney.[74] Importantly, despite persistent intrarenal hypertension, Dworkin et al. found that proteinuria was reduced and glomerular lesions prevented in nifedipine-treated rats.[72] This finding is similar to that of Nickerson,[75] who treated DOC-SALT rats with the structurally related calcium-entry blocker nitrendipine. Although the drug was administered in a dose not associated with a reduction in systemic blood pressure, glomerular injury was reduced in the nitrendipine group. Thus calcium antagonists appear to lessen glomerular injury in models characterized by glomerular capillary hypertension; however, protection does not depend upon an effect of these drugs to decrease glomerular pressure.

One possible explanation for the protective effect of calcium antagonists was advanced by Dworkin and coworkers[76] based upon preliminary studies in which nifedipine was administered to rats after 1 2/3 nephrectomy. Nifedipine not only reduced proteinuria and glomerular sclerosis, but also blocked the hypertrophic response to ablation of renal mass. Thus, kidney weight, glomerular volume, and glomerular capillary radius were all significantly lower in nifedipine-treated rats than in controls or animals treated with enalapril. It was suggested that increased capillary wall tension—due to elevation in glomerular capillary pressure and/or increased glomerular capillary radius—was a key shared mechanism of progressive glomerular sclerosis in this model. Nifedipine, by virtue of its ability to prevent capillary radius from increasing, induced a structurally mediated decline in wall tension similar in magnitude to that produced by agents such as enalapril, which lower tension by reducing glomerular pressure. Of note, there is other experimental evidence to suggest that changes in cytosolic calcium activity may be involved in the regulation of kidney growth.[77] Additionally, administration of verapamil has previously been shown to attenuate the compensatory hypertrophy that follows nephrectomy.[78]

Effects of Antihypertensive Therapy on Progressive Renal Damage in Man

In patients with severe hypertension, pharmacologic reduction in blood pressure preserves kidney function and prolongs life.[79] Control of systemic blood pressure is also felt to be crucial in the management of patients with milder forms of hypertension and renal disease; however, conclusive evidence of a beneficial effect on renal survival in this population has not been provided. Efforts have been hampered by the diversity of renal diseases, difficulty in precisely measuring rates of decline in renal function in patients, and the protracted course many individuals follow from initial diagnosis to end-stage renal failure. Nevertheless, uncontrolled studies suggest that antihypertensive therapy can reduce the rate at which filtration capacity declines.[80]

The most compelling data relating treatment of systemic hypertension to preservation of renal function has come from studies in which antihypertensive agents were administered to patients with diabetic nephropathy. In one series, combination therapy with a beta blocker, vasodilator, and diuretic halved the rate of decline in GFR in patients followed for a 6-year period.[81] In another group of patients treated with a similar combination of drugs for two years, proteinuria was reduced and GFR maintained at baseline levels.[82]

Short- and long-term benefits of antihypertensive therapy have also been reported in hypertensive diabetics treated with angiotensin converting enzyme (ACE) inhibitors. Thus, in patients with overt nephropathy, proteinuria was significantly reduced during 8 weeks of therapy with captopril, at a dose not associated with a reduction in systemic blood pressure.[83] More recently, Bjorck et al.[84] reported on the effects of chronic administration of captopril to patients with diabetic nephropathy, hypertension and kidney failure. Although blood pressure control had been adequate and was not improved by the substitution or addition of captopril, the rate of decline in GFR slowed, from 10.3 to 5.5 cc/yr. Acutely, GFR was unchanged, but renal blood flow increased and filtration fraction declined in these patients. This pattern of perfusion would be observed if captopril selectively decreased efferent arteriolar resistance in these patients. As discussed above, selective efferent vasodilation and resultant reduction in $\overline{\Delta P}$ has been observed in experimental animals treated with CEI.[63] It is attractive to speculate that preservation of filtration function in these captopril-treated diabetic patients resulted from a drug-induced amelioration in glomerular capillary hypertension.

Summary

Our ability to measure the pressures and flows precisely within the glomerular microcirculation has enabled us to begin to unravel the complex relationship between systemic hypertension and kidney disease. Although a number of factors have been implicated in the development of glomerular sclerosis, one consistent finding has been that glomerular injury occurs when elevated pressures are transmitted to the glomerular capillaries. Our current understanding of the relationship between glomerular capillary hypertension, other concomitants of renal functional impairment, and progressive kidney damage is outlined in Figure 7. Reductions in functioning renal tissue, whether the result of surgical ablation of renal tissue or a primary renal disease, are often associated with both systemic hypertension and a decline in preglomerular resistance, a hemodynamic pattern that caused glomerular pressure to rise. Intrarenal hypertension, in conjunction with renal hypertrophy, and, possibly, disturbances of lipid metabolism and blood coagulation, constitute a secondary process by virtue of which those nephrons not severely injured by the primary renal disease are eventually destroyed. Thus, a vicious cycle is set in motion, in which additional nephrons are damaged and, ultimately, all renal function is lost.

The pathophysiologic sequence outlined above is most likely to contribute to progressive glomerular injury in those patients in whom hypertension and mild-to-moderate renal insufficiency coexist. In contrast, by analogy to the intact SHR, afferent vasoconstriction probably protects the glomeruli in most patients with essential hypertension from increased perfusion pressure. Clinically important renal disease is

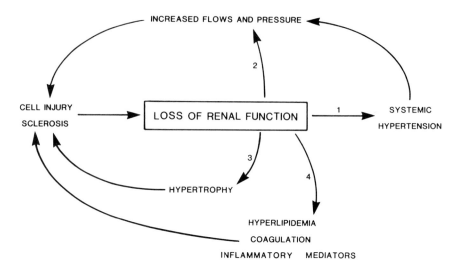

FIGURE 7. As renal function is lost, either by surgical ablation or primary renal disease, systemic and glomerular hypertension and renal hypertrophy develop. Other consequences of renal dysfunction include activation of the coagulation cascade, elevations in blood lipids, and the generation of inflammatory mediators. The cumulative effect is ongoing tissue injury, thus leading to further reduction in renal function and the perpetuation of a vicious cycle that ultimately results in renal failure. Interruption of this process may occur at several points, indicated by numbers (1–4). Traditional antihypertensives (1) act to lower systemic blood pressure. CEI directly lower both systemic (1) and glomerular (2) pressures. Calcium antagonists lower systemic blood pressure (1) and also may inhibit hypertrophy directly (3). Protein restriction lowers glomerular pressures and flows (2) and limits hypertrophy (3). Clofibrate, anticoagulants and thromboxane synthetase inhibitors prevent hyperlipidemia, thrombosis, and inflammation (4).

uncommon in this population. It seems likely that in some patients with diabetes, as yet unidentified factor(s) cause afferent resistance to decrease to the extent that glomerular capillary hypertension develops in the absence of elevation in systemic blood pressures. These patients are at risk to develop overt nephropathy. Finally, although no therapy has been proven to slow the rate of progression to end-stage renal failure in man, studies in experimental models of renal disease have identified a number of extremely promising interventions. These include dietary manipulations, such as protein or salt restriction, and medication, with either converting enzyme inhibitors or calcium antagonists. Widespread application of these therapies to patients with renal disease should await the results of careful clinical trials.

Acknowledgments. During the preparation of this manuscript, Dr. Dworkin was supported by grant DK38157 from the National Institutes of Health as well as grants from the Evans Foundation, the Irma T. Hirschl Memorial Trust, and Pfizer, Inc.

References

1. Mitch WE, Walser M, Buffington GA, Leman J: A simple method for estimating progression of chronic renal failure. Lancet ii:1326–1328, 1976.
2. Addis T: Glomerular Nephritis. Diagnosis and Treatment. New York, Macmillan 1948, p 3.

3. Brenner BM, Dworkin LD, Ichikawa I: Glomerular ultrafiltration. In Brenner BM, Rector FC (ed): The Kidney. Philadelphia, W. B. Saunders, 1986, pp 124–144.

4. Chanutin A, Ferris EB: Experimental renal insufficiency produced by partial nephrectomy in control diet. Arch Intern Med 49:767–787, 1932.

5. Shimamura T, Morrison AB: A progressive glomerulosclerosis occurring in partial five-sixths nephrectomized rats. Am J Path 79:95–106, 1975.

6. Hayslett JP: Functional adaptation to reduction in renal mass. Physiol Rev 59:137-164, 1979.

7. Deen WM, Maddox DA, Robertson CR, Brenner BM: Dynamics of glomerular ultrafiltration in the rat. VII: Response to reduced renal mass. Am J Physiol 223:1184–1190, 1971.

8. Hostetter TH, Olson JL, Rennke HG, Venkatachalam MA, Brenner BM: Hyperfiltration in remnant nephrons: A potentially adverse response to renal ablation. Am J Physiol 241:F85–F93, 1981.

9. Nath KA, Kren SM, Hostetter TH: Dietary protein restriction in established renal injury in the rat: Selective role of glomerular capillary pressure in progressive glomerular dysfunction. J Clin Invest 78:1199–1205, 1986.

10. Meyer TW, Anderson S, Rennke HG, Brenner BM: Reversing glomerular hypertension stabilizes established glomerular injury. Kidney Int 31:751–759, 1987.

11. Gavras H, Brunner HR, Laragh JH, et al: Malignant hypertension resulting from desoxycorticosterone acetate and salt excess. Cir Res 36:300–309, 1975.

12. Hill GS, Heptinstall RH: Steroid induced hypertension in the rat. Am J Path 52:1–20, 1968.

13. Dworkin LD, Hostetter TH, Rennke HG, Brenner BM: Hemodynamic basis for glomerular injury in rats with desoxycorticosterone salt hypertension. J Clin Invest 73:1448–1461, 1984.

14. Feld LG, VanLiew JB, Galeske RG, Boyland JW: Selectivity of renal injury and proteinuria in the spontaneously hypertensive rat. Kidney Int 12:332–343, 1977.

15. Arendshorst WJ, Beierwaltes WH: Renal and nephron hemodynamics in spontaneously hypertensive rats. Am J Physiol 236:F246–F259, 1979.

16. Bank N, Alterman N, Aynedjian HS: Selective deep nephron hyperfiltration in uninephrectomized spontaneously hypertensive rats. Kidney Int 24:191–195, 1983.

17. Dworkin LD, Feiner HD: Glomerular injury in uninephrectomized spontaneously hypertensive rats. A consequence of glomerular capillary hypertension. J Clin Invest 77:797–809, 1986.

18. Zatz R, Brenner BM: Pathogenesis of diabetic microangiopathy: The hemodynamic view. Am J Med 80:443–453, 1986.

19. Mogensen CE: Kidney function and glomerular permeability to macromolecules in early juvenile diabetes. Scand J Clin Lab Invest 28:91–100, 1971.

20. Christensen JS, Gammelgard J, Frandsen M, Parving HH: Increased kidney size, glomerular filtration rate and renal plasma flow in short term insulin dependent diabetics. Diabetologia 20:451–456, 1981.

21. Hostetter TH, Rennke HG, Brenner BM: The case for intrarenal hypertension in the initiation and progression of diabetic and other glomerulopathies. Am J Med 72:375–380, 1980.

22. Mogensen CE, Christensen CK: Predicting diabetic nephropathy in insulin dependent patients. N Engl J Med 311:89–93, 1984.

23. Berkman J, Rifkin H: Unilateral nodular glomerulosclerosis. Metabolism 22:715–722, 1973.

24. Steffes MW, Brown DM, Mauer SM: Diabetic glomerulopathy following unilateral nephrectomy in the rat. Diabetes 27:35–41, 1978.

25. Hostetter TH, Troy JL, Brenner BM: Glomerular hemodynamics in experimental diabetes mellitus. Kidney Int 19:410–415, 1981.

26. Zatz R, Meyer TW, Rennke HG, Brenner BM: Predominance of hemodynamic rather than metabolic factors in the pathogenesis of diabetic glomerulopathy. Proc Nat Acad Sci 82:5963–5967, 1985.

27. Smadel JE, Far LE: Effect of diet on the pathologic changes in rats with nephrotoxic serum nephritis. Am J Path 15:199, 1939.

28. Allison MEM, Wilson CB, Gottschalk CW: Pathophysiology of experimental glomerulonephritis in rats. J Clin Invest 53:1402–1423, 1974.

29. Neugarten J, Feiner H, Schacht RG, Baldwin DS: Amelioration of experimental glomerulonephritis by dietary protein restriction. Kidney Int 24:595–601, 1983.

30. Friend PS, Fernandes G, Good RA, Michael AF, Yunis EJ: Dietary restrictions early and late: effects on nephropathy in NZB X NZW mouse. Lab Invest 38:629–632, 1978.

31. Neugarten J, Kaminetsky B, Feiner H, Schacht RG, Liu DT, Baldwin DS: Nephrotoxic serum nephritis with hypertension: amelioration by antihypertensive therapy. Kidney Int 28:135–139, 1985.

32. Raij L, Azar S, Keane WF: Role of hypertension in immune injury. Hypertension 7:398–404, 1985.

33. Klahr S, Schreiner G, Ichikawa I: The progression of renal disease. N Eng J Med 318:1657–1666, 1988.

34. Klahr S, Heifets M, Purkerson M: The influence of anticoagulation on the progression of renal disease. In Mitch WE, Brenner BM, Stein JH (eds): The Progressive Nature of Renal Disease. New York, Churchill Livingstone, 1986, pp 45–64.

35. Kincaid-Smith P:Coagulation and renal disease, Kidney Int 2:183–190, 1972.

36. Purkerson ML, Joist JH, Yates J, Valdes A, Morrison A, Klahr S: Inhibition of thromboxane synthesis ameliorates the progressive kidney disease of rats with subtotal renal ablation. Proc Nat Acad Sci 82:193–197, 1985.

37. Purkerson ML, Hoffsten PE, Klahr S: Pathogenesis of the glomerulopathy associated with renal infarction in rats. Kidney Int 9:407–417, 1976.

38. Giminez L, Walker WG, Tew WP, Hermann JA: Prevention of phosphate induced progression of uremia in rats by 3-phosphocitric acid. Kidney Int 22:35–41, 1982.

39. Ibels LS, Alfred AC, Haut L, Huffer WE: Preservation of function in experimental renal disease by dietary restriction of phosphate. N Eng J Med 298:122–126, 1978.

40. Lumlertgul D, Burke TJ, Gillum DM, et al.: Phosphate depletion arrests progression of chronic renal failure independent of protein intake. Kidney Int 29:658–666, 1986.

41. Harris DH, Hammond WS, Burke TJ, Schreier RW: Verapamil protects against progression of experimental chronic renal failure. Kidney Int 31:41–46, 1987.

42. Benstein JA, Parker M, Feiner HD, Dworkin LD: Dietary sodium restriction lessens renal hypertrophy and injury without reducing systemic or intrarenal pressure in rats with spontaneous hypertension. Clin Res 36:513A, 1988.

43. Daniels BS, Hostetter TH: Influence of dietary salt on chronic renal injury (abstract). Kidney Int 29:244, 1986.

44. Yoshida Y, Fogo A, Ichikawa I: Glomerular hemodynamic changes vs. hypertrophy in experimental glomerulosclerosis. Kidney Int 35:654–660, 1989.

45. Olivetti G, Anversa P, Rigamonti W, Vitali-Mazza L, Loud AV: Morphometry of the renal corpuscle during normal postnatal growth and compensatory hypertrophy. J Cell Biol 75:573–585, 1977.

46. Moorhead JF, Chan MK, Varghese Z: The role of abnormalities of lipid metabolism in the progression of renal disease. In Mitch WE, Brenner BM, Stein JH (eds): The Progressive Nature of Renal Disease. New York, Churchill Livingstone, 1986, pp 133–148.

47. Keane WF, Kasiske BL, O'Donnell MP: Hyperlipidemia and the progression of renal disease. Am J Clin Nutr 47:157–160, 1988.

48. Nath KA, Hostetter MK, Hostetter TH: Pathophysiology of chronic tubulointerstitial disease in rats. J Clin Invest 76:667–675, 1985.

49. Jamison R: Dietary protein, glomerular hyperemia and progressive renal failure. Ann Intern Med 99:849–851, 1983.

50. Raij L, Chiou XC, Owens R, Wrigley: Therapeutic implications of hypertension induced glomerular injury. Am J Med 79(3C)37–41, 1985.

51. Purkerson ML, Hoffsten PE, Klahr S: Pathogenesis of the glomerulopathy associated with renal infarction in rats. Kidney Int 9:407–417, 1976.

52. Anderson S, Rennke HG, Brenner BM: Therapeutic advantage of converting enzyme inhibitors in arresting progressive renal disease associated with systemic hypertension in the rat. J Clin Invest 77:1993–2000, 1986.

53. Dworkin LD, Feiner HD, Randazza J: Glomerular hypertension and injury in desoxy-corticosterone-salt rats on antihypertensive therapy. Kidney Int 31:718–724, 1987.

54. Fries ED, Ragan DO: Relative effectiveness of chlorothiazide reserpine and hydralazine in spontaneously hypertensive rats. Clin Sci Mol Med 51:6355–6375, 1976.

55. Manhemp JO, Clark SA, Brown WB, Murray GD, Robertson JS: Effect of chlorothiazide on serial measurements of exchangeable sodium and blood pressure in spontaneously hypertensive rats. Clin Sci 69:511–515, 1985.

56. Wallen JD: Antihypertensives and their impact on renal function. Am J Med 75(4A):103–108, 1983.

57. Freis E, Ragan D, Pillsbury H, Matthews M: Alteration of the course of hypertension in the spontaneously hypertensive rat. Circ Res 31:1–7, 1972.

58. Feld LG, Van Liew JB, Brentjens JR, Boyland JW: Renal lesions and proteinuria in the spontaneously hypertensive rat made normotensive by treatment. Kidney Int 20:606–614, 1981.

59. Dworkin LD, Grosser M, Ferner HD, Parker M: Renal vascular effects of antihypertensive therapy in uninephrectomized SHR. Kidney Int 35:790-798, 1989.

61. Okuda S, Onoyamo K, Fujimi S, Oh Y, Nomoto K, Omae T: Influence of hypertension on the progression of experimental autologous immune complex nephritis. J Lab Clin Med 101:461–471, 1983.

62. Edwards, RM: Segmental effects of norepinephrine and angiotensin II on isolated renal microvessels. Am J Physiol 244:F526–534, 1983.

63. Gavras H, Brunner HR, Laragh JH, et al.: Malignant hypertension resulting from desoxycorticosterone acetate and salt excess. Circ Res 36:300–309, 1975.

64. Anderson S, Meyer TW, Rennke HG, Brenner BM: Control of glomerular hypertension limits glomerular injury in rats with reduced renal mass. J Clin Invest 76:612–619, 1985.

65. Feld LG, Springate JE, Van Liew JB: Influence of enalapril on proteinuria in spontaneously hypertensive rats (abstract). Kidney Int 33:295, 1988.

66. Zatz R, Dunn BR, Meyer TW, Anderson S, Rennke HG, Brenner BM: Prevention of diabetic glomerulopathy by pharmacologic amelioration of glomerular capillary hypertension. J Clin Invest 77:1925–1930, 1986.

67. Loutzenhiser R, Epstein M: Effects of calcium antagonists on renal hemodynamics: Am J Physiol 249:F619–629, 1985.

68. Kaplan NM: Clinical Hypertension Baltimore, Williams and Wilkins, 1986, pp 180–272.

69. Ichikawa I, Miele JF, Brenner BM: Reversal of renal cortical actions of angiotensin II by verapamil and manganese. Kidney Int 16:137–147, 1979.

70. Anderson S, Clarey LE, Riley SL, Troy JL: Acute infusion of calcium channel blockers reduces glomerular capillary pressure in rats with reduced renal mass (abstract). Kidney Int 33:370, 1988.

71. Pelayo JC, Harris DCH, Shanley PF, Miller GJ, Schrier RW: Glomerular hemodynamic adaptations in remnant nephrons: effects of verapamil. Am J Physiol 254:F421–425, 1988.

72. Dworkin LD, Benstein JA, Feiner HD, Parker M: Nifedipine prevents glomerular injury without reducing glomerular pressure in rats with desoxycorticosterone-salt hypertension (abstract). Kidney Int 33:374, 1988.

73. Epstein M, Hayashi K, Loutzenhiser R: Nifedipine prevents pressure-induced afferent arteriolar vasoconstriction in isolated perfused hydronephrotic kidneys from hypertensive rats (abstract). Kidney Int 35:427, 1989.

74. Fleming JT, Parekh N, Steinhausen M: Calcium antagonists preferentially dilate pre-glomerular vessels of hydronephrotic kidney. Am J Physiol 253:F1157–1163, 1987.

75. Nickerson PA: A low dose of a calcium antagonist (nitrendipine) ameliorates cardiac and renal lesions induced by DOC in the rat. Exp Mol Path 41:309–320, 1984.

76. Dworkin LD, Parker M, Feiner HD: Nifedipine decreases glomerular injury in rats with remnant kidneys by inhibiting glomerular hypertrophy (abstract). Kidney Int 35:427, 1989.

77. Jobin J, Taylor CM, Caverzasio J, Bonjour JP: Calcium restriction and parathyroid hormone enhance renal compensatory growth. Am J Physiol 246:F685–690, 1984.

78. Jobin JR, Bonjour JP: Compensatory renal growth: modulation by calcium PTH and 1,25-$(OH)_2D_3$ Kidney Int 29:1124–1130, 1986.

79. Mohler ER, Fries ED: Five year survival with malignant hypertension treated with antihypertensive agents. Am Heart J 60:329–335, 1960.

80. Baldwin DS, Neugarten J:Blood pressure control and progression of renal insufficiency. In Mitch WE, Brenner BM, Stein JH (eds): The Progressive Nature of Renal Disease, New York, Churchill Livingstone, 1986, pp 81–110.

81. Mogenson CE: Long-term antihypertensive therapy inhibits progression of diabetic nephropathy. Acta Endocrin S242:31–35, 1981.

82. Parving HH, Andersen AR, Smidt UM, Christensen JS, Oxenboll B, Svendsen PA: Diabetic nephropathy and arterial hypertension: the effect of antihypertensive treatment. Diabetes 32(S2)83–87, 1983.

83. Ishizaki M, Takagashi H, Sekino H, Sasaki Y: Effect of captopril on heavy proteinuria in azotemic diabetics. N Eng J Med 313:1617–1620, 1985.

84. Bjorck S, Nyberg G, Mulec H, Granerus G, Herlitz H, Aurell: Beneficial effects of angiotensin converting enzyme inhibition on renal function in patients with diabetic nephropathy. Br Med J 293:471–474, 1986.

Jules B. Puschett, M.D.

9

Calcium Antagonists and Renal Ischemia

The development of acute renal failure (ARF) in the setting of renal ischemia is a common occurrence in clinical medicine.[1,2] Because this disorder leads to significant morbidity and mortality,[3] strenuous efforts have been undertaken in the past several years to attempt to understand its pathophysiology. Furthermore, studies aimed at developing potential preventive and/or treatment methods have focused on the role of a number of agents in ameliorating both the vascular and metabolic consequences of renal ischemia. The calcium antagonists represent a class of drugs that has received much attention in this regard.[4-6] This review represents an attempt to provide a summary of the current status of the employment of calcium channel inhibitors in the amelioration of experimental ischemic renal failure. No effort will be made to discuss the potential use of these drugs in the other major etiology of ARF—toxic nephropathy. Finally, as with all review articles, it is entirely likely that data developed during the period of publication will provide additional insights into both the pathogenesis and treatment of this vexing clinical and biological problem, especially given the investigative activity in the field.

Pathophysiologic Considerations

Interruption of the blood supply to the kidney leads to a number of important consequences. Primary among these, of course, is the deprivation of the kidney tissue of oxygen and major metabolic substrates and enzymes. Second is the development of alterations in the integrity of the plasma membrane of the renal cell, with the result that potentially noxious substances such as calcium can enter the cytoplasm and, eventually, the mitochondria in toxic amounts.[7] This situation obtains because, in health, the cell membrane maintains the intracellular concentration of calcium at 1/1000th to 1/10,000th that of the extracellular fluid. Third are the problems associated with the re-establishment of blood flow to the ischemic organ. During this period, oxygen-derived free radicals (produced in the ischemic tissue) and calcium in supraphysiological amounts gain access to the cellular contents as part of the postischemic state, contributing to cellular damage.[7-11]

The calcium antagonists were initially employed in models of ischemic damage in an effort to limit or ameliorate the vasoconstriction that attends the hypoxic and ischemic event. Thus, investigations of the ability of this class of drugs to interfere with vascular smooth muscle contraction in the myocardium and in the peripheral vasculature were extended to the kidney.[12] In Figure 1 are presented data from one such representative study. The observations depicted verify the finding that calcium channel blockade reduces afferent arteriolar vasoconstriction due to norepinephrine, resulting in a return of glomerular filtration rate (GFR) toward control levels.[13] This determination is typical of the results obtained in a number of studies in which the effects of calcium channel blockade have been examined.[13-27] They support the thesis that an amelioration of the intensity of attendant vasoconstriction is at least one of the potential benefits of calcium channel antagonism in the setting of ischemia.

More recently, the effects of these agents on cellular metabolism have been examined in an effort to determine whether blockade of calcium uptake by the ischemic cell is an important factor in cell survival. It has been known for some time that "calcium overload" may occur in ischemic cells.[28] Because these phenomena are difficult to study in the whole animal, experiments have been performed in several cell culture systems. Snowdowne and his associates[29] have demonstrated that anoxia and substrate removal for 1 hour result in an increase in intracellular calcium levels by $2\frac{1}{2}$ times over control levels in cultured monkey kidney cells (Fig. 2). Other workers have suggested, however, that the major deleterious effects of increased cellular and mitochondrial calcium on metabolic processes occur in the postischemic period.[7,30] Wilson and his co-workers have found that tissue taken from

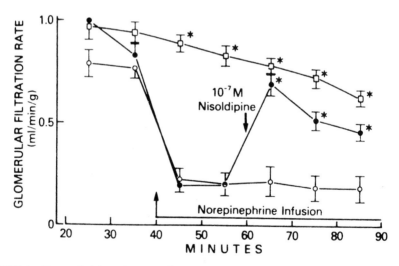

FIGURE 1. Reversal of the reduction in GFR due to vasoconstriction induced by norepinephrine, by the dihydropyridine calcium antagonist nisoldipine. Studies were performed in the isolated perfused kidney. The open squares represent time control observations; open circles = norepinephrine alone; closed circles = norepinephrine infusion followed by a single bolus of nisoldipine (10^{-7}M). Reproduced, with permission, from Loutzenhiser et al, J Pharmacol Exp Ther 232:382–387, 1985.

the kidneys of animals studied after 45 minutes of renal pedicle clamping revealed severely depressed mitochondrial respiration initially, which improved at 1 and 4 hours after reflow, but was again reduced at 24 hours.[31] Mitochondrial calcium content increased early after clamping and rose progressively during the 24-hour period after reflow was established.

That calcium is important in the survival of cells subjected to anoxia is verified by two additional studies. Thus, Wilson and Schrier examined cell survival following the exposure of various rabbit tubular segments to anoxia.[32] Regardless of the nephron segment studied, cell survival was consistently higher when the cells were allowed to recover from the anoxic event in calcium-free medium (Fig. 3). Furthermore, the calcium antagonists, verapamil and nifedipine, improved the survival of cells grown in primary culture in calcium-containing media that were subjected to anoxia.[33] Observations obtained in this system with verapamil are provided in Figure 4. Because of the in vitro methodology employed in the studies just described, the effects of the calcium antagonists could not have been related, of course, to any influence on tissue perfusion. Because there has been no demonstration, thus far, of potential-dependent calcium channels in tubular epithelial cells, the observations reported by Schwertschlag et al. constitute only indirect evidence of their presence.[33]

Therefore, calcium antagonists appear to have (at least) two separate effects on the survival of ischemic tissue: (1) an amelioration of vasoconstriction, and (2) a beneficial effect on cellular (especially, mitochondrial) metabolism, most likely related to a reduction in or the prevention of cellular calcium entry and alterations in calcium release from mitochondria into the cytosol.

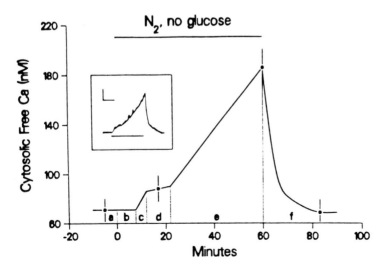

FIGURE 2. Study of the effects of the removal of glucose in the medium and the institution of anoxia (at time zero) on cytosolic calcium in cultured LLC-MK2 cells. Intracellular calcium rose modestly within 20 min, then more steeply, peaking at 60 min. The value then returned to baseline as normal conditions were restored. Reproduced from Snowdowne et al, J Biol Chem 260:11619–11626, 1985, with permission.

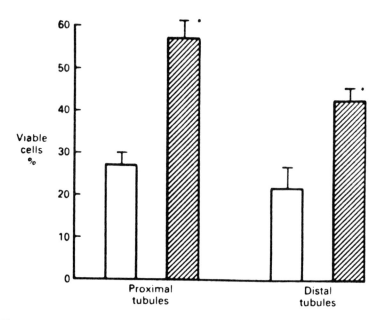

FIGURE 3. Viability of proximal and distal tubular cells in primary culture to the effects of the restoration of oxygen in the atmosphere for 2 hours following 45 minutes of anoxia. Open bars represent media containing calcium and hatched bars media from which calcium had been removed. Reproduced, with permission, from PD Wilson, RW Schrier, Kidney Int 29:1171–1179, 1986.

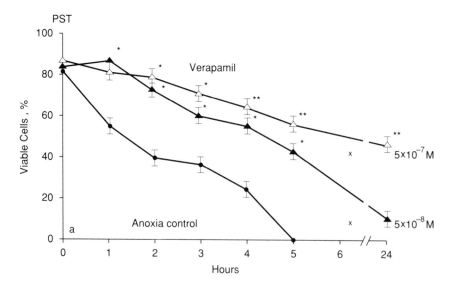

FIGURE 4. Survival of cultured proximal straight tubules subjected to 45 minutes of anoxia with and without the addition of verapamil (5×10^{-7}M, top line; 5×10^{-8}M, middle line) to calcium-containing medium, compared to control observations (bottom curve). Reproduced from Schwertschlag et al, J Pharmacol Exp Ther 238:119–124, 1986.

TABLE 1.   Effects of Verapamil on Experimental Acute Renal Failure Scondary to Renal Ischemia.*

Agent	Experimental Model/Setting	Timing of Administration	Ameliorated/ Prevented Renal Failure	Study
Verapamil	NE* infusion into the renal artery of the rat	Pre-infusion	Yes	Malis et al.[15]
Verapamil	NE infusion into the renal artery of the rat	Post-infusion	No	Malis et al.[15]
Verapamil	NE infusion into the renal artery of the dog	Pre-infusion	Yes	Burke et al.[14]
Verapamil	NE infusion into the renal artery of the dog	Post-infusion	Yes	Burke et al.[14]
Verapamil	NE infusion into rat isolated perfused kidney	Pre-infusion	Yes	Malis et al.[15]
Verapamil	Renal artery clamp in the rat	Pre-clamp	Yes	Goldfarb et al.[18]
Verapamil	Renal artery clamp in the rat	Post-clamp	No	Goldfarb et al.[18]
Verapamil	Renal pedicle clamp in the rat	Pre-clamp	No	Malis et al.[15]
Verapamil	Renal pedicle clamp in the rat	Post-clamp	No	Malis et al.[15]
Verapamil	Renal pedicle clamp in rat isolated perfused kidney	Pre-clamp	No	Malis et al.[15]
Verapamil	Renal pedicle clamp in rat isolated perfused kidney	Post-clamp	No	Malis et al.[15]
Verapamil	Renal pedicle clamp in the dog	Pre-clamp	Yes	Papadimitriou et al.[20]
Verapamil	Renal artery clamp in the dog	Pre-clamp	Yes	Wait et al.[24]
Verapamil	Renal artery clamp in the dog	Immediately Post-clamp	Yes	Wait et al.[24]
Verapamil	Renal artery clamp in the sheep	Pre-clamp	Yes	Woolley et al.[27]
Verapamil	Warm ischemia in isolated perfused rat kidney	Pre-ischemia	Yes	Shapiro et al.[25]
Verapamil	Cold ischemia in isolated perfused rat kidney	Post-ischemia	Yes	Shapiro et al.[25]
Verapamil	Intra-arterial administration of verapamil in the dog prior to nephrectomy, cold ischemia, and autotransplantation	Pre-clamp	Yes	Agatstein et al.[21]

*NE = norepinephrine

Experimental Observations

Investigations of the actions of calcium antagonists in renal ischemia have largely been performed in the experimental animal, whereas only a few studies have been reported in human subjects. In the animal, two models have been employed: (1) interruption of blood flow to the kidney by means of occlusion of the renal artery alone or of the entire renal pedicle, and (2) infusion of vasoconstrictors (especially norepinephrine), usually into the renal artery.

Animal Studies

Tables 1 and 2 summarize the results of those experiments in which the actions of either verapamil (Table 1) or one of the other calcium antagonists (diltiazem, nifedipine, nisoldipine or nitrendipine) (Table 2) have been examined. As is clear from these reports, there is no unanimity of opinion as regards two points: (1) are these agents helpful in averting or minimizing the development of renal failure due to ischemic injury, and (2) if they can be shown to have a protective effect, is it the case that the drug must be given prior to, rather than following, the ischemic event?

With respect to the first of these observations, although there are exceptions, the data strongly argue the view that the calcium antagonists favorably influence renal function in the setting of acute ischemia. This is especially true for verapamil, the most extensively studied drug (Table 1), especially when administration of the drug preceded the experimentally induced ischemia. The single major exception to this otherwise uniform finding is the experimental study reported by Malis and his co-workers.[15] In their experiments, the method by which renal ischemia was produced appears to have been of critical importance. Thus, pretreatment with verapamil successfully mitigated the fall in inulin clearance by 50% in animals subjected to a norepinephrine infusion, whereas the drug had no effect in clamp models, whether given before or after the latter maneuver.[15]

In reference to the second question, as to whether the timing of administration of these agents is crucial, the data are less clear. In roughly an equal number of investigations, verapamil was or was not effective in reducing the incidence or mitigating the severity of ARF when given *after* the renal blood supply had been interrupted (Table 1). As regards the dihydropyridine calcium antagonists and diltiazem (Table 2), their effectiveness appears to depend, in part, on the experimental model. They generally improved GFR when given during a norepinephrine infusion.[13,14,16] However, studies performed in a clamp model in this laboratory demonstrated that protection was provided by nitrendipine only when pretreatment was performed.[19]

TABLE 2. Effects of Calcium Antagonists on Experimental Acute Renal Failure Scondary to Renal Ischemia.

Agent	Experimental Model/Setting	Timing of Administration	Ameliorated/ Prevented Renal Failure	Study
Nifedipine	NE infusion into the renal artery of the dog	Post-infusion	Yes	Burke et al.[14]
Diltiazem	NE infusion into rat isolated perfused kidney	Post-infusion	Yes	Loutzenhiser et al.[16]
Nisoldipine	NE infusion into rat isolated perfused kidney	Post-infusion	Yes	Loutzenhiser et al.[13]
Nitrendipene	Renal pedicle clamp in the rat	Pre-clamp	Yes	Rose et al.[19]
Nitrendipene	Renal pedicle clamp in the rat	Post-clamp	No	Rose et al.[19]

Therefore, the preponderant evidence suggests that calcium channel antagonism is a successful stratagem for ameliorating or preventing ischemic injury to the kidney. Verapamil, the most widely studied agent, appears to be especially effective in this

TABLE 3. Effects of Calcium Antagonists on Clinical Acute
Renal Failure Scondary to Renal Ischemia.

Agent	Clinical Setting	Timing of Administration	Ameliorated/ Prevented Renal Failure	Study
Verapamil	Cadaveric renal transplantation	Infusion of 20 mg verapamil into donor prior to nephrectomy vs. no drug in control subjects	Urine output greater and serum creatinine lower on day 1 in treated group; but no difference on day 7	Duggan et al.[26]
Diltiazem	Cadaveric renal transplantation	Drug was added to Eurocollins solution and recipient received a bolus injection, followed by a 48 hour infusion, then daily oral diltiazem	Controls had higher ATN rate (41%) than treated group (10%)	Wagner et al.[23]

regard. Furthermore, it seems likely that vasoconstrictor infusion and renal artery occlusion are not entirely equivalent models for the production of the ischemic lesion and may have influenced the results obtained, especially as regards the timing of administration of this class of agents. Indeed, there may be additional currently unidentified reasons for the lack of more complete uniformity in the results presented in Tables 1 and 2.

Human Studies

The efficacy of calcium channel blockade in ischemic states in the human subject has thus far been examined in only a limited number of studies (Table 3). Duggan et al. have investigated the effect of 20 mg of verapamil injected intravenously just prior to nephrectomy in 10 kidney donors, compared to 10 controls, randomly selected.[24] They found that urine output was significantly higher and serum creatinine was lower in the treated group at 24 hours post-transplant. However, these differences disappeared at day 7. Furthermore, dialysis requirements for the two groups during the first week post-transplant were not different. Wagner and his colleagues studied 42 consecutive cadaveric renal transplant patients in a prospective randomized investigation in which 20 patients received diltiazem and 22 served as controls.[23] In the treated group, diltiazem (20 mg/L) was added to the Eurocollins solution. The patient also received a bolus injection (0.28 mg/kg) preoperatively, followed by a constant infusion (0.0022 mg/min/kg) for 48 hours, after which oral therapy (at least 60 mg b.i.d.) was provided. They noted a reduction in the incidence of acute tubular necrosis (ATN) in the transplanted kidneys from 41% in the control group to 10% in the treated patients ($P < 0.05$). This difference in acute renal failure was achieved despite the fact that the cyclosporine levels were higher in the diltiazem-treated subjects initially. Finally, in an uncontrolled, retrospective study, the charts of 64 patients undergoing coronary bypass or valve replacement surgery were examined by Hull and Hasbargen.[34] No decrease in the development of ARF was noted in those patients treated preoperatively with calcium antagonists versus those who were not. However, the authors point out that those taking the drug were most likely more severely ill and could have been at increased risk for the development of ATN.

It is difficult to draw conclusions from the human studies thus far reported. Although the data from the carefully controlled investigations are encouraging, more experiments and substantially larger numbers of subjects will be required to settle this issue.

Summary

In conclusion, the data suggest that the calcium antagonists may be effective in ameliorating or preventing experimental acute renal failure due to ischemia, especially if given prior to the ischemic event. Their mechanism of action appears to include not only a beneficial effect on renal blood flow but also on cellular metabolism. Based on these observations, plus the limited number of carefully controlled studies performed in human subjects, it seems clear that additional studies in clinical settings are warranted. Future investigations should help to determine not only whether these drugs are beneficial, but also what the dosing regimen should be.

Acknowledgement.   Supported, in part, by the Veterans Administration. The author thanks Ms. Geri Medock for the production of this manuscript.

References

1. Madius NE, Harrington JT: Postischemic acute renal failure. In Brenner BM, Lazarus JM (eds): Acute Renal Failure. Philadelphia, W. B. Saunders, 1983, pp 235–251.

2. Puschett JB: Non-dialytic therapy of acute renal failure: a review. Int J Artif Organs 8:249–356 1985.

3. Hou SH, Bushinsky DA, Wish JB, Cohen JJ, Harrington JJ: Hospital-acquired renal insufficiency: A prospective study. Am J Med 74:243–248, 1982.

4. Puschett JB: Do calcium channel blockers protect against renal ischemia? Am J Nephrol 7(suppl 1):49–56, 1987.

5. Burnier M, Schrier RW: Protection from acute renal failure. Adv Exptl Med Biol 212:275–283, 1978.

6. Schrier RW, Burke TJ: Calcium-channel blockers in experimental and human acute renal failure. Adv Nephrol 17:287–300, 1988.

7. Cheung JY, Bonventre JV, Malis CD, Leaf A: Calcium and ischemic injury. N Engl J Med 26:1670–1676, 1986.

8. McCord JM: Oxygen-derived free radicals in postischemic tissue injury. N Engl J Med 312:159–163,1985.

9. Malis CD, Bonventre JV: Mechanism of calcium potentiation of oxygen free radical injury to renal mitochondria. J Biol Chem 261: 14201–14208, 1986.

10. Paller MS, Hoidal JR, Ferris TF: Oxygen free radicals in ischemic acute renal failure in the rat. J Clin Invest 74:1156–1164, 1984.

11. Ratych RE, Bulkley GB: Free-radical-mediated postischemic reperfusion injury in the kidney. J Free Radicals Biol Med 2:311–319, 1986.

12. Loutzenhiser R, Epstein M: Effects of calcium antagonists on renal hemodynamics. Am J Physiol 249:F619–F629, 1985.

13. Loutzenhiser R, Epstein M, Horton C, Sonke P: Reversal by the calcium antagonist nisoldipine of norepinephrine-induced reduction of GFR: Evidence for preferential antagonism

of preglomerular vasoconstriction. J Pharmacol Exp Ther 232:382–387, 1985.

14. Burke TJ, Arnold PE, Gordon JA, Bulger RE, Dobyan DC, Schrier RW: Protective effect of intrarenal calcium membrane blockers before or after renal ischemia. J Clin Invest 74:1830–1841, 1984.

15. Malis CD, Cheung JY, Leaf A, Bonventre JV: Effects of verapamil in models of ischemic acute renal failure in the rat. Am J Physiol 245:F735–F742, 1983.

16. Loutzenhiser R, Horton C, Epstein M: Effects of diltiazem and manganese on renal hemodynamics: Studies in the isolated perfused rat kidney. Nephron 39:382–388, 1985.

17. Loutzenhiser R, Epstein M, Horton C: Modification by dihydropyridine-type calcium antagonists of the renal hemodynamic response to vasoconstrictors. J Cardiovasc Pharm 9(suppl 1):S70–S75, 1987.

18. Goldfarb D, Iaina A, Serban I, Gavendo S, Kapuler S, Eliahou HE: Beneficial effect of verapamil in ischemic acute renal failure in the rat. Proc Soc Exptl Biol Med 172:389–392, 1983.

19. Rose H, Philipson J, Puschett JB: Effect of nitrendipine in a rat model of ischemic acute renal failure. J Cardiovasc Pharm 9(suppl 1):S57–S59, 1987.

20. Papadimitriou M, Alexopoulos E, Vargemezis V, Sakellarious G, Kosmidou I, Metaxas P: The effect of preventive administration of verapamil on acute ischaemic renal failure in dogs. Proc EDTA 20:650–655, 1983.

21. Agatstein EH, Farrer JH, Kaplan LM, Randazzo RF, Glassock RJ, Kaufman JJ: The effect of verapamil in reducing the severity of acute tubular necrosis in canine renal autotransplants. Transplantation 44:355–357, 1987.

22. Wagner K, Albrecht S, Neumayer H-H: Prevention of delayed graft function in cadaveric kidney transplantation by a calcium antagonist. Preliminary results of two prospective randomized trials. Transpl Proc 18:510–515, 1986.

23. Wagner K, Albrecht S, Neumayer H-H: Prevention of posttransplant acute tubular necrosis by the calcium antagonist diltiazem: A prospective randomized study. Am J Nephrol 7:287–291, 1987.

24. Wait RB, White G, Davis JH: Beneficial effects of verapamil on postischemic renal failure. Surgery 94:276–282, 1983.

25. Shapiro JI, Cheung C, Itabashi A, Chan L, Schrier RW: The effect of verapamil on renal function after warm and cold ischemia in the isolated perfused rat kidney. Transplantation 40:596–600, 1985.

26. Duggan KA, MacDonald GJ, Charlesworth JA, Pussell BA: Verapamil prevents posttransplant oliguric renal failure. Clin Nephrol 24:289–291, 1985.

27. Woolley JL, Barker GR, Jacobsen WK, et al: Effect of calcium entry blocker verapamil on renal ischemia. Crit Care Med 16:48–51, 1988.

28. Farber JL: The role of calcium in cell death. Life Sci 29:1289–1295, 1981.

29. Snowdowne KW, Freudenrich CC, Borle AB: The effects of anoxia on cytosolic free calcium, calcium fluxes, and cellular ATP levels in cultured kidney cells. J Biol Chem 260:11619–11626, 1985.

30. Schrier RW, Arnold PE, Van Putten VJ, Burke TJ: Cellular calcium in ischemic acute renal failure: Role of calcium entry blockers. Kidney Int 32:313–321, 1987.

31. Wilson DR, Arnold PE, Burke TJ, Schrier RW: Mitochondrial calcium accumulation and respiration in ischemic acute renal failure in the rat. Kidney Int 25:519–526, 1984.

32. Wilson PD, Schrier RW: Nephron segment and calcium as determinants of anoxic cell death in renal cultures. Kidney Int 29:1172–1179, 1986.

33. Schwertschlag U, Schrier RW, Wilson P: Beneficial effects of calcium channel blockers and calmodulin binding drugs on in vitro renal cell anoxia. J Pharmacol Exp Ther 238:119–124, 1986.

34. Hull RW, Hasbargen JA: No clinical evidence for protective effects of calcium-channel blockers against acute renal failure. N Engl J Med 313:1477–1478, 1985.

Ulrich F. Michael, M.D.
Stanley M. Lee, M.D.

10

The Role of Calcium Antagonists in Nephrotoxic Models of Renal Failure

Renal tubular cell necrosis may occur following exposure to a wide variety of diverse chemical agents and ultimately results in the clinical syndrome of acute renal failure (ARF). Various segments of the nephron appear to be sensitive to particular toxins, and a variety of factors may influence the development of renal cell injury. Recently much attention has been focused on the role of calcium as a mediator of cell death. Although histologically recognizable tissue calcification usually indicates tissue necrosis, there is no correlation between total calcium content and cellular viability.

It has been proposed that uncontrolled calcium entry into the cell is the final common pathway in the process of cell death (for references see ref.[18]). In early studies, Schanne and coworkers showed that when hepatic cells were incubated with various membrane toxins, the presence of calcium in the medium greatly enhanced cell death.[32] However, using freshly isolated hepatocytes, Smith and his collaborators exposed these cells to organic toxins including carbon tetrachloride and bromobenzene.[37] They demonstrated that cell death occurred in the absence of calcium in the medium, thereby attempting to counter the hypothesis that exogenous calcium was a necessary element in the death throes of the cell.

It is evident that the distribution of intracellular calcium and the maintenance of cell membrane integrity are intimately related, and are necessary for normal cell metabolism. Humes has reviewed the importance of calcium in the pathogenesis of ARF and details the role of calcium distribution and cellular function.[18] There is normally an extracellular (EC) to intracellular (IC) calcium gradient, with an EC free-ionized calcium concentration of 10^{-3}M, and an IC concentration of 10^{-7}M. This gradient is maintained by several transport systems in the plasma membrane, with a Ca-Mg ATPase exerting control at low basal cytosolic Ca^{++} concentrations, whereas a Na–Ca exchanger becomes involved in situations where intracellular calcium is increased. Within the cell, calcium is sequestered in various organelles, bound to intracellular membranes, or lies "free" in the cytosol. Estimation of calcium in viable kidney tubular cells by electron probe x-ray microanalysis (EPXMA) has yielded values of 3.8 mmol/kg dry weight or 5.4 nmol/mg protein.[27] Although earlier measurements of the calcium content in mitochondria concluded that about 60–70% of IC calcium was contained in these structures,[18] more recent and refined measurements by EPXMA have resulted in an estimate of 20–25% of IC calcium being contained in viable mitochondria.[27] The remainder is associated with the endoplasmic reticulum, bound to the IC proteins calmodulin and troponin, bound to phosphate, and existing as free-ionized calcium.

Tissue injury is associated with a complex series of events, with loss of cell membrane integrity signaling the initial phase of cell death. Malfunction of the plasma membrane calcium transport systems permits influx of calcium into the cell and may override the systems that control the IC calcium distribution. Mitochondrial overloading is an early event, because of their strong avidity for calcium, and mitochondrial dysfunction ultimately disrupts cell respiration and energy production. In addition, increased free cytosolic calcium activates a calcium-dependent phospholipase, leading to cell membrane dissolution and release of free fatty acids and lysophospholipids that are toxic to the cell. Other enzymes may be activated in a similar manner, including proteases and nucleases, which contribute to cytosolic disintegration.[9]

It should be emphasized, however, that increased cell calcium may play a physiologic role in certain situations. With the advent of modern techniques capable of measuring cytosolic free calcium directly in normal cells, it has been shown that physiological processes such as cell fertilization and hormonal stimulation are associated with remarkable increases in free cytosolic calcium (25- and 8-fold, respectively). These physiological increases are much larger than the two-fold rise of cytosolic calcium observed in cells subjected to hypoxia or metabolic blockade.[9]

Numerous studies have delineated the beneficial effects of calcium antagonists in *ischemic* tissue injury. These agents have been shown to offer protection against ischemic damage in the heart, central nervous system and the kidney. The prevention of IC calcium accumulation during reperfusion is thought to play a critical role in this setting, although the influence of calcium antagonists on free-radical production and scavenging remains an additional factor.[36] Loutzenhiser and Epstein have demonstrated in elegant experiments with the isolated rat kidney[28] that calcium antagonist–induced vasodilation depends crucially on the underlying vascular tone and the mode of action of the vasoconstrictor involved. Vasoconstriction associated with KCl-induced depolarization was completely reversed by the calcium antagonist nitrendipine, whereas similar degrees of vasoconstriction induced by norepinephrine or angiotensin II were only partially reversed.[28] The possible modes of action of calcium antagonists in ischemic acute renal failure have recently been reviewed.[31,34]

The role of calcium antagonists in *nephrotoxic* renal failure is not well defined. There are a large number of chemical agents with varying degrees of nephrotoxicity and different mechanisms of action that affect specific portions of the nephron. Their precise onset of action is not always known. Certain toxins have multiple actions, such as the glycerol-myoglobinuria model, which has both toxic and hemodynamic effects in the kidney. In addition, receptors for calcium antagonists have not been demonstrated on renal tubular epithelial cells.[34] However, several models of nephrotoxic injury have been studied in detail, in particular the renal injury caused by aminoglycoside antibiotics. The relationship between cellular calcium content, the IC distribution of calcium, and cellular dysfunction have been well described.[18] Humes has summarized the available literature, and concludes that calcium-mediated cell injury is mediated via activation of phospholipases, subsequently leading to the deterioration of mitochondrial structure and function.[18]

We will review the data (at times conflicting) on the effects of calcium antagonists on some nephrotoxic models of renal failure and conclude with some recent speculations concerning the mechanism of nephrotoxic cell injury, as well as the possible mode(s) of action of calcium antagonists in this setting.

Effects of Calcium Antagonists in Four Animal Models of Nephrotoxicity

The effects of calcium antagonists in experimental nephrotoxic renal failure are summarized in Table 1.

Myohemoglobinuric Acute Renal Failure

This model of ARF is induced by intravenous injection of methemoglobin or by intramuscular administration of hypertonic glycerol to dehydrated animals.[16] Renal failure develops in almost all cases if the animals are volume depleted, whereas less than half develop ARF if they are well-hydrated. The pathophysiology of the ARF in this model is complex. Glycerol causes a significant decrease in cardiac output, which leads to a decline in renal blood flow. Glycerol also promotes fluid sequestration at the injection site, contributing to diminished plasma volume and further compromising renal blood flow. The release of "toxic" tissue metabolites presumably leads to

TABLE 1. Summary of Calcium Antagonist Effects in Experimental Nephrotoxic Renal Failure*

Experimental Method	Experimental Animal	Drug admin.	Drug Protection	Ref.
Glycerol ARF	rat	Diltiazem p.o. and i.p. prior and after glycerol.	Partial protect. of CIN and of morph. structure.	(24)
Gentamicin ARF	rat	Verapamil p.o. prior to and during genta-micin.	No protection	(42)
Gentamicin ARF	rat	Nitrendipine p.o. prior to and during gentamicin.	Mitigated fall of CIN and pre-served morph. structure	(25)
Cyclosporin A ± ischemia	rat	Verapamil p.o. post ischemia/ together with	Partial protect. of CCr & of FENa and FEK.	(19)
Cyclosporin A	rat	Verapamil i.v. prior to CyA	Partial protect. of CIN & CPAH	(2)
Cyclosporin A	rat (isol. kidney)	Verapamil in perfusate toge-ther with CyA	Mitgated fall of CIN & RPF	(39)
Diatrizoate meglumine	dog	Verpamil diltiazem	Mitgated fall of CIN.	(1)

*Abbr.: CCr, CIN, CPAH: clearances of creatinine, inulin and para-amino hippurate; FENa, FEK: fractional excretion of sodium, potassium; RPF: renal perfusate flow; ARF, acute renal failure.

renal tubular injury. The initial hemodynamic perturbations are associated with renal vasoconstriction and ischemia, and this sets the stage for secondary tubular toxic injury.[16] Evidence that hydroxyl radical might be involved in the pathogenesis of this form of ARF was recently presented by Shah and Walker.[35] They demonstrated that dimethylthiourea, a hydroxyl radical scavenger, as well as deferoxamine (DFO), an iron chelator, provided significant protection of the animals pretreated with them. The DFO presumably prevents the iron-dependent conversion of hydrogen peroxide into the much more aggressively injurious hydroxyl radical by the Fenton reaction. Volume repletion, or failure to dehydrate the animals, also will abrogate the initial hemodynamic alteration. Thus, myoglobinuric ARF occupies a transitional position between ischemic and toxic renal failure.

Involvement of the renin-angiotensin system in the pathogenesis of glycerol-induced renal injury was suggested by the observation that prior saline loading could prevent the development of ARF.[16] However, studies utilizing angiotensin II antagonists, or the angiotensin-converting enzyme (ACE) inhibitor (SQ 20881), in glycerol renal failure showed that these agents could increase renal blood flow, but there was little influence on the glomerular filtration rate (GFR).[20] These observations were confirmed in a recent experimental study by our laboratory using captopril, another ACE inhibitor.[24] This drug was given to rats for 3 days prior to the glycerol and was continued up to 4 weeks after the acute injury. Captopril had no effect on renal function or the extent of renal tubular cell injury.

In the same model of ARF, diltiazem, a benzothiazepine calcium channel blocker, significantly reduced the severity of the renal injury, decreased the extent of tubular cell necrosis, and was associated with a more rapid histologic (Fig. 1) and functional (Fig. 2) recovery.[24] Microangiography of the kidneys in this study showed improved visualization of the microvasculature at 1 and 2 weeks after the glycerol injection in diltiazem-treated rats.

At 4 weeks after the acute glycerol injury, all the animals exhibited significant microangiographic abnormalities, including the captopril and diltiazem groups. This occurred at a time when there was evidence of complete functional and histologic recovery and, in this model of acute renal injury suggested a lack of correlation between function and histology on the one hand and microangiographic perfusion patterns on the other. It also suggested that subtle microvascular alterations may persist following ARF and are not prevented by a relatively short course of diltiazem.[24]

In summary, although modulation of the renin-angiotensin system by means of the prophylactic application of ACE inhibitors appears incapable of protecting or restoring GFR in the glycerol-induced ARF of rats, diltiazem administered prophylactically has been shown to be protective, as judged by functional as well as morphological parameters. Similar functional protection was provided by the administration of dimethylthiourea (a hydroxyl radical scavenger) and of deferoxamine (an iron chelator that prevents the formation of hydroxyl radical) before and during the glycerol exposure.

Aminoglycoside-induced ARF

Aminoglycosides are the mainstay in the treatment of gram-negative infections, despite their well recognized nephrotoxicity. The incidence of renal dysfunction in patients receiving aminoglycosides approximates 10–20%, even when drug levels are

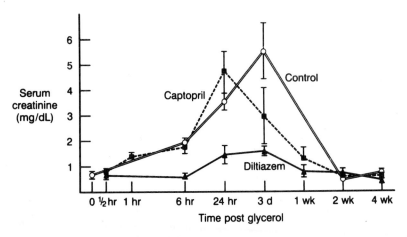

FIGURE 1. The effects of captopril and diltiazem on the acute renal failure induced by glycerol in rats. Pretreatment with diltiazem blunted the rise of serum creatinine in response to glycerol. Modified from Lee et al.[23]

well monitored.[10] The role of calcium antagonists in this model of renal failure is not completely understood, but understanding may be facilitated by some knowledge of the pharmacology and renal handling of the aminoglycosides. The unbound drug is freely filtered across the glomerular capillary and absorbed by the convoluted and straight segments of the proximal tubule. Reabsorption results from a charge interaction between the cationic aminoglycoside and anionic phospholipid receptors on the brush border of the tubular cell, and is related in part to the number of amino groups on the drug. The aminoglycoside accumulates in the renal tubular cell, causing disruption of intracellular membrane structures and ultimately inhibiting cell respiration. Increased tissue calcium content has been demonstrated in the renal cortex of animals with aminoglycoside nephrotoxicity,[17] although administration of a calcium-enhanced diet has been shown to protect the kidney against gentamicin injury.[10] The relationship between these observations remains undefined, as does the mechanism by which dietary calcium acts in this setting.

Attempts to analyze the effects of calcium antagonists in experimental amino-glycoside nephrotoxicity are confounded by several problems: the drug dose, duration of treatment, frequency and route of administration, and the sex of the animal may all influence the ultimate outcome.[10] Intercurrent illness in the animals, gram-negative infection, potassium and/or magnesium depletion, and the diet may alter drug toxicity.[3,22,43] In addition there are significant strain and species differences with regard to susceptibility to aminoglycoside toxicity. Hence it is difficult to compare the various reported studies.

Effects of Verapamil. Only one study has addressed the utility of verapamil in gentamicin-induced ARF.[42] Watson and coworkers employed Sprague-Dawley rats and administered a high dose of gentamicin, namely 120 mg/kg/day for either 6 days or 9 days. Different groups of animals were given verapamil in the drinking water at a dose of 10 mg/dl. There was no evidence that verapamil protected against the nephrotoxic

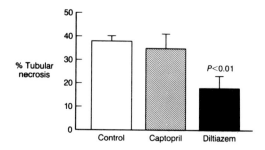

FIGURE 2. The effects of captopril and diltiazem on the degree of tubular necrosis in rats 24 hours after glycerol administration. The ordinate axis indicates the percentage of necrotic tubules throughout the renal cortex. Diltiazem treated rats (n = 6) had significantly less necrosis than the captopril (n = 5) and non-drug-treated (n = 6) animals (means ± SE). Modified from Lee et al. [23]

effect of gentamicin; in fact serum creatinine and tissue calcium levels were slightly higher in the verapamil-treated animals.

In interpreting the above study, it should be noted that work undertaken by Giuliano and colleagues[13] demonstrated fundamentally different behavior after gentamicin loading with high or low doses. When given in a "low" dose (10 mg/kg), there was regression of drug-induced changes in the absence of any sign of necrosis regeneration. At the "high" dose (140 mg/kg), there was relentless progression towards cell death. Therefore, it is not inconceivable that the high dose of gentamicin used by Watson could have obscured any potential beneficial effect of verapamil.

Effects of Nitrendipine. Nitrendipine, a dihydropyridine-derived calcium antagonist, was studied in our laboratory with regard to its protective effects against gentamicin nephrotoxicity.[25,26] Fischer rats were utilized in these studies, and a "moderate" dose of gentamicin was employed, namely 40 mg/kg/day for periods up to 14 days. Oral nitrendipine was given in a dose of 25–30 mg/kg/day ("high" dose) or 10 mg/kg/day ("low" dose), and was initiated 3 days prior to the gentamicin. It was observed that nitrendipine offered significant histologic and functional protection. Tubular cell necrosis was diminished in the nitrendipine groups, both by morphometric histopathologic analysis and indirectly by a reduction in urinary enzyme { N-acetyl-glucosaminidase [NAG] and beta-glucosidase} excretion. Glomerular filtration rate was increased (Fig. 3) but not normalized in "high" dose nitrendipine-treated animals, although para-aminohippurate (PAH) clearance (a measure of renal plasma flow) was not enhanced by nitrendipine. When nitrendipine was initiated several days after gentamicin dosing, the protective effects of the calcium antagonist were still evident but not as marked as when the drug was started at the same time or prior to the aminoglycoside. In these latter studies gentamicin in a dose of 40 mg/kg BW/day i. m. was given to Fischer rats starting on day 0 and continued for 12 days. On day 5 nitrendipine (suspended in 0.05% polyethylene glycol) in a dose of 30 mg/kg BW/day by gavage was added to the regimen. Urinary excretion of N-acetyl glucosaminidase (NAG) was examined on days 0, 3, 6, 9 and 12. Kidneys were harvested at the end of 12 days for histological evaluation and for determination of gentamicin content of the renal cortex. There was no statistically significant difference in the cortical gentamicin

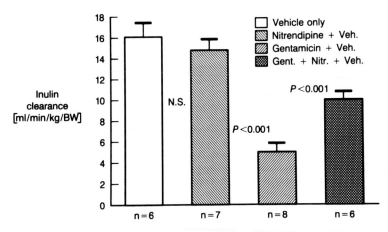

FIGURE 3. The effect of nitrendipine on the acute renal failure induced by gentamicin in rats. The vehicle for the nitrendipine was 0.05% polyethylene glycol. Pretreatment with nitrendipine partially restored the glomerular filtration rate in these animals (means ± SE). Reproduced with permission, from Lee and Michael.[24]

content among the different groups studied. However, severity of injury, judged by histological criteria, was not more extensive when the nitrendipine was started 5 days after the initiation of gentamicin rather than 3 days before. The urinary excretion of N-acetyl glucosaminidase was also less in the animals protected by high dose nitrendipine started on day 5 (Lee et al: unpublished observations) (Fig. 4).

In summary, divergent results were obtained in three studies evaluating the protective role of prophylactic calcium antagonists in gentamicin-induced ARF in rats. Verapamil, a phenylalkylamine type antagonist, was incapable of preventing the very severe renal damage induced by a very high dose (120 mg/kg/day) of gentamicin. In contrast, nitrendipine, a dihydropyridine calcium antagonist, substantially protected rats with a moderate dose (40 mg/kg/day) of gentamicin ARF. It is most plausible that the difference of gentamicin dose and the resulting difference of the severity of ARF explain the different findings in these studies. However, the observation that another dihydropyridine Ca^{++} antagonist, nifedipine, was shown to have a more profound ability to scavenge reactive oxygen species than verapamil might be of significance.[36]

Cyclosporin A Nephrotoxicity

Cyclosporin A (CsA) is a potent immunosuppressive agent that has assumed a central role in the management of renal, hepatic and cardiac transplants. It is also being utilized in the treatment of certain autoimmune disorders, including diabetes mellitus and rheumatoid arthritis. The major limiting factor with cyclosporin A is its nephrotoxicity. In man, the early renal histologic changes are subtle and nonspecific, involving both tubular and vascular elements, although they can generally be distinguished from acute rejection. Chronic CsA toxicity leads to chronic interstitial nephritis, usually accompanied by hypertension. In experimental animal studies, higher drug

Urinary NAG Excretion

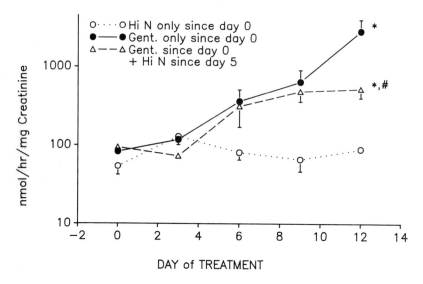

FIGURE 4. The effect of 30 mg/kg BW/day of nitrendipine started 5 days after initiating 40 mg/kg BW/day of gentamicin on urinary excretion of N-acetyl-glucosaminidase (NAG). * = $p < 0.025$ (comparison to nitrendipine control); # = $p < 0.05$ (comparison to gentamicin alone). ($n = 6$/group, means ± SE.) Unpublished observations by Lee et al.

doses are usually employed and tubular lesions, acute hypertension, and systemic effects can be observed.[2,5,14,19,39] The interpretation of studies using high-dose CsA in experimental animals, and how this relates to clinical transplantation, should be appropriately tempered. For a detailed consideration of CsA nephrotoxicity see Chapter 14.

Iaina and colleagues utilized Sprague-Dawley rats and produced a combination ischemic-toxic model of ARF, perhaps attempting to simulate renal transplantation.[19] The animals underwent right nephrectomy, followed by clamping of the left renal pedicle for 20 minutes, and were given intraperitoneal cyclosporin in a dose of 60 mg/kg for 4 days. Verapamil was administered in the drinking water in a concentration of 10 mg/100 ml. Verapamil was significantly protective in animals that had undergone both pedicle clamping and CsA treatment. Their creatinine clearance was higher, the BUN was diminished, and the fractional excretion of sodium, potassium and water was substantially lower, indicating preservation of tubular function. Verapamil was less effective in animals given CsA alone (without pedicle clamping), suggesting that it primarily attenuated the ischemic component of the combined renal injury.

Barros and coworkers using Munich-Wistar rats, studied glomerular hemodynamics in animals given CsA (50mg/kg) intravenously as a single dose.[2] Besides measurements of GFR and renal blood flow (RBF) these studies allow the estimation of vascular resistance in the afferent and efferent arteriolar beds of the kidney and the calculation of the glomerular ultrafiltration coefficient. (The glomerular ultrafiltration coefficient [k_f] is the product of glomerular capillary hydraulic conductance [L_p] and the capillary area [A] available for filtration.) CsA caused a decrease of GFR (from 0.96 ± 0.04 to 0.47 ± 0.07 ml/min) and renal plasma flow (from 2.91 ± 0.19 to 1.30 ± 0.23 ml/min). Total arteriolar resistance rose from 39 ± 3 to 129 ± 40 mmHg·min/ml, and glomerular capillary pressure was increased from 45 ± 1 to 55 ± 4 mmHg, while the ultrafiltration coefficient K_f declined by 70%. In additional studies, verapamil was administered as an intravenous infusion at 20 micrograms/kg/min. After obtaining baseline measurements, CsA in the above dose was infused in addition to verapamil. Verapamil attenuated the CsA induced decline in glomerular filtration (0.92 ± 0.06 to 0.65 ± 0.06 ml/min) and plasma flow (from 2.91 ± 0.29 to 2.31 ± 0.17 ml/min) by preventing the CsA-induced increase of vascular resistance (from 34 ± 3 to 38 ± 3 mmHg·min/ml). It was of interest that the ACE inhibitor captopril exerted similar protective effects, whereas indomethacin was without activity.

Sumpio and colleagues employed an isolated perfused kidney preparation from Holtzman rats.[39] With the addition of CsA to the perfusate in a concentration of 500 ng/ml, they observed a reduction of inulin clearance (Fig. 5), renal perfusate flow, urine production, and fractional water reabsorption. Verapamil in the perfusate at 1.0 microgram/ml, reversed these functional changes and actually increased renal perfusate flow and urine output (Fig. 6) to levels exceeding those of the control group.

Wagner and colleagues examined the effects of diltiazem in patients undergoing cadaveric renal transplantation.[40] In a prospective trial, they perfused the graft with diltiazem prior to implantation and treated the recipients with intravenous, followed by oral, diltiazem in a dose of 60 mg bid. In the diltiazem-treated patients, the incidence of postoperative ARF was reduced from 41 to 10%, and there were less (.75 vs 2.3%) acute rejection episodes during the first month. Diltiazem altered the pharmacokinetics of CsA, leading to higher blood levels, such that a 30% reduction of the CsA dose provided comparable therapeutic blood levels. It was concluded by the authors that diltiazem may have attenuated CsA nephrotoxicity, although the evidence for this is somewhat indirect.

In summary, studies in experimental animals as well as recent clinical studies have indicated that calcium antagonists confer protection from cyclosporine nephrotoxicity. Additional studies will be needed to elucidate the mode of action by which calcium antagonists provide this protective effect.

Radiocontrast–induced Renal Injury

Intrarenal infusion of radiocontrast medium causes prolonged vasoconstriction and a decreased glomerular filtration rate in laboratory animals. Individuals with underlying renal insufficiency associated with nephrosclerosis and diabetic nephropathy, and patients with dysproteinemic syndromes such as multiple myeloma, represent a special high risk group when subjected to radiographic contrast agents. They may develop acute deterioration in renal function with only partial reversibility.

It is therefore of interest, that Bakris and Burnett[1] demonstrated in dogs that radiocontrast-induced renal vasoconstriction was amenable to calcium antagonist modulation. They measured GFR utilizing inulin clearances and renal blood flow by electromagnetic flow probe, following administration of diatrizoite meglumine to anesthetized dogs. Both verapamil and diltiazem, as well as the nonspecific calcium

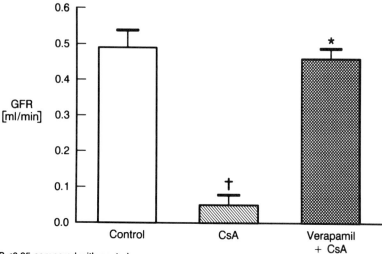

†= $P<0.05$ compared with control
*= $P<0.05$ compared with CsA

FIGURE 5. The effect of cyclosporine A (CsA) with and without verapamil on GFR in the isolated perfused kidney. Values are mean ± SE of 6 kidneys in each group. Pretreatment with verapamil prevented the CsA induced drop of GFR. Modified from Sumpio et al.[35]

chelator ethyleneglycol-bis-N, N´-tetraacetic acid (EGTA) diminished the extent of the decrement of GFR (see Fig. 3 in Chapter 17, p. 280). The beneficial effect on renal blood flow was less marked.

In summary, two different calcium antagonists, verapamil and diltiazem, were shown to provide protection from the radiocontrast-induced renal vasoconstriction in dogs.

Discussion

It has been proposed to divide the time course of ARF into a (vascular) initiation phase and a (tubular) maintenance phase. The maintenance phase, which is always preceded by a period of diminished glomerular filtration, depends on the severity of the tubular epithelial damage, which in turn determines the extent of tubular obstruction by cast of cell debris and the magnitude of tubular back leak. In contrast to the onset of ischemic ARF, which can be rather well timed under most clinical and experimental circumstances, the timing of the onset of nephrotoxic ARF remains frequently quite poorly defined. Although it is intuitively easier to envision a vascular initiating event in ischemic ARF (severe preglomerular and glomerular vasoconstriction by shock, norepinephrine, angiotensin II or ADH), it is more difficult to do so in the case of nephrotoxic renal failure.

It is intriguing to speculate that **tubuloglomerular feedback** might initiate glomerular vasoconstriction in the event of primary tubular damage caused by a nephrotoxin. Bell and and co-workers[4] have demonstrated that cytosolic calcium plays a role in the transmission of feedback signals both at the macula densa and at the site of the afferent arteriole (as well as the glomerular mesangium?) constitutes the final common pathway, which is amenable to calcium channel blockade. Preservation of glomerular filtration in the face of nephrotoxic injury (which would be expected to increase macula densa sensed osmolality or NaCl concentration and therefore glomerular mesangial contraction and afferent arteriolar vasoconstriction) by paralyzing the tubuloglomerular feedback loop, either by chronic sodium loading or by calcium antagonists, might be essential in the clinical prevention of tubular obstruction, which induces the maintenance phase of ARF (vide supra). It has been demonstrated that significant histological injury can be present in the absence of clinical renal failure,[16] possibly by exclusion of tubuloglomerular feedback by chronic saline loading of rats prior to the nephrotoxic injury. Since the clinical/experimental sequelae of prolonged glomerular vasoconstriction by means of *prolonged* inhibition of the cytosolic calcium-modulating mechanisms (calmodulin, cAMP, etc.) have not been determined, the invocation of this tubuloglomerular pathway in the initiation of the vascular phase of nephrotoxic renal injury must remain hypothetical.

It also needs to be stressed that inactivation of the tubuloglomerular feedback mechanism by medical intervention might be detrimental to the kidney in the setting of ARF. This cautionary note relates to the precarious state of oxygenation of parts of the kidney that are receiving borderline amounts of blood flow in the face of high metabolic activity (i.e., the medullary thick limb of the loop of Henle [mTAL]). Although this situation was initially observed (in vitro) in the isolated kidney, where necrotic lesions in the mTAL are regularly seen (unless they are prevented by inhibition of metabolic activity in this segment[7]), susceptibility of this segment of the kidney to nephrotoxic damage can also be demonstrated in vivo.[15] It could be argued that allowing tubular solutes that were not reabsorbed in the proximal nephron due to nephrotoxic damage to overtax the metabolic capacity of the mTAL by interrupting tubuloglomerular feedback might result in necrotic damage of this latter segment as well, unless an increased blood flow to this segment was facilitated simultaneously. Bird and coworkers have provided experimental evidence that maneuvers to increase nephron filtration rate (possibly by interruption of tubuloglomerular feedback) might indeed have resulted in more severe tubular injury by placing increased metabolic demands upon nephron segments further "downstream." They did their study in a model of ischemic injury in rats treated with the antioxidant probucol.[6]

The role of **prostaglandins and other arachidonic acid derivatives**, in ARF is difficult to assess due to many conflicting reports in the literature.[38] The consensus appears to be that there is a delicate balance of vasodilatory (PGE_2, PGI_2) and vasoconstrictive (TxA_2) prostaglandins in the kidney. The overall effect on kidney function will depend on the disturbance of this balance by nephrotoxins as well as by drugs intended to ameliorate the renal damage resulting either in a vasoconstrictor or vasodilator preponderance. Busse and coworkers have described the release of prostacyclin (PGI_2), a vasodilatory prostaglandin from cultured endothelial cells under the influence of fendiline, a dihydropyridine-derived calcium antagonist.[8]

The role of *free-radical induced* renal damage mediated by lipid peroxidation in nephrotoxic and even in postischemic renal failure is still controversial.[12,29,30,35,41] However, this does not exclude a detrimental effect of reactive oxygen species on other cellular processes.[41] Shah and Walker have elegantly demonstrated that hydroxyl radical scavengers as well as iron chelators are capable of ameliorating both gentamicin- as well as glycerol-induced ARF in rats.[35,41] (Iron is required for the generation of hydroxyl radical from hydrogen peroxide in the Fenton reaction.) In contrast, Gamelin and Zager were not able to reproduce the beneficial effects of some antioxidants (allopurinol, superoxide dismutase on ischemic renal failure in rats[12]; these antioxidants were alleged to be beneficial previously.[29] Nevertheless, if there is a role for free radicals in nephrotoxic renal failure, calcium antagonists might have a beneficial effect under those circumstances. Shridi and Robak have found that diltiazem, fendiline, nifedipine and verapamil all had some antioxidant activity; however, only nifedipine scavenged superoxide anions both in an enzymic and nonenzymic generating system.[36]

Diminution of the glomerular ultrafiltration coefficient (K_f) might be the only abnormality in mild and easily reversible renal failure, whereas widespread tubular obstruction and tubular back-leak are features of severe nephrotoxic renal failure.[16] A reversal of the renal vascular actions (including a diminution of K_f) of angiotensin II by the calcium antagonist verapamil has been demonstrated.[21] The possibility that calcium antagonists might reverse more severe tubular changes leads to the question: Is there a role for calcium entry blockers beyond that on vascular smooth muscle cells? Schrier and coworkers have speculated that there might be a means for calcium antagonists to attach to tubular epithelial cells, despite the latter's lack of receptors, and that such an attachment might be facilitated by the depolarization of these cells due to the loss of K^+ ions from the cell.[34] The postulation of a direct protective effect of calcium antagonists on tubular epithelium, diminishing widespread tubular necrosis, is particularly attractive in view of the improved histopathologic appearance of the tubules observed in the studies from our laboratory.[24–26] It may therefore be speculated that some calcium antagonists either are capable of limiting the uptake of the nephrotoxin into tubular cells or of preventing their destructive influence within the tubular cell.

Conclusions

We have reviewed the effects of calcium antagonists on several forms of nephrotoxic renal failure. The conflicting observations of their utility, particularly in aminoglycoside-induced renal failure, indicate that important details need to be worked out before these drugs can find clinical application for the prevention of aminoglycoside-induced nephrotoxic renal failure in man. Overall, there should be optimism that the elucidation of the pathogenetic mechanisms of the role of calcium, arachidonic acid derivatives, and free radicals in the causation of nephrotoxic renal failure by further experimentation will ultimately lead to this goal. The data obtained in patients with renal transplants receiving cyclosporin A do suggest a protective role of calcium antagonists in this situation.

Acknowledgment: This work was supported in part by a Merit Review Program Grant from the Veterans Administration.

References

1. Bakris GL, Burnett JC: A role for calcium in radiocontrast- induced reductions in renal hemodynamics. Kidney Int 27:465–468, 1985.

2. Barros EJG, Boim MA, Ajzen H, Ramos OL, Schor N: Glomerular hemodynamics and hormonal participation on cyclosporine nephrotoxicity. Kidney Int 32:19–25, 1987.

3. Beauchamp D, Poirier A, Bergeron M: Increased nephrotoxicity of gentamicin in pyelonephritic rats. Kidney Int 28:106–113, 1985.

4. Bell PD: Calcium antagonists and intrarenal regulation of glomerular filtration rate. Am J Nephrol 7(suppl 1):24–31, 1987.

5. Bennett WM: Comparison of cyclosporine nephrotoxicity with aminoglycoside nephrotoxicity. Clin Nephrol 25 (suppl 1):S126–S129, 1986.

6. Bird JE, Milhoan K, Wilson CB, et al: Ischemic acute renal failure and antioxidant therapy in the rat: The relation between glomerular and tubular dysfunction. J Clin Invest 81:1630–1638, 1988.

7. Brezis M, Rosen S, Silva P, Epstein FH: Transport activity modifies thick ascending limb damage in the isolated perfused kidney. Kidney Int 25:65–72, 1984.

8. Busse R, Lückhoff A, Winter I, Mülsch A, Pohl U: Fendiline and calmidazolium enhance the release of endothelium-derived relaxant factor and of prostacyclin from cultured endothelial cells. Naunyn Schmiedebergs Arch Pharmacol 337:79–84, 1988.

9. Cheung JY, Bonventre JV, Malis CD, Leaf A: Calcium and ischemic injury. N Engl J Med 314:1670–1676, 1986.

10. Coggins CH, Fang LS-T: Acute renal failure associated with antibiotics, anesthetic agents, and radiographic contrast agents. In Brenner BM, Lazarus JM (eds): Acute Renal Failure. Philadelphia, WB Saunders Co, 1988, p 295.

11. Evan AP, Huser J, Avasthi PS, Luft FC: Gentamicin induced glomerular injury. Antimicrob Agents Chemother 19:933–940, 1979.

12. Gamelin LM, Zager RA: Evidence against oxidant injury as a critical mediator of postischemic acute renal failure. Am J Physiol 255:F450–F460, 1988.

13. Giuliano RA, Paulus GJ, Verpooten GA, et al: Recovery of cortical phospholipidosis and necrosis after acute gentamicin loading in rats. Kidney Int 26:838–847, 1984.

14. Hay R, Tammi K, Ryffel B, Mihatsch MJ: Alterations in molecular structure of renal mitochondria associated with cyclosporine A treatment. Clin Nephrol 25 (suppl 1):S23–S26, 1986.

15. Heyman SN, Brezis M, Reubinoff CA, et al: Acute renal failure with selective medullary injury in the rat. J Clin Invest 82:401–412, 1988.

16. Hostetter TH, Brenner BM: Renal circulatory and nephron function in experimental acute renal failure. In Brenner BM, Lazarus JM (eds): Acute Renal Failure. Philadelphia, WB Saunders Co, 1988, p 67.

17. Humes HD, Weinberg JM, Knauss TC: Clinical and pathophysiologic aspects of aminoglycoside nephrotoxicity. Am J Kidney Dis 2:5–29, 1982.

18. Humes HD: Role of calcium in pathogenesis of acute renal failure. Am J Physiol 250:F579–F589, 1986.

19. Iaina A, Herzog D, Cohen D, et al: Calcium entry-blockade with verapamil in cyclosporin A plus ischemia induced acute renal failure in rats. Clin Nephrol 25 (suppl 1):S168–S170, 1986.

20. Ishikawa I, Hollenberg NK: Pharmacologic interruption of the renin-angiotensin system in myohemoglobinuric acute renal failure. Kidney Int 10 (suppl 6):S183–S190, 1976.

21. Ichikawa I, Miele JF, Brenner BM: Reversal of renal cortical actions of angiotensin II by verapamil and manganese. Kidney Int 16:137–147, 1979.

22. Klotman PE, Boatman JE, Volpp BD, Baker JD, Yarger WE: Captopril enhances aminoglycoside nephrotoxicity in potassium-depleted rats. Kidney Int 28:118–127, 1985.

23. Leahy AL, Fitzpatrick JM, Wait RB: Variable results of calcium blockade in postischemic renal failure. Eur Urol 14:222–225, 1988.

24. Lee SM, Hillman BJ, Clark RL, Michael UF: The effects of diltiazem and captopril on glycerol-induced acute renal failure in the rat. Invest Radiol 20:961–970, 1985.

25. Lee SM, Michael UF: The protective effect of nitrendipine on gentamicin acute renal failure in rats. Exp Mol Pathol 43:107–114, 1985.

26. Lee SM, Pattison ME, Michael UF: Nitrendipine protects against aminoglycoside nephrotoxicity in the rat. J Cardiovasc Pharmacol 9 (suppl 1):S65–S69, 1987.

27. LeFurgey A, Ingram P, Mandel LJ: Heterogeneity of calcium compartmentation: Electron probe analysis of renal tubules. J Membrane Biol 94:191–196, 1986.

28. Loutzenhiser R, Epstein M: Modification of the renal hemodynamic response to vasoconstrictors by calcium antagonists. Am J Nephrol 7 (suppl 1):7–16, 1987.

29. Paller MS, Hoidal JR, Ferris TF: Oxygen free radicals in ischemic acute renal failure in the rat. J Clin Invest 74:1156–1164, 1984.

30. Paller MS, Hebbel RP: Ethane production as a measure of lipid peroxidation after renal ischemia. Am J Physiol 251:F839–F843, 1986.

31. Puschett JB: Do calcium channel blockers protect against renal ischemia? Am J Nephrol 7 (suppl 1):49–56, 1987.

32. Schanne FAX, Kane AB, Young EE, Farber JL: Calcium dependence of toxic cell death: A final common pathway. Science 206:700–702, 1979.

33. Schor N, Ichikawa I, Rennke HG, Troy JL, Brenner BM: Pathophysiology of altered glomerular function in aminoglysoside-treated rats. Kidney Int 19:288–296, 1981.

34. Schrier RW, Arnold PE, Van Putten VJ, Burke TJ: Cellular calcium in ischemic acute renal failure: Role of calcium entry blockers. Kidney Int 32:313–321, 1987.

35. Shah SV, Walker PD: Evidence suggesting a role for hydroxyl radical in glycerol-induced acute renal failure. Am J Physio 255:F438–F443, 1988.

36. Shridi F, Robak J: The influence of calcium channel blockers on superoxide anions. Pharm Res Comm 20:13–21, 1988.

37. Smith MT, Thor H, Orrenius S: Toxic injury to isolated hepatocytes is not dependent on extracellular calcium. Science 213:1257–1259, 1981.

38. Stoff JS, Clive DM: Role of arachidonic acid metabolites in acute renal failure. In Brenner BM, Lazarus JM (eds): Acute Renal Failure. Philadelphia, WB Saunders Co, 1988, p 143.

39. Sumpio B, Baue AE, Chaudry IH: Treatment with verapamil and adenosine triphosphate-$MgCL_2$ reduces cyclosporine nephrotoxicity. Surgery 101:315–322, 1987.

40. Wagner K, Albrecht S, Neumayer H-H: Prevention of posttransplant acute tubular necrosis by the calcium antagonist diltiazem: A prospective randomized study. Am J Nephrol 7:287–291, 1987.

41. Walker PD, Shah SV: Evidence suggesting a role for hydroxyl radical in gentamicin-induced acute renal failure in rats. J Clin Invest 81:334–341, 1988.

42. Watson AJ, Gimenez LF, Klassen DK, Stout RL, Whelton A: Calcium channel blockade in experimental aminoglycoside nephrotoxicity. J Clin Pharmacol 27:625–627, 1987.

43. Zager RA, Prior RB: Gentamicin and gram-negative bacteremia: A synergism for the development of experimental nephrotoxic acute renal failure. J Clin Invest 78:196–204, 1986.

Friedrich C. Luft, M.D.
Myron H. Weinberger, M.D.

11
Calcium Antagonists and
Renal Sodium Homeostasis

Calcium antagonists are gaining rapid acceptance in the treamtment of hypertension.[1] Their potent relaxing effect on vascular smooth muscle accounts for much of their efficacy in lowering total peripheral resistance.[2] However, increasing evidence suggests that calcium antagonists exert important effects upon the kidney that may also contribute to the reduction in blood pressure.[3] Contrary to other vasodilatory drugs that foster salt and water retention, calcium antagonists may facilitate the removal of salt and water from the body in a fashion not dissimilar to the action of diuretics.[4]

The action of calcium antagonists on renal function has been the subject of several recent reviews.[3-5] A number of features have been emphasized, including effects of calcium antagonists on renal blood flow, glomerular filtration rate, glomerular mesangial function, tubuloglomerular feedback and sodium transport, renin release, prostaglandin secretion, and aldosterone production. The natriuresis and diuresis observed with the calcium antagonists may be related to some of the above effects.

Several balance studies have been reported, which support the notion that the natriuretic action of calcium antagonists may be relevant to their blood pressure reducing effects.[6-8] Natriuresis may account in part for the apparent increased efficacy of calcium antagonists during the ingestion of a high-salt diet.

Acute Effects of Calcium Antagonists
on Sodium Excretion

A number of animal investigations have been performed evaluating the direct effect of calcium antagonists administered to experimental animals. In these studies, renal blood flow (RBF), glomerular filtration rate (GFR), and urinary sodium excretion (UNaV) were monitored (Table 1). An increase in UNaV was a prominent feature in all the studies.[9-16] RBF increased in most, whereas GFR increased in only half of the studies. These findings indicate that the localized renal effects of calcium antagonists,

203

TABLE 1. Effect of Calcium Blockers on Renal Function and Sodium Homeostasis in Animals*

Reference	Drug	BP ↓ (%)	RBF ↑ (%)	GFR ↑ (%)	UNaV ↑ (fold)
Abe	Nicardipine	none	30	17	6
Roy	Verapamil	none	16	42	4
Bell	Verapamil	none	11	75	20
Bell	Nifedipine	12	29	50	24
Yamaguchi	Diltiazem	none	11	17	2.6
Abe	Verapamil	none	39	none	4.5
Dietz	Verapamil	none	10	none	6
Dietz	Nifedipine	20	none	none	2.8
Burke	Verapamil	none	45	none	3.6
DiBona	Felodipine	10	none	none	2.4

*BP = blood pressure, RBF = renal blood flow, GFR = glomerular filtration rate, and UNaV = timed sodium excretion.

characterized by a systematic increment in RBF and UNaV, can be dissociated from increases in GFR. The increases in sodium excretion were observed despite decreases in blood pressure, which would ordinarily favor increased sodium reabsorption by reducing renal blood flow. In some of the investigations, RBF and GFR were controlled by renal artery clamping.[13] Nevertheless, natriuresis was persistently demonstrable. These observations suggest that, contrary to earlier points of view, the natriuretic effects of calcium antagonists cannot be solely attributed to hemodynamic effects.

The acute animal investigations also stress the importance of endogenous vasoconstrictors in adjusting vascular tone, and the subsequent vascular responses to the calcium antagonists. For instance, some of the studies have shown that calcium antagonists are capable of impeding the renal constrictor autoregulatory response induced by increases in perfusion pressure.[17,18] Other investigations have shown that the response to calcium antagonists is enhanced under circumstances when renal sympathetic tone is stimulated, or when endogenous circulating vasoconstrictor substances are likely to be present.[19,20] Calcium antagonists regularly increase RBF and GFR when the renal vasculature has been previously constricted with angiotensin II.[21] Such an effect is generally, but not invariably, observed with norepinephrine.[5,21] Variability in these factors can account for some of the variability observed in many of the experiments.

A series of investigations on the acute natriuretic effects of calcium antagonists has been performed in human subjects with or without hypertension. These investigations are briefly reviewed in Table 2. All classes of currently utilized calcium antagonists have been investigated. A decrease in blood pressure was uniformly observed in patients with hypertension, although in normotensive subjects this effect was not always demonstrable.[22-27] RBF and GFR were reported to increase in less than half of the studies. Nevertheless an increase in UNaV was observed in almost all of the studies in hypertensive subjects, and in most of the studies in normal subjects. Since natriuresis occurred often without demonstrable changes in renal blood flow or glomerular filtration rate, these observations suggest that the natriuretic responses may occur independent of intrarenal hemodynamic effects.

TABLE 2. Effects of Short-term Calcium Blockers on Renal Function and Sodium Homeostasis in Man*

Author	Drug	BP ↓ (%)	RBF ↑ (%)	GFR ↑ (%)	UNaV ↑ (fold)
(Hypertensive)					
Sakurai	Diltiazem	5	11	15	2.6
Leonetti	Verapamil	20	—	none	none
Leonetti	Nifedipine	30	—	none	2
Yokoyama	Nifedipine	3	45	46	1
Van Schaik	Nicardipine	5	—	11	3.3
(Normotensive)					
Leonetti	Verapamil	none	—	none	none
Leonetti	Nifedipine	none	—	none	none
Yokoyama	Nifedipine	4	2	6	0.1
Van Schaik	Nicardipine	5	—	none	3
Wallia	Nitrendipine	none	none	none	2.23
Luft	Nifedipine	none	none	none	0.3

*BP = blood pressure, RBF = renal blood flow, GFR = glomerular filtration rate, and UNaV = timed sodium excretion.

The mechanisms by which calcium antagonists induce natriuresis have not been completely elucidated. Clearly, hemodynamic effects within the kidney play a role. The effects of calcium antagonists on glomerular function are largely determined by pre-existing vascular tone. Loutzenhizer and Epstein conducted an illuminating series of investigations.[5] In isolated perfused kidney, diltiazem reversed the renal vasoconstriction induced by potassium chloride, an endoperoxide analog, or angiotensin II. The glomerular vasoconstrictor effect of norepinephrine was influenced as well, but to a lesser degree.

The effects of calcium antagonists on glomerular function may be in part related to their effects upon the glomerular mesangium. For instance, verapamil reduced deposition of macromolecules into the mesangium. The mesangium may play a regulatory role in long-term glomerular function and in that way may influence sodium homeostasis.[28–30]

Calcium antagonists may exert an effect on natriuresis by influencing the distribution of renal blood flow. Important effects on renal interstitial pressure and papillary plasma flow have been reported following calcium antagonist administration under a variety of experimental circumstances.[31] Some of these effects may be related to a redistribution of renal blood flow similar to that induced by acetylcholine or bradykinin. Calcium antagonists may also serve to influence the tubuloglomerular feedback mechanism.[32] Such a mechanism could be operative, particularly in situations featuring an increased afferent arteriolar tone resulting from altered regulation of cytosolic calcium in the macula densa.[33] Under such conditions, calcium antagonists could reset the mechanism regulating intrarenal perfusion pressure.

It is likely that calcium antagonists also exert direct tubular effects. Precisely how such effects relate to tubular cell cytosolic calcium is uncertain. Windhager and colleagues[34] presented a body of evidence that an increase in cytosolic calcium activity leads to a net inhibition of sodium transport. Thus, a decrease of cytosolic calcium by calcium blocking drugs would be expected to enhance renal tubular sodium reabsorption. Conceivably, calcium antagonists effect epithelial sodium transport by other mechanisms as well. For instance, calcium antagonists may bind to calmodulin,[35] which functions to regulate cyclic AMP levels by stimulating phosphodiesterase activity without affecting adenylate cyclase activity.[36] Such an action could influence the regulatory effects of calmodulin on intracellular cyclic AMP stores, and thus influence overall cellular energy metabolism. Further, sodium reabsorption by renal epithelium is influenced by renal nerves and involves adrenergic receptors.[37] Calcium blocking drugs may influence the actions of adrenergic mediators of tubular function by influencing the uptake and release of norepinephrine. A decrease in intracellular calcium would be expected to favor the re-uptake of norepinephrine by synaptic vesicles and thereby decrease its effects on post-synaptic receptors.[38]

DiBona and Sawin performed both clearance and micropuncture studies to elucidate the renal tubular site of action of felodipine.[16] In the clearance experiments, felodipine had no effect on arterial pressure or glomerular filtration rate, but significantly increased urinary flow rate, sodium, and potassium excretion. In re-collection micropuncture experiments, felodipine decreased mean arterial pressure but did not affect renal blood flow, renal vascular resistance, or glomerular filtration rate. Absolute and fractional urinary excretion of sodium and water, but not potassium, were increased. Proximal tubular and loop of Henle sodium, potassium, and water reabsorption were not affected, whereas distal tubular and collecting duct sodium and water reabsorption were decreased by felodipine. These effects indicate that felodipine decreased distal tubular and collecting duct sodium and water reabsorption while concomitantly decreasing arterial pressure.

Nagao et al.[39] contributed additional important information elucidating the actions of calcium antagonists on renal tubular epithelium by examining the effect of diltiazem on the urinary bladder of the bullfrog, a model of distal tubular function. When applied to the serosal surface, diltiazem suppressed short-circuit current. A weak, but reproducible, inhibition was also observed when diltiazem was applied to the mucosal surface. These results contrast to those observed with the diuretics hydrochlorothiazide and furosemide, which have selective effects on the mucosal surface. Ethacrynic acid, on the other hand, exerts selective serosal effects. The results support a direct effect of diltiazem on the distal tubule. Verapamil has also been reported to inhibit short-circuit current in amphibian bladders.[40]

In summary, acute and short-term experiments clearly demonstrate a natriuretic effect of calcium channel blocking drugs. The effect may be in part attributed to the actions of calcium antagonists on intrarenal hemodynamics and neural and hormonal mediators. However, a direct effect of calcium-blocking drugs on tubular epithelium appears likely. Indirect clearance methodology suggests that such an effect occurs in the proximal tubule, whereas micropuncture studies and short-circuit current experiments suggest a distal tubular effect. The potential significance of these effects is illustrated by long-term investigations in experimental animals and man.

Long-Term Effects on Renal Function and Salt Regulation

Guyton and co-workers developed a model of renal sodium cybernetics, in which the kidney functions as the final common pathway in blood pressure control through its regulation of salt and water excretion.[41] They described a fundamental relationship between renal salt and water excretion and blood pressure termed the "renal function curve." An ideal antihypertensive drug should restore that relationship to more normal values. The long-term antihypertensive effect of such an agent should feature renal function that is no different from that found in normal subjects. Moreover, the kidney's ability to regulate salt and water homeostasis, and eventually blood pressure, should be preserved over a wide range of dietary salt intake. Abnormal renal function curves have been defined in secondary forms of hypertension, and their restoration to a normal relationship has been described following operative intervention.[42] Antihypertensive drugs are not generally studied at several fixed, known levels of salt intake. However, several investigators have conducted studies examining the long-term effects of calcium antagonists on renal function. Most of these investigations indicate that renal function is preserved. Chronic treatment with diltiazem in doses ranging from 30 to 120 mg/day for 1 week to 3 months resulted in a persistent increase in RBF, often accompanied by increases in GFR. The administration of 120 to 240 mg of diltiazem twice daily for 8 weeks was effective in normalizing blood pressure in patients with essential hypertension while maintaining renal function in the normal range.[43] In this study, renal vascular resistance appeared to be reduced. Verapamil had no deleterious effects on renal function in patients with hypertension who were given the drug for as long as 12 months.[44] Verapamil had no effect on serum electrolytes, plasma volume or body weight in these studies. Similar results were reported for nitrendipine and nifedipine, although occasional decreases in renal function have been reported in some individuals.[45]

Collectively, most of the studies of the long-term effects of calcium antagonists indicate that elevated blood pressure can be reduced without impairing renal hemodynamics or renal excretory function. However, it is not known to what degree long-term treatment influences the kidney's ability to adjust to alterations in dietary salt intake. To effectively delineate this issue, a study would require different levels of known dietary salt intake coupled with detailed balance investigations in which all urine made is collected until homeostasis is achieved. Such studies have not been done for any antihypertensive agent. However, balance studies have been performed with calcium antagonists in which dietary salt intake was known and cumulative sodium balance was examined. In addition, a number of investigations have been reported in which the antihypertensive effect of calcium antagonists has been examined at different levels of dietary salt intake.

Huelsemann et al.[46] examined the effects of nitrendipine on a rat model of experimental hypertension induced by the chronic infusion of angiotensin II with implanted minipumps. The animals were maintained in metabolism cages. They received a known dietary salt intake, and 24-hour urine collections were made daily. With the administration of nitrendipine, blood pressure of rats receiving angiotensin II decreased rapidly to control values. Concomitantly, urine sodium excretion increased as blood pressure decreased, until balance was re-established.

Thananopavarn et al.[6] gave nitrendipine 20 to 40 mg daily to eight men with essential hypertension and observed them for 2 weeks. There was an increase in sodium excretion during the first 5 days of therapy despite a persistent antihypertensive effect of the drug. The natriuresis did not appear to be caused by either an increase in glomerular filtration rate or effective renal blood flow. A similar experience was reported by de Leeuwe and Birkenhager, who observed a diuresis and natriuresis in subjects who collected their urine for 7 days while ingesting verapamil.[6] The natriuresis and diuresis occurred in the face of a reduction in blood pressure.

We conducted a similar study of 8 normal and 8 mildly hypertensive subjects who were given a constant, 150 mmol/d sodium intake.[8] The subjects received all their meals in the Clinical Research Center and ingested precisely the same diet for a 2-week period. All urine made was collected. The study included a 7-day placebo period and a 7-day period during which the subjects received nitrendipine 20 mg daily. Nitrendipine resulted in a decrease in blood pressure in the hypertensive subjects and engendered approximately a 1 kg weight loss in both groups. Both normal and hypertensive subjects experienced a natriuresis of several days duration. The total amount of negative sodium balance amounted to about 150 mmol in both normal and hypertensive subjects and is not dissimilar to values quoted for thiazide diuretics in the treatment of patients with essential hypertension.[47] An increase in potassium excretion was not observed. Renin values in both groups of subjects, as well as plasma norepinephrine concentrations, increased significantly with the administration of nitrendipine. An increase in renin release is known to occur with a reduction of cytosolic calcium concentration in juxtaglomerular cells.[48] We attributed the modest increase in plasma norepinephrine concentrations to the effects of volume contraction. Interestingly, plasma aldosterone values did not increase in our subjects, even in the face of higher renin values. Calcium antagonists are known to suppress the renin-angiotensin II induced release of aldosterone from the adrenal gland.[49] This uncoupling of renin from aldosterone may work to the patient's advantage by inhibiting the secondary aldosteronism usually accompanying the administration of drugs that are natriuretic. Other investigators have confirmed the renin and aldosterone effects that we observed with long-term calcium antagonist administration.[50]

Curiously, the action of calcium antagonists on blood pressure does not appear to be enhanced by dietary salt restriction.[51] Morgan et al.[52] reported on 78 patients with mild essential hypertension who were randomized to no treatment, thiazide diuretics, centrally acting antisympathetic drugs, beta blockers, or calcium antagonists. The groups were then counseled to reduce their dietary salt intake, as verified by 24-hour urinary sodium excretion. Blood pressure remained the same in a nontreated, non-salt restricted control group. Salt restriction alone lowered blood pressure. Diuretics, centrally acting drugs, and beta blockers were all more effective when combined with reduced dietary salt intake. Interestingly, the blood pressure of patients receiving calcium antagonists actually increased during salt restriction.

MacGregor and colleagues[53] evaluated the effects of salt intake on the response to nifedipine, both as a single dose and in a longer protocol. In their single-dose study, they found that the decrease in blood pressure in hypertensive patients following a single 5-mg dose of nifedipine was greater when a diet containing 350 mmol/d sodium was ingested than when the intake was 150 mmol/d or 10 mmol/d. Initial blood pressure values were also greater at the higher two levels of salt intake. These results were corroborated in a 15-day study period.[54]

Nicholson et al.[55] gave 8 patients low (10 mmol/d) or high (200 mmol/d) salt diets, and found that the decrease in blood pressure of their subjects following three doses of verapamil was greater at the higher level of salt intake than at the lower level of salt intake. These results were corroborated in a longer term study in which

8 patients received nitrendipine for 1 month.[56] The drug was more effective when dietary salt intake was generous (sodium excretion 250 mmol/d) compared to when salt intake was reduced (sodium excretion 50 mmol/d).

As indicated previously, calcium antagonists do not cause weight gain and are natriuretic. Thus, contrary to drugs that promote sodium retention, such as the direct-acting vasodilators, they may not require diuretics or salt restriction to exert a maximum effect. Further, if salt-sensitive hypertension is indeed mediated by an inhibitor of sodium transport that is responsible for an increase in cytosolic calcium, calcium antagonists should be more effective under conditions when such a circulating inhibitor is most active. A diet rich in salt would promote high levels of such a natriuretic material. Verapamil binds to alpha-2 receptors on platelets and in that way may compete with alpha-2 receptor agonists for these sites.[57] Alpha-2 receptor number has been found to increase in salt-sensitive individuals with ingestion of a high-salt diet.[58] It is possible that verapamil may impede alpha-2 receptor activation at high levels of salt intake in such subjects.

The effect of salt restriction on treatment with calcium antagonists is incompletely defined, as it is for all of the antihypertensive drugs currently employed.[51] The studies available are short-term, lacking in statistical power, and are not generally directed at pathophysiologic mechanisms. Additional balance studies at more than one known level of salt intake are warranted to delineate the effects of calcium antagonists on the hypertensive renal function curve. In that regard, a comparison of calcium antagonists to conventional diuretic agents would be informative.

References

1. Bühler FR, Hulthen L: Calcium channel blockers: a pathophysiologically based antihypertensive treatment concept for the future? Euro J. Clin Invest 12:1–3, 1982.

2. Fleckenstein A: History of calcium antagonists. Circ Res 52(Suppl I):3–16, 1983.

3. Romero J, Raij L, Granger JP, Ruilope LM, Rodicio JL: Multiple effects of calcium entry blockers on renal function in hypertension. Hypertension 10:140–151, 1987.

4. Luft FC: Calcium channel blocking drugs and renal sodium excretion. Am J Nephrol 1988 (in press).

5. Loutzenhiser R, Epstein M: Effects of calcium antagonists on renal hemodynamics. Am J Physiol 249:F619–F629, 1985.

6. de Leeuwe PW, Birkenhager WH: Effects of verapamil in hypertensive patients. Acta Med Scand 681(Suppl):125–128, 1984.

7. Thananopavarn C, Golub H, Eggena P, Barrett J, Sambhi MP: Renal effects of nitrendipine monotherapy in essential hypertension. J Cardiovasc Pharmacol 6(Suppl): 125–128, 1985.

8. Luft FC, Aronoff GR, Sloan RS, Fineberg NS, Weinberger MH: Calcium channel blockade with nitrendipine: effects on sodium homeostasis, the renin-angiotensin system, and the sympathetic nervous system in humans. Hypertension 7:438–442, 1985.

9. Abe Y, Komori T, Miura K, et al.: Effects of the calcium antagonist nicardipine on renal function and renin release in dogs. J Cardiovasc Pharmacol 5:254–259, 1983.

10. Roy MW, Guthrie GP, Holladay FP, Kotchen TA: Effects of verapamil on renin and aldosterone in the dog and rat. Am J Physiol 245:E410–E416, 1983.

11. Bell AJ, Linder A: Effects of verapamil and nifedipine on renal function and hemodynamics in the dog. Renal Physiol 7:329–343, 1984.

12. Yamaguchi J, Ikezawa K, Takada T, Kiyomoto A: Studies on a new 1,5 benzothiazepine derivative (CRD-401): VI. Effects on renal blood flow and renal function. Jpn J Pharmacol 24:511–522, 1974.

13. Abe Y, Yukimura T, Iwao H, Mori N, Okahara T, Yamamoto K: Effects of EDTA and verapamil on renin release in dogs. Jpn J Pharmacol 33:627–622, 1983.

14. Dietz JR, Davis JO, Freeman RH, Villarreal D, Echtenkamp SF: Effects of intrarenal infusion of calcium entry blockers in anesthetized dogs. Hypertension 5:482–488, 1983.

15. Burke TJ, Arnold PE, Gordon JA, Bulger RE, Dobyan DC, Schrier RW: Protective effect of intrarenal calcium membrane blockers before or after renal ischemia: functional, morphological, and mitochondrial studies. J Clin Invest 74:1830–1841, 1984.

16. DiBona GF, Sawin LL: Renal tubular site of action of felodipine. J Pharmacol Exp Ther 228:420–424, 1984.

17. Ono H, Kokubun H, Hashimoto K: Abolition by calcium antagonists of the autoregulation of renal blood flow. Naunyn Schmiedebergs Arch Pharmacol 285:201–207, 1974.

18. Cohen AJ, Fray JCS: Calcium ion dependence of myogenic renal plasma flow autoregulation: evidence from the isolated perfused rat kidney. J Physiol (Lond) 330:449–460, 1982.

19. Pelletier CL, Shepherd JT: Relative influence of carotid baroreceptors and muscle receptors in the control of renal and hindlimb circulations. Can J Physiol Pharmacol 53:1042–1049, 1975.

20. Ishikawa H, Matsushima M, Matsui H, et al: Effects of diltiazem hydrochloride on renal hemodynamics of dogs. Arzneimittleforsch Drug Res 28:402–406, 1978.

21. Goldberg JP, Schrier RW: Effect of calcium membrane blockers on in vivo vasoconstrictor properties of norepinephrine, angiotensin II and vasopressin. Mineral Electrolyte Metab 10:178–183, 1984.

22. Sakurai T, Kurita T, Nagano S, Sonoda T: Antihypertensive vasodilating and sodium diuretic actions of D-cis isomer of benzothiazepine derivative (CRD-401). Acta Biol Jpn 18:695–701, 1972.

23. Leonetti G, Cuspidi C, Sampiere L, Terzoli L, Zanchetti A: Comparison of cardiovascular, renal, and humoral effects of acute administration of two calcium channel blockers in normotensive and hypertensive subjects. J Cardiovasc Pharmacol 4(Suppl 3):319–323, 1982.

24. Yokoyama S, Kaburagi T: Clinical effects of intravenous nifedipine on renal function. J Cardiovasc Pharmacol 5:67–71, 1983.

25. Van Schaik BAM, Van Nistelrooy AEJ, Geyskes GG: Antihypertensive and renal effects of nicardipine. Br J Clin Pharmacol 18:57–63, 1984.

26. Wallia R, Greenberg A, Puschett JB: Renal hemodynamic and tubular transport effects of nitrendipine. J Lab Clin Med 105:498–503, 1985.

27. Luft FC, Aronoff GR, Weinberger MH: Effect of oral calcium, potassium, nifedipine, and digoxin on natriuresis in normal man. Am J Hypertens 2: 14-19, 1989.

28. Michael AF, Deane WF, Raij L, Vernier RL, Mauer SM: The glomerular mesangium (editorial). Kidney Int 17:141–154, 1980.

29. Raij L, Michael AF: Immunologic aspects of kidney disease. In Parker CW (ed): Clinical Immunology Vol 2. Philadelphia, Saunders, 1980, pp 1051–1087.

30. Raij L, Keane WF: Glomerular mesangium: Its function and relationship to angiotensin II. Am J Med 5:254–259, 1985.

31. Abe Y, Okahara T, Yamamoto K: Effect of D-3-acetoxy-2, 3-dihydro-5-2-(dimethylamino) etyl-2-(P-methoxyphenyl)-1, 5-benzothiazepine-4 (5H)-one-hydrochloride (CRD) on renal function in the dog. Jpn Circ J 36:1002–1003, 1972.

32. Mueller-Suur R, Gutsche HU, Schurek HJ: Acute and reversible inhibition of tubuloglomerular feedback mediated afferent vasoconstriction by the calcium antagonist verapamil. Curr Probl Clin Biochem 6:291–297, 1976.

33. Bell PD, Navar, LG: Cytoplasmic calcium in the mediation of macula densa tubuloglomerular feedback responses. Science 215:670–673, 1982.

34. Windhager E, Frindt G, Yang JM, Lee CO: Intracellular calcium ions as regulators of renal tubular sodium transport. Klin Wochenschr 64:847–852, 1986.

35. Bronstrom SL, Ljung B, Mardh S, Forsen S, Thulin E: Interaction of the antihypertensive drug felodepine with calmodulin. Nature 292:777–778, 1981.

36. Morgan D, Kim S, Campbell BJ, Cheung WY, Lynch T: Purification and characterization of calmodulin from porcine renal medulla. Arch Biochem Biophys 205:510–519, 1980.

37. DiBona GF: Neural mechanisms of volume regulation. Ann Intern Med 98(Part 2):750–759, 1983.

38. Blaustein MP, Hamlyn JM: Sodium transport inhibition, cell calcium, and hypertension. Am J Med 77(Suppl):45–59, 1984.

39. Nagao T, Yamaguchi I, Narita H, Nakajima H: Calcium entry blockers: antihypertensive and natriuretic effects in experimental animal models. Am J Cardiol 65:56H–61H, 1985.

40. Bently PJ: Effects of verapamil on the short-circuit current of an epithelial membrane; the toad urinary bladder. J Pharmacol Exp Ther 189:563–569, 1974.

41. Guyton AC, Coleman TG, Cowley AW, Scheel KW, Manning RD, Norman RA: Arterial pressure regulation: overriding dominance of the kidneys in long-term regulation and in hypertension. Am J Med 52:584–594, 1972.

42. Kimura G, Saito F, Kohma S, et al.: Renal function cure in patients with secondary forms of hypertension. Hypertension 10:11–15, 1987.

43. Sunderrajan S, Reams G, Bauer JH: Renal effects of diltiazem in primary hypertension. Hypertension 8:238–242, 1986.

44. Erne P, Bolli P, Bertel O, et al: Factors influencing the hypertensive effects of calcium antagonists. Hypertension 5(Suppl II):II97–II102, 1983.

45. Diamond JR, Cheung JY, Fang LST: Nifedipine-induced renal dysfunction: alterations in renal hemodynamics. Am J Med 77:905–909, 1984.

46. Huelsemann JL, Sterzel RB, McKenzie DE, Wilcox CS: Effects of a calcium entry blocker on blood pressure and renal function during angiotensin-induced Hypertension. 7:374–379, 1985.

47. Freis ED, Wanko A, Wilson IM, Parish AE: Chlorothiazide in hypertensive and normotensive patients. Ann NY Acad Sci 71:450–455, 1958.

48. Kurtz A: Intracellular control of renin release: an overview. Klin Wochenschr 64:838–846, 1986.

49. Guthrie GP, McAllister RG, Kotchen TA: Effects of intravenous and oral verapamil upon pressure and adrenal steroidogenic responses in normal man. J Clin Endocrinol Metab 57:339–343, 1983.

50. Pedrinelli R, Fouad FM, Tarazi RC, Bravo EL, Textor SC: Nitrendipine, a calcium entry blocker: renal and humoral effects in human hypertension. Arch Intern Med 146:62–65, 1986.

51. Luft FC, Weinberger MH: Review of salt restriction and the response to antihypertensive drugs. Hypertension 11 (suppl 4): I-229-232, 1988.

52. Morgan T, Anderson A, Wilson D, Myers J, Murphy J, Nowson C: Paradoxical effect of sodium restriction on blood pressure in people on slow-channel calcium blocking drugs. Lancet 1:793, 1986.

53. MacGregor GA, Cappuccio FP, Markandu ND: Sodium intake, high blood pressure, and calcium channel blockers. Am J Med 82(Suppl 3b):16–22, 1987.

54. Cappuccio FP, Markandu ND, MacGregor GA: Calcium antagonists and sodium balance. J Pharmacol Cardiovasc (in press).

55. Nicholson JP, Pickering TG, Resnick LM, Laragh JH: The hypotensive effect of calcium channel blockade with verapamil is enhanced by increased dietary sodium intake. Clin Res 32:245A, 1984.

56. Nicholson JP, Resnick LM, James GD, Jennis R: Sodium restriction and the antihypertensive effect of nitrendipine. Clin Res 34:404A, 1986.

57. Motulsky HJ, Smavely MD, Hughes RJ, Insel PA: Interaction of verapamil and other calcium channel blockers with alpha-1 and alpha-2 adrenergic receptors. Circ Res 52:226–231, 1983.

58. Skrabal F, Kotanko P, Meister B, Doll P, Gruber G: Up regulation of alpha-2 adrenoceptors and down regulation of beta-2 adrenoceptors by high salt diet in normotensives: enhanced up regulation of "operative (a-2/b-2) adrenoceptor ratio" predicts salt sensitivity. J Hypertens 4(Suppl 6):S136–S139, 1986.

Graham A. MacGregor, M.A., FRCP

12

Sodium Balance and Calcium Antagonists in Hypertension

There is now much circumstantial and some direct clinical evidence to suggest that a high intake of salt predisposes patients to the development of essential hypertension.[1] The recent INTERSALT study, in which carefully controlled measurements of blood pressure and urinary electrolytes were done in 52 communities around the world, has clearly demonstrated that salt intake is related to blood pressure both across different communities and within many individual communities.[2] In those communities where salt intake was low there was no hypertension. This study therefore confirms previous less rigorous studies that had suggested that a high salt intake is an important factor in the development of essential hypertension.

Potential Mechanisms

Although a high intake of salt predisposes towards the development of high blood pressure, the mechanism underlying the rise in pressure is not known. One possibility is that there is a renal defect either inherited or acquired that may impair the kidney's ability to excrete sodium.[3] On a high sodium intake this would lead to extracellular volume expansion and eventually by autoregulation to the development of an increase in peripheral resistance, and thereby an increase in blood pressure. However, a major problem with this concept is the lack of substantial evidence indicating extracellular volume expansion in patients with essential hypertension. Indeed, total plasma volume in most patients is either normal or, indeed, low. However, patients with essential hypertension may have a reduction in venous compliance and thereby a reduction in the capacitance of the circulatory system, with a shift of blood towards the thorax.[4] Therefore, the measurement of total plasma volume would not then be a reliable index of whether the kidney is tending to retain sodium.

Cross-transplantation experiments clearly demonstrate that the kidneys play a major role in the development of high blood pressure in rats with inherited hypertension.[4] Studies from human renal transplants also suggest that there might be an inherited abnormality in the kidney responsible for the development of essential hypertension.[5]

If a subject inherited a kidney that was less able to excrete sodium on a high salt intake, there would be a tendency towards sodium retention, which would stimulate various mechanisms to increase sodium excretion. The recent finding that plasma levels of atrial natriuretic peptides are elevated in many patients with established hypertension indirectly may support this concept.[6] Previous work has also shown that in many patients with essential hypertension there is inhibition of the sodium potassium pump on the cell membrane and that this inhibition, particularly that found in the white cells, may be due to a circulating plasma factor.[7] Cross-incubation experiments with white cells from normotensive subjects that were incubated in hypertensive plasma acquired the same reduction in sodium transport as the hypertensives' own white cells. However, the exact nature and structure of this sodium transport inhibitor remains to be clarified.

If there is an increase in circulating sodium transport inhibitor in essential hypertension, there are several potential mechanisms whereby this inhibitor could increase vascular reactivity. For instance, inhibition of sodium transport across arteriolar smooth muscle cells could lead to a decrease in membrane potential, making depolarization of arteriolar smooth muscle cells more likely. If it worked in a similar way to ouabain, it is possible that it could enhance release of noradrenaline from sympathetic ganglia and at the same time might reduce the reuptake of noradrenaline leading to an increase in sympathetic tone and, thereby, a rise in blood pressure. Blaustein suggested another potential mechanism whereby inhibition of the sodium pump by an increase in intracellular sodium could inhibit sodium calcium exchange, leading to an increase in intracellular calcium.[8] At the same time there is accumulating evidence of independent abnormalities of calcium binding and calcium transport across the arteriolar smooth muscle cell in essential hypertension independent of any changes in the sodium potassium pump.[9]

Calcium Antagonists

The calcium antagonists were first used in the 1960s without clear therapeutic indications. Their mode of action was not fully understood. They were then found to dilate coronary arteries, and it was felt they might be useful in patients with angina. Fleckenstein, in pioneering studies, showed that both verapamil and nifedipine inhibited calcium-dependent excitation contraction of isolated cardiac capillary muscle, and it became apparent that at least in part the action of the calcium entry antagonists was through inhibition of calcium flux across the cell membrane.[10] Studies with verapamil and nifedipine in the late 1960s and 1970s clearly demonstrated that both drugs could lower blood pressure when it was raised, and there was little effect of either drug on blood pressure in normotensive subjects. This important therapeutic indication was not realized, as it was felt that the fall in blood pressure that was seen was likely to lead to a complication of a drug that was then being found increasingly useful in patients with angina.

Subsequent studies have shown that the fall in blood pressure with the calcium antagonists is due to peripheral vasodilation with no long-term change in cardiac output or heart rate, although nifedipine acutely can cause transient increases in heart rate and cardiac output.[11] Fleckenstein was the first to show with verapamil and subsequently with nifedipine that they both caused a reduction in the uptake of radiolabeled calcium into cardiac cells and that inhibition of muscle contraction that occurred could be overcome by increasing extracellular calcium.[10] It was assumed, therefore, that the overall effect of nifedipine was due to a reduction in intracellular calcium in arteriolar smooth muscle and this presumably led to vasodilation of the arteriole.

Independent studies by Robinson[12] and Buhler's group[13] showed that infusion of verapamil into the brachial artery caused a greater increase in forearm blood flow in hypertensive subjects compared to normotensive subjects. This difference in response to verapamil was more impressive if the results were compared to those obtained with nitroprusside. Indeed, Robinson was able to show that the increase in forearm blood flow with verapamil relative to nitroprusside was greater the higher the blood pressure[9] (Fig. 1). This latter finding makes it unlikely that a structural alteration in the arteriole could account for the greater response to verapamil. Buhler's group subsequently confirmed that nitrendipine, a dihydropyridine derivative similar to nifedipine, also caused the same enhanced vasodilation in the forearm, suggesting that the blood pressure fall with the calcium-entry antagonists is at least in part determined by a functional abnormality of arteriolar smooth muscle as blood pressure increases. Several early studies suggested that the higher the pretreatment blood pressure, the greater the decrease in blood pressure following treatment with nifedipine, but these studies looked at absolute rather than percentage changes in blood pressure, and the normotensive subjects tended to be younger than the hypertensive subjects.[14,15]

Blaustein's hypothesis suggests that the more severe the hypertension, the more intracellular calcium in arteriolar smooth muscle may be raised. We therefore decided to re-examine the acute effect of nifedipine in a group of age-matched, normotensive and hypertensive subjects.[16] Blood pressure was measured before and at 30 min and 2 hr after a single 5 mg capsule of nifedipine. At 30 min the hypertensive patients demonstrated a significantly greater decrease in mean blood pressure (10.4%) com-

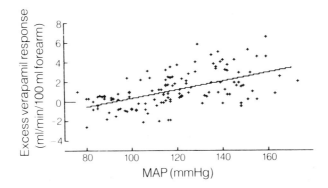

FIGURE 1.   Relationship between mean arterial pressure (MAP) and responsiveness of resistant vessels of the forearm to verapamil in 127 men, including both normal subjects and patients with essential hypertension. The dilatory response to verapamil has been normalized by relating the response to sodium nitroprusside in the same subject ($r = 0.55$) ($P < 0.001$). For further details see ref. 9. Reproduced with permission from Robinson BF, Hypertens, 1984.[9]

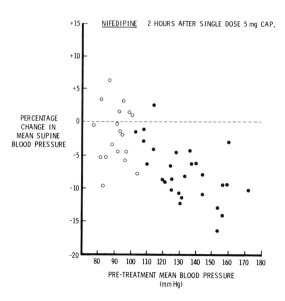

FIGURE 2.   The percentage change in mean supine blood pressure 2 hr after the administration of a single 5 mg capsule of nifedipine in a group of normotensive and hypertensive subjects who were age and sex matched.

pared with the normotensive subjects (4.7%) (P < 0.001). The same difference in response was observed after 2 hr and, as seen in Figure 2, the fall in blood pressure tended to be greater the higher the blood pressure before nifedipine was given. However, one problem in interpreting these studies is that when the fall in blood pressure is calculated the pretreatment blood pressure is used. This can give rise to misleading correlations, making it difficult to interpret whether the pretreatment blood pressure is an important predictive factor or not. However, these statistical problems can be overcome by plotting the pretreatment blood pressure against the posttreatment blood pressure, and then examining the slope of the line that is obtained against the line of identity. Using these methods, and particularly when the blood pressure is plotted on a log scale so that the percentage or ratio change in blood pressure is examined, it is clear that the higher the blood pressure, the greater the percentage or ratio fall in blood pressure with nifedipine[17] (Fig. 3), indicating that, with higher blood pressure in the hypertensive subjects, the functional abnormality of the smooth muscle cell that is revealed with the forearm studies does appear to become greater. These changes in blood pressure with nifedipine contrast with those that we have found in similar studies with beta-blockers and converting enzyme inhibitors.[18]

Buhler and colleagues have claimed that there may be other predictive factors to the fall in blood pressure with calcium antagonists, particularly age and renin,[19] and others more recently have claimed evidence that black patients may respond better. However, none of these studies has allowed for the importance of the severity of blood pressure before treatment. It remains unclear, therefore, whether, if the severity of hypertension is allowed for, other factors such as age, renin or race make any difference in the response to calcium antagonists. Evidence in animals also supports the concept that the calcium antagonists have a greater effect the higher the blood

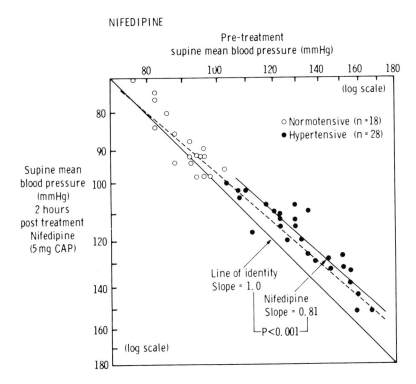

NIFEDIPINE

FIGURE 3. Relationship between pretreatment mean supine blood pressure in 18 normotensive and 28 hypertensive subjects vs. mean supine blood pressure 2 hr after the administration of a single 5 mg capsule of nifedipine (note log scale). The slopes of the correlation line for the hypertensive patients (—) and the group of patients as a whole (---) are significantly less than the slope of the line of identity, indicating that nifedipine becomes more effective the higher the blood pressure. Reproduced with permission from MacGregor et al, Lancet, 1985.[17]

pressure, in contrast to some other drugs. For instance studies with nitrendipine compared to hydralazine have shown that in the spontaneously hypertensive rat nitrendipine caused a greater fall in blood pressure in the hypertensive rat compared to the normotensive rat, whereas hydralazine caused a similar fall in blood pressure in both hypertensive and normotensive rats.[20]

Response to Nifedipine When Sodium Intake is Altered

The effects of most antihypertensive agents are potentiated by a reduction in salt intake, and their blood pressure lowering effect is blunted by a high intake of salt. The Blaustein hypothesis predicts that a high salt intake might increase intracellular calcium.[8] This raises the possibility that the calcium entry antagonists might be more effective with patients on a high salt intake. We therefore studied the acute effect of nifedipine in patients with essential hypertension receiving various amounts of salt in their diet.[21]

Ten patients with essential hypertension were studied on their normal diet with a sodium intake of approximately 150 mmols/day. The patients were then given a high sodium diet of 350 mmols/day for 5 days, followed by 5 days of a low sodium diet of 10 mmols/day. A single capsule of nifedipine was given orally on the 5th day of each diet, and blood pressure was measured before and 30 min after the capsule was given. There were significant falls in blood pressure in patients on all three diets with nifedipine. However, the decrease in blood pressure on the high sodium diet (10.7%) was significantly greater than the decrease in patients receiving the normal diet[21] ($P < 0.05$)(Fig. 4). Subsequently seven patients with essential hypertension were studied in a double-blind, randomized, crossover study. They received a similar sequence of normal, high, and low sodium diets, but this time they were given either placebo throughout the 15 days of the diet or nifedipine tablets 20 mg twice a day for the 15 days. The difference in blood pressure between those on placebo and nifedipine was greater on the high sodium diet than on the low sodium diet, but this difference failed to reach statistical significance.[21]

Studies with verapamil have also shown that the blood pressure fall tends to increase on a high sodium intake.[22] The finding, therefore, that a high sodium intake appears at the very least not to blunt the effect and may possibly enhance the effect of the calcium antagonists is of interest. The studies, however, do not provide any evidence as to what the possible mechanism for this effect could be. It is possible that salt loading is associated with a higher level of a sodium transport inhibitor, which could give rise to an increase in the calcium concentration in arteriolar smooth muscle, thereby enhancing the hypertensive effect of nifedipine. It is also possible that the natriuretic and diuretic effects of nifedipine may play a role in determining these results, although this is less likely when examining acute changes in blood pressure. Whether these acute results that have been found with both nifedipine and verapamil apply to more chronic therapy is not clear, but the intriguing possibility is suggested that in hypertensive patients on long-term treatment with a calcium entry antagonist, salt restriction may not be additive. As yet no studies have examined this important question.

Nifedipine and Diuretics

In Europe in the late 1970s and early 1980s nifedipine was increasingly being used as a third-line agent in patients with resistant hypertension. As nifedipine was regarded as an arteriolar vasodilator, it was assumed by most investigators that it would be additive to the combination of a beta-blocker and a diuretic in a similar way to hydralazine and minoxidil. However, out studies, in which we had altered salt intake and looked at the acute effect of nifedipine, suggested the possibility that diuretics might not be so effective in the presence of nifedipine. A study by Rosenthal and colleagues had shown to their surprise that, when nifedipine and a thiazide diuretic were combined, there was no greater effect on blood pressure than with either drug alone.[23] To examine this question further we conducted two separate studies, one where patients were given bendrofluazide first and then nifedipine was added, and a separate study where nifedipine was given first and bendrofluazide was then added to the regimen.[24]

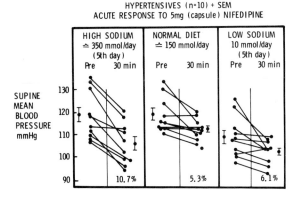

FIGURE 4. Changes in mean supine blood pressure before and 30 min after a 5 mg capsule of nifedipine in 10 patients with essential hypertension who were studied on the 5th day of a high, normal and low sodium diet.

Patients and Methods

Twenty-four patients with essential hypertension who had been referred to the Blood Pressure Unit by local general practitioners were studied. They had been seen regularly every 2–4 weeks for at least 2 months before entering the study and had either not received previous treatment or, if they had, it was stopped at least 2 weeks before the study. Diuretics were stopped at least 4 weeks prior to the study. Patients were then entered into the study if, after a further month's observation on no treatment, their supine diastolic pressure was greater than 95 mmHg. Patients were excluded if there was evidence of renal failure, ischemic heart disease, or cerebrovascular disease, or if they were taking any oral contraceptive or other medications. All patients were studied on their normal diet and no dietary advice was given.

First Study

Twelve patients (9 men, 3 women; 7 white, 5 black; mean age 50 ± 3 yrs) were studied. Average supine blood pressure after 1 month's observation on no treatment was 170/108 ± 8/3 mmHg. Bendrofluazide 5 mg once daily was given for a month and nifedipine tablets 20 mg twice daily were then added to the diuretic for 2 weeks.

Second Study

Twelve patients (6 men, 6 women; 9 white, 3 black; mean age 53 ± 3 yrs) were studied. Average supine blood pressure was 169/106 ± 4/2 mmHg after 1 month's observation on no treatment. Nifedipine tablets 20 mg twice daily were given for a month, and bendrofluazide 5 mg once daily was then added to the nifedipine for an additional month.

During both studies, patients were seen every 2 weeks in the Blood Pressure Unit between 9–10 a.m.; each patient was seen on the same day of the week by the same nurse in the same room, and blood pressure was measured in the arm by nurses using a semiautomatic ultrasound sphygmomanometer (Arteriosonde) with attached recorders. Measurements were therefore free from observer bias. Supine and standing blood pressures were the means of five readings taken at 1- to 2-min intervals with the patient in the corresponding position.

In the first study, bendrofluazide caused a significant fall in blood pressure; mean blood pressures fell by 7.1% (P < 0.01). The addition of nifedipine tablets showed a further significant fall in blood pressure of approximately 10% (P < 0.001), resulting in a fall in mean blood pressure compared with the pretreatment blood pressure of 17% (Fig. 5).

In the second study, when nifedipine alone was given first, there was a highly significant fall in blood pressure; mean blood pressures fell by 14.1% (P < 0.001). The addition of bendrofluazide for a 2nd month did not cause any further significant fall in blood pressure (Fig. 5). In both studies there was the expected fall in plasma potassium and increase in uric acid seen with the use of the diuretic.

These findings have given rise to some controversy. A study from Kenya did show an additional effect of a diuretic when it was added to patients already on nifedipine.[25] Clearly, at present the number of studies published on this interesting question is small and the results may well depend on inter-individual differences and particularly compliance with the nifedipine regimen. Although it is difficult at present to draw an overall consensus, there would appear little to be gained by adding a diuretic to nifedipine therapy, as at the very least the blood pressure lowering effect appears to be blunted and the diuretics may cause adverse metabolic effects as well as serious side effects.[26] In a double-blind study where patients were already on nifedipine and atenolol, we were unable to find any additional effect of a diuretic on blood pressure,[27] but whether this applies to patients on the combination of nifedipine and a converting-enzyme inhibitor is not clear.

Nifedipine and Sodium Excretion

Several studies have demonstrated that nifedipine acutely causes an increase in sodium and water excretion.[28,29] Intriguingly, one study demonstrated that this acute increase in sodium and water excretion is greater in patients with high blood pressure compared to normotensive subjects.[30] The mechanism whereby nifedipine causes a natriuresis is not clear. Initially it was thought to be due to changes in renal hemo-dynamics, but recent studies with felodipine have shown that this dihydropyridine derivative has a direct tubular effect on sodium excretion and that the changes that are seen in glomerular filtration rate and renal blood flow are probably either too small or too inconsistent for the natriuresis to be explained (see also Chapter 11).[31]

However, it was not clear from these studies whether the loss of sodium was maintained in the longer term, and most investigators had assumed that, although there was a transient loss of sodium, sodium balance came back to the same level with long-term therapy. To examine this further we studied the effect of the withdrawal of nifedipine on sodium balance in patients who had been on it long-term.[24] So far, 6 patients (3 black, 3 white; 2 women, 4 men; mean age 58 yrs) with essential

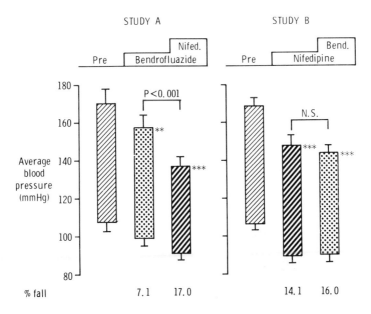

FIGURE 5. Study A: Average systolic and diastolic blood pressure changes in 12 patients on no treatment after 1 month of bendrofluazide 5 mg a day and then after a further month of nifedipine 20 mg twice daily combined with the bendrofluazide. Study B: Average systolic and diastolic blood pressures in 12 patients on no treatment after 1 month of nifedipine tablets 20 mg twice daily and after 1 month of the combination of nifedipine with 5 mg of bendrofluazide added. ** = $P < 0.01$; *** = $P < 0.001$ for the difference of mean blood pressure as compared with pretreatment values. Reproduced with permission from MacGregor et al, Am J Nephrol, 1987.

hypertension who had been on treatment with nifedipine retard tablets 20 mg twice a day for at least 6 weeks (range 6–45 wks) have been studied. Patients were placed on a constant dietary intake of sodium 150 mmols/day and potassium 80 mmols/day. All food and drink were supplied by the metabolic kitchen. The patients were studied as outpatients and seen daily in the hospital. After a control period on this diet nifedipine was stopped and replaced by matching placebo tablets in a single-blind fashion for 7 days. Daily measurements were made of 24-hr urinary sodium excretion, blood pressure and weight. During the control phase of the study (that is, when patients remained on nifedipine), the mean urinary sodium excretion was 137 ± 14 mmols/24 hrs. This fell significantly to 64 ± 8 mmols on the first day after nifedipine withdrawal ($P < 0.02$), and during the second day the urinary sodium excretion was 98 ± 13 mmols. The mean cumulative positive sodium balance for 7 days off nifedipine was 132 ± 39 mmols.

    Changes in cumulative sodium balance and weight in a representative patient are illustrated in Figure 6. In this particular patient nifedipine tablets were resumed 1 week after stopping them, and it can be seen from the changes in sodium balance that there was a subsequent loss of sodium when nifedipine was restarted, associated with a reduction in weight as well. Although these studies are in a small number of patients, they do suggest that nifedipine does have a long-term effect on sodium balance (see Chapter 13). In other words, the acute loss of sodium is maintained in the

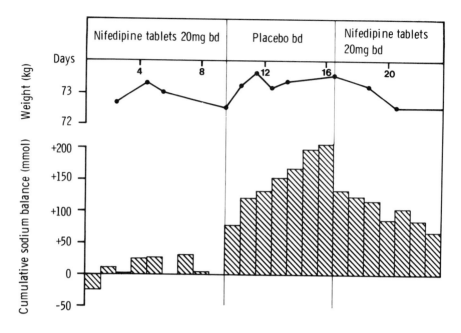

FIGURE 6. Changes in cumulative sodium balance and body weight in a patient who had been on long-term nifedipine treatment. Nifedipine was stopped for 7 days and then restarted. Reproduced with permission from MacGregor et al, Am J Nephrol, 1987.

longer term in a similar way to that which occurs with a thiazide diuretic. This could play an important additive role in its blood pressure lowering effect and contrasts with other peripheral arteriolar vasodilators such as minoxidil and hydralazine, where there is invariably sodium retention. Nifedipine can, in some patients, cause edema of the ankles and legs, but this does not appear to be associated with sodium retention and is more likely related to a change in capillary hemodynamics. The mechanism for the natriuresis caused by nifedipine is of some interest, since this effect appears to be without metabolic effects in contrast to thiazide diuretics.

Nifedipine in Combination with Other Drugs

Beta-blockers

Many studies have shown that nifedipine has an additive effect on blood pressure when combined with a beta-blocker, irrespective of the order in which the drugs are given. Combination of a beta-blocker with nifedipine may possibly reduce the acute vasodilating symptoms attributable to the nifedipine. Certainly, when the beta-blocker is added, there is a similar fall in heart rate to that seen for the beta-blocker alone (for review see McCarthy et al. [32]). A recent large study in a general practice setting showed that nifedipine and atenolol had an additional effect on blood pressure compared to either drug alone.[33] Several studies have demonstrated in patients with more resistant hypertension that the addition of nifedipine to a beta-blocker causes a further fall in blood pressure, often with good control of blood pressure in the long term.[34]

Nifedipine and Converting-enzyme Inhibitors

Several reports have suggested that nifedipine and converting-enzyme inhibitors have an additive effect on blood pressure. Nifedipine is known at least acutely to cause a rise in renin release and therefore angiotensin II, and most long-term studies have also shown a small but significant increase in plasma renin activity (see Chapter 7). In patients with moderate hypertension we demonstrated an additive effect of captopril to nifedipine and an additive effect of nifedipine to captopril.[35] However, the effect of this combination was relatively short-acting. One advantage of using the combination of a calcium antagonist and converting-enzyme inhibitor is that patients with more severe hypertension can be controlled without the need for large doses of diuretic.

References

1. MacGregor GA: Sodium is more important than calcium in essential hypertension. Hypertension 7:628–637, 1985.

2. The INTERSALT Cooperative Research Group: INTERSALT, An international study of electrolyte excretion and blood pressure. 12th Scientific Meeting of the International Society of Hypertension Tokyo, Japan. Abstract No. 0001, 1988.

3. Borst JGG, Borst de Geus A: Hypertension explained by Starling's theory of circulatory homeostasis. Lancet i:667–682, 1963.

4. de Wardener HE, MacGregor GA: The relation of a circulating transport inhibitor (the natriuretic hormone?) to hypertension. Medicine 62:310–326, 1983.

5. Curtis JJ, Luke RG, Dustan HP, et al: Remission of essential hypertension after renal transplantation. N Engl J Med 309:1009–1015, 1983.

6. Sagnella GA, Markandu ND, Shore AC, MacGregor GA: Raised circulating levels of atrial natriuretic peptides in essential hypertension. Lancet ii:179–181, 1986.

7. Gray HH, Hilton PJ, Richardson PJ: Effect of serum from patients with essential hypertension on sodium transport in normal leucocytes. Clin Sci 70:583–586, 1986.

8. Blaustein MP: Sodium ions, calcium ions, blood pressure regulation and hypertension: a reassessment and a hypothesis. Am J Physiol 232:C165–C173, 1977.

9. Robinson BF: Altered calcium handling as a cause of primary hypertension. J Hypertens 2:453–460, 1984.

10. Fleckenstein A: History of calcium antagonists. Circ Res 52(suppl 1):3–16, 1983.

11. Lederballe-Pedersen O, Mikkelsen E: Acute and chronic effects of nifedipine in arterial hypertension. Eur J Clin Pharmacol 14:375–381, 1978.

12. Robinson BF, Dobbs FJ, Bayley S: Response of forearm resistance vessels to verapamil and sodium nitroprusside in normotensive and hypertensive men: evidence for a functional abnormality of vascular smooth muscle in primary hypertension. Clin Sci 63:33–42, 1982.

13. Hulthen UL, Bolli P, Amann FW, Kiowski W, Buhler FR: Enhanced vasodilation in essential hypertension by calcium channel blockade with verapamil. Hypertension 4(suppl 2):26–31, 1982.

14. Corea L, Miele N, Bentivoglio M, Boschetti E, Agabiti-Rosei E, Muiesan G: Acute and chronic effects of nifedipine on plasma renin activity and plasma adrenaline and noradrenaline in controls and hypertensive patients. Clin Sci 57:115S–117S, 1979.

15. Lederballe-Pedersen O, Christensen JJ, Ramsch KD: Comparison of acute effects of nifedipine in normotensive and hypertensive man. J Cardiovasc Pharmacol 2:357–366, 1980.

16. MacGregor GA, Markandu ND, Rotellar C, Smith SJ, Sagnella GA: The acute response to nifedipine is related to pre-treatment blood pressure. Postgrad Med J 59(suppl 2):91–94, 1983.

17. MacGregor GA, Sagnella GA, MacRae KD: Misleading paper about misleading statistics. Lancet i:926–92, 1985.

18. MacGregor GA, Rotellar C, Markandu ND, Smith SJ, Sagnella GA: Contrasting effects of nifedipine, captopril and propranolol in normotensive and hypertensive subjects. J Cardiovasc Pharmacol 4:S358–S362, 1982.

19. Erne P, Bolli P, Bertel O, et al: Factors influencing the hypertensive effect of calcium antagonists. Hypertension 5:97–102, 1983.

20. Knorr A, Garthoff B: Differential influence of the calcium antagonist nitrendipine and the vasodilator hydralazine on normal and elevated blood pressure. Arch Int Pharmacodyn Ther 269:316–322, 1984.

21. Cappuccio FP, Markandu ND, MacGregor GA: Calcium antagonists and sodium balance: Effect of changes in sodium intake and of the addition of a thiazide diuretic on the blood pressure lowering effect of nifedipine. J Cardiovasc Pharmacol 10:S57–S60, 1987.

22. Nicholson JP, Resnick LM, Laragh JH: The antihypertensive effect of verapamil at extremes of dietary sodium intake. Ann Intern Med 107:329–334, 1987.

23. Rosenthal J: Antihypertensive effects of nifedipine, mefruside and a combination of both substances in patients with essential hypertension. In Kaltenback M, Neufeld HN (eds): New Therapy of Ischaemic Heart Disease and Hypertension. Amsterdam, Excerpta Medica, 1982, pp 175–181.

24. MacGregor GA, Pevahouse JB, Cappuccio FP, Markandu ND: Nifedipine, sodium intake, diuretics and sodium balance. Am J Nephrol 7(suppl 1):44–48, 1987.

25. Poulter N, Thompson AV, Sever PS: A double-blind, placebo-controlled, crossover trial to investigate the additive hypotensive effect of a diuretic (mefruside) to that produced by nifedipine. J Cardiovasc Pharmacol 10(suppl 10):S53–S56, 1987.

26. Medical Research Council Working Party on Mild to Moderate Hypertension: Adverse reactions to bendrofluazide and propranolol for the treatment of mild hypertension. Lancet 2:539–543, 1981.

27. Cappuccio FP, Markandu ND, Tucker FA, Shore AC, MacGregor GA: A double-blind study of the blood pressure-lowering effect of a thiazide diuretic in hypertensive patients already on nifedipine and a beta-blocker. J Hypertens 5:733–738, 1987.

28. Klutsch K, Schmidt P, Grosswendt J: Der Einfluss von Bay A 1040 auf die Nieren-funktion des Hypertonikers. Arzneimittel-Forsch 22:528, 1972.

29. Yokoyama S, Kaburagi T: Clinical effects of intravenous nifedipine on renal function. J Cardiovasc Pharmacol 5:67–71, 1983.

30. Leonetti G, Cuspidi C, Sampieri L, Terzoli L, Zanchetti A: Comparison of cardiovascular, renal and humoral effects of acute administration of two calcium channel blockers in normotensive and hypertensive subjects. J Cardiovasc Pharmacol 4:S319–S324, 1982.

31. DiBona GF: Effects of felodipine on renal function in animals. Drugs 29:168–175, 1985.

32. MacCarthy EP: Dihydropyridines and beta-adrenoceptor agonists as combination treatment in hypertension. J Hypertens 5(suppl 4):S133–S137, 1987.

33. Heagerty AM, Swales J, Baksi A, et al: Nifedipine and atenolol singly and combined for treatment of essential hypertension: comparative multicentre study in general practice in the United Kingdom. Br Med J 296:468–472, 1988.

34. Bayley S, Dobbs RJ, Robinson BF: Nifedipine in the treatment of hypertension: report of a double-blind controlled trial. Br J Clin Pharmacol 14:509–512, 1982.

L. M. Ruilope, M.D.
B. Miranda, M.D.
J. L. Rodicio, M.D.

13

Characterization of the Long-Term Natriuretic Effects of Calcium Antagonists

Calcium antagonists are potent pharmacologic agents that are gaining wide acceptance for the treatment of arterial hypertension. The primary pharmacologic action of these compounds is to decrease peripheral vascular resistance. However, these agents also have potent renal actions that have been recently reviewed.[1-3] Calcium antagonists are consistently reported to cause an acute increase in the urinary output of sodium[1-3] (see Chapter 11). In contrast, the long-term natriuretic effects of calcium antagonists have not been well characterized. Furthermore, the mechanism(s) underlying the natriuretic effects of calcium antagonists, and its relevance to the control of blood pressure by these agents, remain a matter of debate. In this chapter, we summarize our findings characterizing the natriuretic effects of calcium antagonists in normotensive volunteers and essential hypertensive patients during the short- and long-term administration of three different types of dihydropiridine derivatives: nifedipine, nitrendipine, and nisoldipine.

Short-term Studies

Since the initial description of Leonetti et al.,[4] it has been amply recognized that the short-term administration of calcium antagonists is accompanied by a diuresis and natriuresis (see Chapter 11). These effects persist during the first few days of administration of the drug, as suggested by the negative sodium balance and the decrease of body weight observed both in normotensive volunteers and in essential hypertensive patients.[5-7] Table 1 contains the values of systolic and diastolic blood pressures, body weight, glomerular filtration rate, renal plasma flow, and the 24-hour sodium secretion of six normotensive volunteers and six essential hypertensive patients who received a 4-day course of either placebo or nisoldipine (10 mg/day) while on a constant sodium intake of 150 mEq/day. As can be seen, in response to 4 days of therapy, blood pressure fell in hypertensive patients but not in normal

225

TABLE 1. Values of Systolic (SBP), Diastolic (DBP), Body Weight (BW), Glomerular Filtration Rate (GFR), Renal Plasma Flow (RPF), and 24-hour Natriuresis (Na_u) Obtained in Normotensive Volunteers and Essential Hypertensive Patients after a Four-day Course of Placebo (P) and Nisoldipine (Ns) Sodium Intake Maintained ad libitum

		Normotensives			Hypertensives		
		Day 0	Day 4	P	Day 0	Day 4	P
SBP	P	118 ± 4	117 ± 9	NS	171 ± 9	172 ± 8	NS
(mmHg)	Ns	119 ± 10	118 ± 9	NS	170 ± 11	156 ± 12**	<0.001
DBP	P	70 ± 4	69 ± 9	NS	101 ± 6	100 ± 8	NS
(mmHg)	Ns	70 ± 4	70 ± 6	NS	100 ± 9	91 ± 8**	<0.001
BW	P	69 ± 8	69 ± 7	NS	73 ± 8	73 ± 7	NS
(kg)	Ns	70 ± 8	69 ± 10	<0.05	74 ± 9	73 ± 5	<0.05
GFR	P	99 ± 8.9	99 ± 7.4	NS	86 ± 14	85 ± 17	NS
(ml/min)	Ns	96 ± 9.4	109 ± 10.1*	<0.05	85 ± 13	88 ± 15	NS
RPF	P	560 ± 84	561 ± 86	NS	380 ± 61	383 ± 60	NS
(ml/min)	Ns	564 ± 81	662 ± 110*	<0.05	376 ± 70	391 ± 69	NS
Na_u	P	178 ± 24	184 ± 31	NS	189 ± 41	194 ± 49	NS
(mEq/24 h)	Ns	181 ± 29	199 ± 29*	<0.01	195 ± 58	230 ± 39*	<0.01

*$p < 0.05$ vs. P
**$p < 0.01$ vs. P

subjects. Both groups, however, exhibited an increase in 24-hour urinary sodium output and a fall in body weight in the absence of significant changes of renal plasma flow and glomerular filtration rate. After the first week of treatment, the natriuretic effect of the calcium antagonist subsides in the balance studies, probably due to the attainment of a steady state.

We have demonstrated that the short-term administration of nifedipine improves the ability of the kidney to excrete an acute volume load.[3] The urinary sodium excretory rate was measured in five essential hypertensive patients and in five normotensive patients during 4 hours of isotonic saline infusion (500 ml/hour). Paired measurements were obtained in the absence of any medication and after a single 20 mg oral dose of nifedipine. Our findings are summarized in Figure 1. Nifedipine significantly increased cumulative sodium excretion in both groups to similar extents. In the lower panel of Figure 1, the rates of urinary sodium excretion are plotted against mean arterial pressure. As depicted, nifedipine induced increases in urinary sodium excretion in hypertensive patients and was accompanied by a decrease in mean systemic pressure. Thus, nifedipine potentiated the natriuresis in hypertensive subjects even though renal perfusion pressure decreased.

To determine if this effect would occur with another calcium antagonist, a similar study was carried out using the dihydropyridine derivative, nisoldipine[8] in normotensive volunteers and essential hypertensive patients.[6] All underwent a 4-day course of therapy of placebo and nisoldipine while on a sodium intake of 150 mEq/day. They were then challenged with a saline volume load (500 ml/hr) for 4 hours. As can be seen in Figure 2, nisoldipine also enhanced the renal capacity to excrete the intravenous sodium load in both groups. The enhanced sodium output was also accompanied by a diminution in the renal perfusion pressure in the hypertensive group.

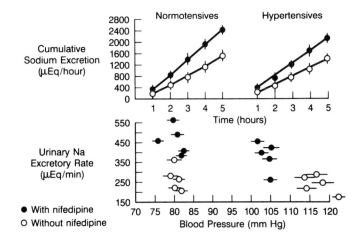

FIGURE 1. Top panel: Average cumulative rates of urinary sodium excretion (U_{NA}) in five normotensive subjects and five subjects with hypertension during infusion of isotonic saline before (O) and after (●) administration of a single 20 mg oral dose of nifedipine. Bottom panel: U_{Na} secretory rates during each of the 5 hours of sodium overload plotted against averages of mean arterial pressure recorded during the same hours. Bars represent SEM. Reproduced with permission from Romero et al., Hypertension, 1987.[3]

The mechanism(s) responsible for this augmentation of volume-induced natriuresis by calcium antagonists has not been fully defined. A renal hemodynamic component is possible, since calcium antagonists can be demonstrated to increase GFR in some settings. However, the ability of the calcium antagonists to dilate renal vasculature and to increase glomerular filtration rate is largely determined by the pre-existing vascular tone[1-3] (also see Chapter 1). The capacity of the kidney to respond to fluctuations in the level of sodium chloride intake depends, in part, on renal hemodynamic adjustments largely due to the activation of the renin-angiotensin and the sympathetic nervous systems.[9] Calcium antagonists may modify the renal hemodynamic response to such compensatory adjustments.

In order to evaluate the influence of changes in the renal vascular tone on the natriuretic effect of calcium antagonists, we have investigated the natriuretic properties of nisoldipine during dietary sodium restriction. Table 2 summarizes the values for blood pressure, body weight, and renal function in six normotensive volunteers and six essential hypertensive patients who received placebo or nisoldipine while on a low sodium-intake (20 mEq/day). In contrast to the effects during high sodium intake, GFR and RPF increased significantly during sodium restriction in response to the administration of the calcium antagonists. Figure 3 depicts the cumulative urinary sodium excretion attained during the administrations of an intravenous sodium load. The rate of urinary sodium excretion is plotted against the mean arterial pressure recorded during the same period. As depicted in Figure 3, sodium depletion did not prevent the increase in the urinary sodium excretion following nisoldipine. Furthermore, the enhanced natriuresis occurred in the group of hypertensive patients even though renal perfusion pressure decreased.

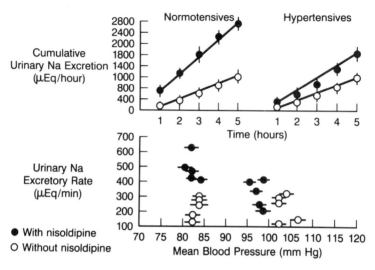

FIGURE 2. Top panel: Average cumulative rates of urinary sodium excretion (U_{Na}) in six normotensive subjects and six subjects with hypertension during infusion of isotonic saline before (O) and after (●) a 4-day course of therapy with nisoldipine (19 mg/day). The intake of sodium was 150 mEq/day along the study. Bottom panel: U_{Na} secretory rates during each of the 5 hours of sodium overload plotted against averages of mean arterial pressure recorded during the same hours. Bars represent SEM. Reproduced with permission from Ruilope et al., J Cardiovasc Pharmacol, 1989.[14]

In addition to inducing a natriuresis, the acute intravenous or intrarenal arterial administration of calcium antagonists also results in an increased excretion of calcium and, more variably, potassium.[4,10–14]

The natriuretic effect of calcium antagonists observed during short-term studies may be partly attributed to the actions of the drugs on intrarenal hemodynamics. In addition, these agents may also interact with neural and hormonal mediators.[1–3,15] The increase in sodium excretion, however, can occur without alterations of renal hemodynamics, and a direct action of calcium antagonists on the tubular transport of sodium has been proposed to account for the increase of sodium excretion in such circumstances[1,3,12,14] (also see Chapter 11).

Long-term Studies

The acute stimulation of sodium excretion upon the initial administration of calcium antagonists has been a consistent finding[15] (see Chapter 11). With time, however, the rate of sodium excretion usually returns to pretreatment values,[15] suggesting that calcium antagonists may not have a sustained action on renal sodium handling. Nevertheless, if calcium antagonist therapy is abruptly terminated, a post-therapy period of positive sodium balance has been observed[16] (see Chapter 12). In concert, these observations imply that calcium antagonists may exert long-term effects on sodium homeostasis, which may be masked by normal compensatory mechanisms.

TABLE 2. Values of Systolic (SBP) and Diastolic Blood Pressure (DBP), Body Weight (BW), Glomerular Filtration Rate (GFR), Renal Plasma Flow (RPF), and 24-hour Natriuresis (Na_u) Obtained in Normotensive Volunteers and Essential Hypertensive Patients after Four Days of Placebo and Nisoldipine (N) (Sodium Intake Maintained Constant at 20 mEq/day)

		Normotensives (Diet 20mEq MaDay)			Hypertensives (Diet 20mEq Na/Day)		
		Day 0	Day 4	P	Day 0	Day 4	P
SBP	P	113 ± 8	113 ± 9	NS	165 ± 6	165 ± 7	NS
(mmHg)	N	112 ± 6	113 ± 6	NS	160 ± 17	148 ± 14**	<0.001
DBP	P	66 ± 6	70 ± 6	NS	101 ± 6	100 ± 6	NS
(mmHg)	N	65 ± 4	64 ± 4	NS	100 ± 8	90 ± 6**	<0.001
BW	P	69.3 ± 7.2	69.4 ± 7.3	NS	68.2 ± 7.0	68.2 ± 7.1	NS
(kg)	N	69.6 ± 7.1	68.7 ± 6.7*	<0.05	68.1 ± 7.0	67.8 ± 6.9*	<0.01
GFR	P	92.6 ± 12.8	92.6 ± 12.8	NS	84.9 ± 16.2	85.3 ± 14.8	NS
(ml/min)	N	90.1 ± 8.1	106.1 ± 14.9*	<0.01	84.6 ± 13.5	94.1 ± 13.0*	<0.01
RPF	P	461 ± 89	457 ± 86	NS	349 ± 81	365 ± 73	NS
(ml/min)	N	450 ± 85	601 ± 161*	<0.05	365 ± 73	403 ± 69*	<0.05
Na_u	P	24.3 ± 3.8	22.4 ± 3.1	NS	22.3 ± 3.7	25.6 ± 4.3	NS
(mEq/24h)	N	20.6 ± 3.9*	22.78 ± 4.7	<0.05	22.4 ± 3.1	29.6 ± 2.2*	<0.01

from Yokoyama S, Kaburagi T[13] with permission.
*p<0.5 vs. P; **p<0.01 vs. P.
P = placebo; N = nisoldipine; NS = not significant.

In other words, during chronic administration of calcium antagonists, a new steady-state is established in which other factors override the natriuretic actions of calcium antagonist therapy, and sodium balance returns at a reduced set-point. Such a long-term action of calcium antagonists should be unmasked by maneuvers designed to perturb the steady state of sodium homeostasis, such as acute volume expansion.

In order to test the persistence of the natriuretic effect of calcium antagonists during chronic administration, we have studied the sequential administration of a simi-

TABLE 3. Cumulative Sodium Excretion (μEq/min×hour) Before and After 1, 8, and 24 Weeks of Treatment with Nitrendipine During the Intravenous Infusion of Saline

Time (hr)	Initial	1 Week	8 Weeks	24 Weeks
0	96.3 ± 74.1	146.4 ± 107.2	181.5 ± 59.3*	259.2 ± 162.1**
1	306.2 ± 260.1	439.7 ± 236.6	518.8 ± 257.3*	631.7 ± 255.1**
2	557.4 ± 456.7	1024.8 ± 691.3*	881.7 ± 481.4*	1137.2 ± 427.6***
3	1003.2 ± 698.6	1559.6 ± 1142*	1374.7 ± 681.9*	1571.6 ± 544.6**
4	1397.3 ± 82.5	2031.5 ± 1322.4*	1982.5 ± 881.8**	2213.8 ± 637.8***
5	1767.6 ± 930.0	2549.8 ± 1534.8*	2456.7 ± 951.8**	2730.7 ± 743.7***

from Ruliope et al., J Cardiovasc Pharmacol, 1989[17], with permission.
± 50 *p<0.05; **p<0.02 vs. INITIAL; and ***p<0.001.

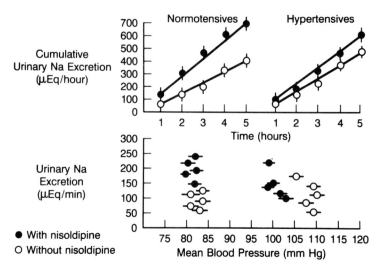

FIGURE 3. Top panel: Average cumulative rates of urinary sodium excretion (U_{Na}) in six normotensive subjects and six subjects with hypertension during infusion of isotonic saline before (O) and after (●) a 4-day course of therapy with nisoldipine (19 mg/day). The intake of sodium was 20 mEq/day along the study. Bottom panel: U_{Na} secretory rates during each of the 5 hours of sodium overload plotted against averages of mean arterial pressure recorded during the same hours. Bars represent SEM. Reproduced with permission from Ruilope et al, J Cardiovasc Pharmacol, 1989.[14]

lar intravenous sodium load during the long-term administration of nitrendipine.[17] As can be seen in Table 3, the cumulative sodium excretion during an intravenous infusion of saline was significantly higher after 1 week of nitrendipine therapy and remained enhanced after 8 and 24 weeks of treatment. These observations confirm that the natriuretic effect of this calcium antagonist persisted after chronic therapy. During the follow-up study at 6 months, the glomerular filtration rate as measured by the creatinine clearance did not change.[17] The absence of variations in glomerular filtration rate suggests a predominance of a tubular effect of nitrendipine in the maintenance of the natriuretic effect after several months of therapy.

The investigation of the long-term effects of isradipine, a new dihydropiridine derivative, on renal hemodynamics and excretory function in essential hypertensive patients has been carried out by Krusell et al.[18] These investigators found that the morning dose of isradipine after 3.5 months of therapy induced a 40% increase in sodium excretion and a diuresis. The changes in blood pressure correlated significantly with the changes in absolute proximal reabsorption of sodium and inversely with the excretion of sodium.

These results suggest that calcium antagonists exert long-term effects on sodium homeostasis with a persistent natriuretic effect. This natriuretic effect is not always apparent because steady state is attained after the initial days of therapy. A direct tubular effect of the calcium antagonists appears to constitute the main determinant of the natriuretic effect.

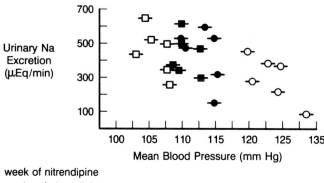

FIGURE 4. Urine sodium secretory rates before and during the 5 hours of sodium overload plotted against averages of mean arterial pressure recorded during the same hours before (O) and after 1(●), 8(■) and 24(□) weeks of nitrendipine administration. Bars represent SEM. Reproduced with permission from Ruilope et al, J Cardiovasc Pharmacol, 1989.[17]

Summary

In summary, our experience and the data in the literature indicate that calcium antagonists have natriuretic properties that are manifested by an increase in the 24-hour urinary output of sodium during the first days of therapy. Thereafter a steady state is attained and body weight remains constant during long-term treatment.[16] The persistence of the natriuretic capacity of these drugs is indicated by the maintenance of an increased renal capacity to excrete an intravenous sodium load, by the enhancement of sodium clearance after several months of therapy,[18] and also by the gain in body weight that is observed after the withdrawal of the drug at a time when sodium intake is maintained constant.[16] It indicates that the natriuretic properties of the calcium antagonists are important in the long-term control of blood pressure. The persistence of the natriuretic effect of calcium antagonists may have important implications from the clinical point of view, since the natriuretic effect may obviate the need for combination therapy with a diuretic agent.[19]

References

1. Loutzenhiser R, Epstein M: Effects of calcium antagonists on renal hemodynamics. Am J Physiol 249:F619–F629, 1985.

2. Loutzenhiser R, Epstein M: Modification of the renal hemodynamic response to vasoconstrictors by calcium antagonists. Am J Nephrol 7(suppl 1):7-16, 1987.

3. Romero JC, Raij L, Granger JP, Ruilope LM, Rodiocio JL: Multiple effects of calcium entry blockers on renal function in hypertension. Hypertension 10:140–151, 1987.

4. Leonetti C, Cuspide C, Sampieri L, Terzoli L, Zanchetti A: Comparison of cardiovascular, renal and humoral effects of acute administration of two calcium channel blockers in normotensive and hypertensive subjects. J Cardiovasc Pharmacol 4(suppl 3):S319–S324, 1982.

5. Thananopavarn C, Bolub M, Eggena P, Barrett JD, Sambhi MP: Renal effects of nitredipine monotherapy in essential hypertension. J Cardiovasc Pharmacol 6(suppl 7):S1032–S1026, 1986.

6. Ruilope LM, Miranda B, Garcia Robles R, et al.: Natriuretic properties of nisoldipine in essential hypertension. J Hypertension 4(suppl 5):S469-S470, 1986.

7. Luft FC, Arnoff GR, Sloan RS, Fineberg NS, Weinberger MH: Calcium channel blockade with nitrendipine: effect on sodium homeostasis, the renin-angiotensin system, and the sympathetic nervous system in humans. J Hypertension 7:438–442, 1985.

8. Kazda S, Knorr A, Towart R: Common properties and differences between various calcium antagonists. Prog Pharmacol 5:86–116, 1983.

9. Arendshorst WJ, Navar LG: Renal circulation and glomerular hemodynamics: In Schrier RW, Gottchalk CW (eds): Diseases of the Kidney. Boston, Little Brown, 1988, p 65.

10. Bell AJ, Lindner A: Effects of verapamil and nifedipine on renal function and hemodynamics in the dog. Renal Physiol 7:329–343, 1984.

11. Marse M, Misumi J, Raemsch K, De Corvol P, Menard J: Diuretic and natriuretic effect of nifedipine on isolated perfused rat kidney. J Pharmacol Exp Ther 223:263–270, 1982.

12. Wallia R, Greenberg A, Puschett JB: Renal hemodynamic and tubular transport effects of nitrendipine. J Lab Clin Med 105:498–503, 1985.

13. Yokoyama S, Kaburagi T: Clinical effects of intravenous nifedipine on renal function. J Cardiovasc Pharmacol 5:67–71, 1983.

14. Ruilope LM, Garcia-Robles R, Miranda B, et al.: Effect of nisoldipine on renal function in normal volunteers and essential hypertensive patients. J Cardiovasc Pharmacol, 13:90-93, 1989.

15. Luft FC: Calcium-channel-blocking drugs and renal sodium excretion. Am J Nephrol 7(suppl 1):39–43, 1987.

16. MacGregor GA, Pevahouse JB, Cappuccio FP, Markandu ND: Nifedipine, sodium intake, diuretics and sodium balance. Am J Nephrol 7(suppl 1):44–48, 1987.

17. Ruilope LM, Miranda B, Oliet A, Alcazar JM, Bigorra J, Rodicio JL: Persistence of the natriuretic effect of calcium entry blockers. J Cardiovasc Pharmacol, 12(suppl 4): S136 S139, 1988.

18. Krussell LR, Jespersen LT, Schmnitz A, Thomsen K, Pedersen OL: Repetitive natriuresis and blood pressure. Long-term calcium entry blockade with Isradipine. Hypertension 10:577–581, 1987.

19. Epstein M, Oster JR: Role of calcium channel blockers in the treatment of hypertension. In Epstein M, Oster JR (eds): Hypertension: Practical Management. Miami, Battersea Medical Publishers, 1988, pp 114–125.

Ingemar Dawidson, M.D., Ph.D.
Pål Rooth, Ph.D.

14

Effects of Calcium Antagonists in Ameliorating Cyclosporine A Nephrotoxicity and Post-transplant ATN

Cyclosporine A (CsA), a cyclic polypeptide, consists of an 11-amino-acid sequence. It is insoluble in water, but soluble in organic solvents and lipids. CsA, isolated from a strain of fungi imperfecti, *Tolypocladium inflatum gams*, was shown to have strong immunosuppressive properties and was introduced to clinical transplantation in the late 1970s.[1] Variable and incomplete intestinal absorption, as well as multiple organ toxicity, have made its clinical application difficult and challenging. Nevertheless, CsA has truly revolutionized organ transplantation, in that not only has the cadaver kidney 1-year graft survival rate increased by 20%—to about 75%[2]—but other organ transplant procedures, such as livers[3] and hearts,[4] also have a success rate approaching that of kidney transplantation.

Recently, CsA has been used with increasing frequency for treatment of autoimmune diseases such as ocular inflammatory disorders,[5] rheumatoid arthritis,[6] Type I diabetes,[7] and multiple sclerosis.[8] As the clinical applications for CsA increase in number, the search for an effective means to circumvent CsA-induced nephrotoxicity has intensified. Recent evidence suggests that calcium antagonists (CATs) may prove to be an effective pharmacologic means of reducing the severity and incidence of CsA-induced nephrotoxicity.

Cyclosporine A (CsA) Nephrotoxicity

Mechanisms

The nephrotoxicity of CsA is a serious and well-documented problem,[9,10] which has somewhat tempered initial enthusiasm for the drug. The pathophysiology of CsA-induced acute nephrotoxicity is not fully understood, but animal studies[11-15] as well as clinical data,[9,16-18] strongly suggest glomerular hypoperfusion, secondary to vasospasm, as a contributing factor. A dose-related increase in serum creatinine,[10,19] and up to 50% reduction in glomerular filtration rate (GFR),[9] as well as renal blood flow inhibition,[9-11,12,17,18] have been well-documented and are features more characteristic for acute CsA nephrotoxicity. The nature of chronic CsA nephrotoxicity is harder to delineate because of the often concomitant chronic rejection. Features associated with chronic CsA nephrotoxicity include hypertension, tubular dysfunction, and interstitial fibrosis.[9,10]

CsA and Renal Blood Flow. Since the clinical entity of CsA-induced acute nephrotoxicity is similar to that of post-transplant ischemia, CATs have been used in an attempt to prevent CsA nephrotoxicity. Using in vivo fluorescence microscopy, Rooth and Dawidson demonstrated a dose-related CsA-induced decrease in renal subcapsular microcirculation after both bolus (18–19 mg/kg) and 1-hr continuous infusions[11,12](Fig. 1). Flow inhibition occurred after a 15–20 min delay, suggesting as a causative agent the appearance of a metabolite or attenuation of a protective mechanism such as the prostaglandin system. The decreased renal blood flow seen in animal models after CsA administration was also observed in patients receiving cadaver renal transplants.[17] In ten study patients, systolic and diastolic main artery and parenchymal blood flow velocity were measured via Duplex Doppler ultrasonography (Fig. 2). On the first day of CsA therapy, diastolic parenchymal flow decreased 70%, from 10.3 ± 2.2 to 3.2 ± 3.5 cm/sec ($p < 0.001$)(Fig. 2B). Parenchymal blood flow gradually returned to normal, despite continued CsA therapy.

CsA and Renal Histopathology. In addition to vasospasm, CsA induces several histological changes, including direct tubular cell damage, and, particularly, prominent vacuole formation in proximal tubules.[20] Even so, no correlation between these lesions and functional changes has been established.[21]

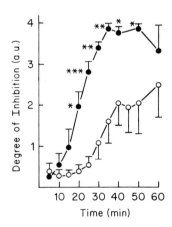

FIGURE 1. Inhibition of subcapsular renal blood flow at two different rates of CsA infusion, in relation to time. At higher CsA infusion rates (0.8–2.0 mg/kg/min; ●—●; N = 12), flow inhibition was seen after 15 min and became progressively more pronounced within 30 min. At lower infusion rates (0.15-0.23 mg/kg/min; ○—○; n = 7), inhibition was delayed to 25 min, significantly less than with the larger CsA dose (mean ± SEM:* p ‹ 0.05,** p ‹ 0.01,*** p ‹ 0.001). Reproduced with permission from Transplantation 45:433, 1988.

CsA nephrotoxicity is difficult to differentiate from the coexistence of acute rejection. Using nine histologic parameters, Sibley found CsA nephrotoxicity to be associated with mononuclear cellular infiltrates within dilated peritubular capillary lumens rather than in the interstitial tissue, which is more typical of rejection.[22] The acute nephrotoxicity of CsA usually is reversible by decreasing the CsA dose.

The chronic form of CsA nephrotoxicity is even less well-defined histologically, again obscured by the concomitant chronic rejection. Usually one sees in the affected tubules severe atrophy and thickened basement membranes. The most prominent feature is interstitial fibrosis. Other common findings include focal hyalinosis of small arteries and arterioles, and sclerosis of glomeruli, possibly secondary to compromised blood vessels and ischemia.[9] CsA nephrotoxicity seems to be more readily reversible with cessation of CsA therapy during the first 6 months post-transplant. Long-term CsA therapy that results in nephrotoxicity is less likely to be reversible and may, in fact, contribute to late renal allograft loss.

The presence of renal vasoconstriction or renal ischemia may exacerbate the nephrotoxic actions of CsA. In rats, for instance, CsA has been shown to induce more severe damage when given after an episode of ischemia.[23] Even a low (5 mg/kg) dose caused GFR to drop from 290 to 20 μl/min/100g bwt, when given after 45 min of warm ischemia. In contrast, doses of CsA of up to 20 mg/kg, when administered to normal kidneys, had no detrimental effect on GFR.[23] These experimental data are supported by the clinical observation that CsA causes an increased incidence of ATN and renal graft loss when compared with those patients treated with ALG and AZA, but not CsA.[24,25]

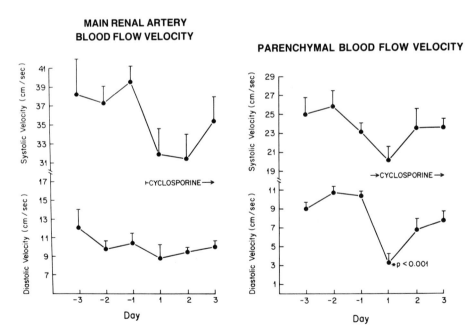

FIGURE 2. Parenchymal diastolic and systolic blood flow velocities before and during cyclosporine A administration to ten cadaver transplant recipients. Reproduced with permission of Trans Proc 20(3):222, 1988.

Acute CsA nephrotoxicity produces a clinical picture similar to that of acute tubular necrosis (ATN) after renal transplantation (i.e., ischemic injury), both entities possibly caused by the same mechanism—vasospasm. When CsA is given i.v., nephrotoxicity often manifests itself by a decrease in glomerular filtration rate (GFR) and an increase in serum creatinine. Oliguria and, occasionally, anuria may also occur, lasting for days or weeks.

Methods of Decreasing CsA Nephrotoxicity

The increased use of CsA in organ transplantation, as well as for autoimmune disorders, has prompted an intensive search for methods of ameliorating CsA nephrotoxicity. Several approaches have led to a reduction in the incidence and severity of CsA-induced nephrotoxicity, including dose adjustments, intraoperative blood volume expansion, and the use of renal vasodilating drugs.

Changing the Immunosuppressive Protocol. The frequency of CsA-induced nephrotoxicity is related to the dosage administered and the underlying renal status. The incidence of CsA-induced nephrotoxicity has been reduced by a concerted effort to achieve immunosuppression at the lowest effective CsA dosage. In recent years, most renal transplant centers have decreased the initial daily dose from 20–25 to 8–12 mg/kg/day. Furthermore, due to increased absorption of CsA with time after transplantation, smaller doses are used to avoid toxicity. The distribution of multiple smaller doses throughout the day may also decrease toxic effects. By using "triple therapy" (the addition of azathioprine to CsA and corticosteroids), the CsA dose can be further reduced with maintenance of immunosuppression. "Quadruple induction therapy" is often employed to avoid the initial toxic effects of CsA.[20] This method uses antithymocyte or antilymphocyte globulin instead of CsA for the first 5–14 days after transplantation. Once adequate renal function has been established, CsA is initiated. The rationale is that CsA seems to be more damaging to kidneys that have been subjected to an ischemic insult such as occurs with procurement and transplant procedures.[24,25] Converting to azathioprine in order to decrease chronic nephrotoxicity has been associated with an increased incidence of rejection and graft loss,[26] and therefore is not feasible. Finally, the development of alternate immunosuppression drugs with less nephrotoxicity has not been forthcoming.

Intravascular Volume Expansion and Acute Tubular Necrosis (ATN). The typical scenario in the development of classic ATN is the presence of hypovolemia, which leads to renal hypoperfusion and ischemia. It is not surprising, therefore, that strict control of the blood volume has been shown to affect the post-transplant incidence of ATN.

Surgery and Intravascular Colloid Losses. There are three phases of renal transplantation that may induce vasospasm. First, during procurement, low circulating blood volume and surgical dissection of the kidneys may cause vasospasm. Secondly, the duration of warm and cold ischemia and the use of cold (4°C) perfusion solutions containing high KCl (80–100 mEq) may further induce vasospasm. Finally, during organ procurement and implantation, plasma proteins—predominantly albumin—are lost secondary to bleeding and increased vascular permeability. During a transplant procedure, an average loss of 1 g/kg bwt, corresponding to a plasma volume loss of 20 ml/kg (1400 ml in a 70 kg man), is usually observed.[27] It is conceivable that a blood volume loss of this magnitude could induce vasospasm, which would further worsen function in a kidney that has already been subjected to ischemia during the various procurement phases.

Intraoperative blood volume expansion. Aggressive intravascular volume expansion with albumin and electrolyte solutions during transplantation restores blood volume and improves post-transplant kidney function at five levels of analysis: (1) earlier onset of urine production and larger urine volumes; (2) improved kidney function, with lower creatinines at one week; (3) decreased incidence of post-transplant ATN; (4) greater graft survival; and (5) greater patient survival.[28]

Blood volume expansion with albumin (0.4 g/kg) completely restored CsA-impaired renal microcirculation in mice.[29] Similarly, in clinical renal transplantion, volume expansion with albumin (1–1.6 gm/kg), along with electrolyte solutions (50 cc/kg), decreased post-transplant ATN from 36% to 6%.[28] Colloids appear to be particularly effective. This was documented for both azathioprine and CsA-treated patients (Fig. 3). In our cadaver kidney transplant recipients from 1982–1987 (n = 311), early (3-month) mortality rates have shown a linear decrease from 10% when no intraoperative albumin is given, to 0% when 1.2-1.6 g/kg is infused (Dawidson, unpublished data).

Renal Vasodilators. Several pharmacologic agents with known intrarenal activity have been used in an attempt to prevent or decrease CsA nephrotoxicity. These include α-blocking agents, converting enzyme inhibitors (CEIs), prostaglandin synthesis inhibitors, β-blocking agents, and others.

There are conflicting data in the literature regarding the effect of α-blocking agents on CsA-induced vasoconstriction.[11,14,15,30] Although Murray found phenoxybenzamine and prazosin effective in rats in averting the CsA-induced decreased blood flow,[14,15] Rooth, with mice,[11] and Diepirink, with rats,[30] did not. These differences may reflect species-specific effects, or the dosage and timing of CsA and/or the α-blocking drug. In addition to the beneficial

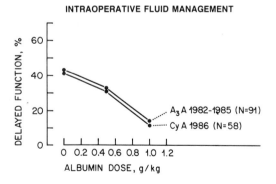

INTRAOPERATIVE FLUID MANAGEMENT

FIGURE 3. Increasing doses of intraoperative albumin offers protection against post-transplant delayed function or ATN in patients immunosuppressed with both azathioprine (AZA) and CsA. (Dawidson, unpublished data)

effect of an α-blocking agent (phenoxybenzamine), Murray also demonstrated that renal denervation prevented the CsA-induced decreased renal blood flow in rats.

In several studies,[14,30] CEIs such as captopril failed to improve CsA-impaired renal hemodynamics. This suggests that the decreased vasospasm was not mediated by angiotensin II, even though CsA increases renin in vivo.[14] The increased renin angiotensin from CsA may be a result of the decreased blood flow. The fact that angiotensin acts mainly on the efferent, and CsA on the afferent, arterioles may explain the lack of effect from captopril. CATs, on the other hand, exert their vasodilation predominantly on the preglomerular arterioles, also the site of CsA-induced vasospasm.

Prostaglandins seem to play a protective role in CsA-induced vascular spasm. Meclofenamate, a prostaglandin synthesis inhibitor, does not in itself affect renal blood flow in control animals.[14] CsA (10 mg/kg), however, in rats caused worsening vasoconstriction when given in combination with meclofenamate.

Calcium Antagonists and CsA Nephrotoxocity

Verapamil's vasodilatory effect on the ischemic myocardium has been known for more than 20 years. More recently, calcium antagonists (CATs) have been shown to exert profound effects on renal hemodynamics. These aspects are discussed in detail in Chapter 3.

Calcium Antagonists and Acute Tubular Necrosis

There are numerous experimental studies demonstrating renal protection against ischemia by CATs. The effects are usually more pronounced if the CATs are given prior to the ischemic insult. Verapamil, when given to dogs prior to induction of cold ischemia, afforded protection against post-transplant ATN, as well as greater renal function.[31] Furthermore, ATP and total nucleotide levels were higher in kidneys pretreated with verapamil in a 40-minute warm-ischemia model in rats. A larger (100 μM/100 ml) concentration of verapamil offered greater protection than less (2.5–5 μM/100 ml).

The protective effect on organ-function parameters such as inulin clearance and sodium reabsorption was lost when verapamil was administered after a period of cold ischemia, although there was still a significant increase in renal blood flow. This dissociation of the vasodilatory effect of verapamil from its effect on organ function suggests more than one protective mechanism.[32] Such possible mechanisms include diminished vascular smooth muscle contraction (or vasodilatation), protection of cell membranes from destruction by phospholipid breakdown, hindrance of the decrease in cell-membrane ATP levels after ischemic injury, and, finally, inhibition of platelet activity. The protective effect of CATs against warm ischemia also has been demonstrated in large animal models.[33] Recently, in a clinical study, Neumayer and Wagner demonstrated a significant decrease (from 44% to 10%) in the incidence of delayed function when both the cadaver donor and the kidney transplant recipient were treated with diltiazem. This effect was lessened when only the transplant recipient was so treated.[34]

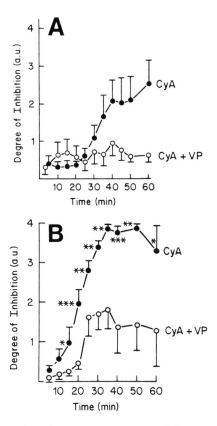

FIGURE 4. Pretreatment with a calcium antagonist, verapamil (0.35 mg/kg), markedly improved the kidney subcapsular blood flow at different infusion rates of CsA. At low infusion rates (0.18-0.22 mg/kg/min; N = 10; [A]), inhibition was completely prevented; at higher infusion rates (0.9-2.4 mg/kg/min; N = 13; [B]), the effect was partial (mean ± SEM). Reproduced with permission of Transplantation 45:433, 1988.

Calcium Antagonists Abolish CsA-induced Blood Flow Inhibition

The site of action for CsA-induced renal vasospasm is the preglomerular arteriole. Theoretically, CATs, especially those belonging to the dihydropyridine group, should be ideal, from a pharmacological standpoint, in preventing this detrimental hemodynamic event.[35-37] In fact, Rooth and Dawidson found that pretreatment with verapamil (0.35 mg/kg) or isradipine (0.18 μg/kg) completely blocked the unfavorable effect of CsA when verapamil was given in a dose of up to 13 mg/kg.[11,12] Therefore, CsA-induced vasospasm seems to represent calcium channel–mediated vasoconstriction. At very large (54–144 mg/kg) CsA doses, however, verapamil offered partial renal protection, suggesting still another mechanism for vasospasm, possible α-receptor mediated[14,15] (Fig. 4). Also, the dose of verapamil may have been insufficient with this large a dose of CsA. The protective effect of verapamil on renal blood flow probably is representative of this class of vasodilators, since other CATs, such as diltiazem, nicardipine, nitrendipine, and isradipine, exert similar effects.[12,35-37]

Calcium Antagonists in Clinical Renal Transplantation

It is likely that CATs would optimize early kidney function after transplantation by preglomerular vasodilatation, similar to that achieved with intravascular volume expansion. We have observed that intraarterial injection of verapamil (2.5–10 mg) to ten kidney recipients during the transplant procedure resulted in immediate improvement in color and turgor, as well as urine production. Currently, using both intraoperative volume expansion (albumin; 1–1.4 gm/kg bodyweight) and intraarterial verapamil, post-transplant incidence of delayed function is 0% (0/10) versus 18% (5/28) without intraoperative verapamil (Dawidson, unpublished data).

Similar data are presented by Neumayer and Wagner with an ATN rate of 10% (2/20) when both donors and recipients were pretreated with diltiazem. In contrast, 45% (9/20) of control patients experienced delayed function. Furthermore, diltiazem-treated patients had significantly better GFR and blood flow 4 and 7 days post-transplant.[37] Diltiazem had less effect when only the recipients were treated.

Salutary Effects of CATs. Encouraged by the effects of verapamil on CsA-induced decreased renal blood flow in mice,[11,12] and the observed CsA-induced decline in renal blood flow in post-transplant cadaver recipients,[17] we have initiated a randomized clinical study of verapamil. The immunosuppressive regimen includes ALG (15 mg/kg) for 5 days, overlapping 1 day with CsA (7 mg/kg), started on day 5, and increasing to 12 mg/kg on day 6. Using Duplex Doppler scanning, main renal artery and parenchymal systolic and diastolic blood flow velocities are obtained daily after transplantation.

In the first ten consecutive pilot patients, parenchymal diastolic blood flow velocity decreased by 70% on day 1 of CsA therapy.[17] Blood flow gradually returned to normal after 2–3 days despite continued CsA therapy (Fig. 2). When verapamil was given 2 days prior to initiation of CsA, patients with initially low (1.6 ± 2.6 cm/sec) or indetectible parenchymal diastolic flow velocity had prompt return of blood flow to levels observed in kidneys with good function (10.0 ± 1.4 cm/sec). Patients not given verapamil significantly differed from this pattern (p < 0.008) (Fig. 5). Kidneys with parenchymal diastolic flow rate of 9 cm/sec or more were not affected by verapamil.[17,18,18a] These findings are consistent with the concept that the effect of CATs depends upon the underlying vascular tone.[35-37] In other words, only when vasospasm and decreased flow are present would CATs be expected to be beneficial to renal hemodynamics.

Verapamil (120 mg t.i.d.) also prevented the decrease in renal blood flow seen on day 1 of CsA therapy, significantly different from the effect seen in patients who had not received verapamil, (p < 0.001) (Fig. 6). In fact, with continued administration of verapamil, blood flow patterns continued to improve during CsA therapy. With verapamil treatment, nadir serum creatinine values 1 week after CsA administration were slightly lower (1.31 ± 0.39 mg%) compared with controls (1.65 ± 0.54 mg%) (p = 0.053), despite significantly higher whole blood CsA levels (203 ± 74 vs. 125 ± 64 ng/ml, respectively) (p < 0.05). Finally, and more importantly, only 2

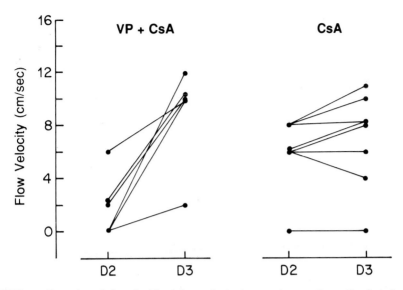

FIGURE 5. Parenchymal diastolic blood flow velocity improved promptly on the first day of verapamil (VP)(D3), especially when the blood flow velocity was low (< 8 cm/sec) prior to administration of VP (p < 0.001).

of 15 patients randomized to verapamil were treated for rejection within 4 weeks of transplantation, in contrast to 8 of 14 who received no verapamil (p < 0.02). A decreased incidence in rejections was observed also with diltiazem in Neumayer's study[34] and with nifedipine in a retrospective study by Feehally.[38]

Calcium Antagonists and CsA Blood Levels

In a randomized prospective study, Dawidson found significantly higher CsA blood levels (203 ± 74 vs. ng/ml) in patients receiving verapamil compared to 125 ± 64 ng/ml (p < 0.05) in controls, despite the same CsA dose.[18] When verapamil was discontinued after 10 days, according to the study protocol, CsA levels became similar in both patient groups (Fig. 7). The higher CsA levels observed in our patients treated with verapamil have been reported with other CATs (i.e., diltiazem, nicardipine, and nifedipine).[34,39–42] The increased CsA blood levels are most likely secondary to interaction between CATs and CsA at the cytochrome P-450 enzyme level. CATs such as verapamil and diltiazem inhibit the cytochrome P-450–dependent biotransformation. Since CsA is also metabolized through the P-450 enzyme system, CATs appear to be competitive inhibitors of CsA metabolism.[43] Despite the significantly higher CsA levels observed in our patients, nephrotoxicity did not occur, as evidenced by serum creatinine levels. In fact, kidney function, as determined by GFR, improved by 29.2 ± 12.5 ml/min in verapamil-treated patients, from day 1 to day 7, significantly more than that seen without verapamil, or 11.8 ± 14.9 ml/min (p < 0.008) (Fig. 8). Others have observed a similar lack of CsA toxicity with CATs.[34,38] The increased CsA levels could be the result of an increased concentration of the less nephrotoxic, but pharmacologically active, metabolite #17.[44]

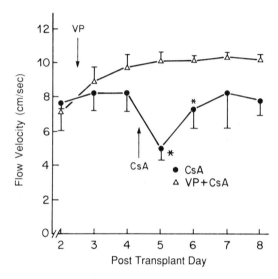

FIGURE 6. Parenchymal diastolic blood flow velocity improved on the first day of verapamil (VP) treatment and continued to increase during CsA therapy, significantly different from that seen with CsA alone ($p < 0.001$). Mean ± SEM.

Interaction of CATs on CsA-induced Immunosuppression

The decreased incidence of early rejection episodes in cadaver kidney recipients who receive calcium antagonists emphasizes still another potential use for CATs in human organ transplantation—enhanced immunosuppression and graft survival and decreased nephrotoxicity.[18,34,38] Extracellular calcium plays an important role in the regulation of cellular functions, including proliferation, secretion, and contraction.[45] Furthermore, there is evidence that an increment of intracellular calcium concentration may be the signal that initiates T-lymphocyte mitosis. Also, interaction between calcium and the intracellular protein, calmodulin, may play an important role in modulating lymphocyte immune responses.[46]

Because cytosolic calcium acts as an important messenger in lymphocyte regulation, calcium and CATs have been used in an attempt to modify the immune response. Three different calmodulin inhibitors were shown to inhibit lymphocyte proliferation in mixed lymphocyte reaction.[47] Furthermore, McMillen demonstrated that verapamil decreases calcium uptake in lymphocytes and inhibits lymphocyte proliferation in vitro. Preliminary data indicate that other calcium blockers have the same effect.[47] The same authors also reported a potentiation of CsA immunosuppression by verapamil in vitro.[48] While the effects of CATs are more limited to calcium transport and metabolism, the exact mechanism or site of their interaction with CsA is less clear. Calmodulin, the intracellular calcium-interacting protein necessary for lymphocyte proliferation, binds to and is inhibited by CsA and constitutes one possible mechanism for CAT and CsA interaction.[49,50]

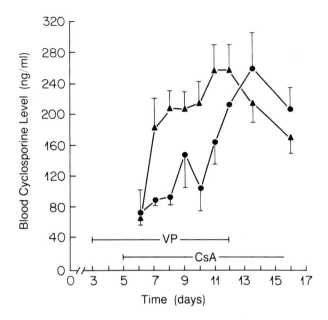

FIGURE 7. CsA whole blood levels (HPLC) were significantly higher during VP therapy than in patients receiving only CsA (p < 0.01). Mean ± SEM.

In vitro and animal studies have shown that verapamil does not alter cell or tissue uptake or release of CsA, suggesting that its action must involve disruption of an intracellular pathway of lymphocyte activation.[51] Somewhat contradictory to this is the overwhelming evidence of increased blood CsA concentration associated with CATs.[18,38-43]

Other possible mechanisms of CsA and verapamil interactions may involve inhibition of the transmembrane calcium transport. One theory is that CATs interact with CsA at the level of the lymphocyte protein kinase activations that induce the production of interleukin II.[51,52]

These in vitro studies are consistent with experimental results showing prolonged graft survival with verapamil (10 mg/kg) in rat heterotopic cardiac allograft transplants.[53] Furthermore, these data are also supported by significantly fewer rejections in clinical renal transplantation, with both verapamil[18] and diltiazem.[34]

Summary and Prospects

Animal research and clinical studies of transplant recipients strongly suggest hypoperfusion secondary to vasoconstriction as a causative factor in acute CsA nephrotoxicity. After organ transplantation, CATs improve blood flow in kidneys with low flow, thereby protecting from ischemia and resulting in decreased incidence of post-transplant ATN. Additionally, CATs given prior to CsA prevent a CsA-induced inhibition in renal blood flow. CATs also seem to reduce the number of early rejection episodes, suggesting a synergistic effect with CsA immunosuppression. Further exper-

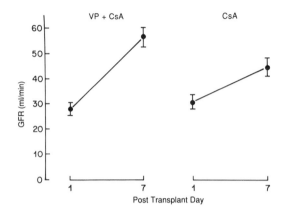

FIGURE 8. Glomerular filtration rate (GFR) increased significantly more between days 1 and 7 with VP, compared to CsA alone, especially when the initial GFR on day 1 was below 45 ml/min ($p < 0.008$). Mean ± SEM.

imental and clinical studies are needed to more clearly define the role of CATs in post-transplant renal function and rejection.

A future role for CATs in the prevention of chronic CsA nephrotoxicity is an exciting possibility. Further studies are needed of the interactions between calcium antagonists and cyclosporine A, a drug that has dramatically improved the outcome of kidney transplantation, making liver and heart transplantation procedures life-saving for thousands of patients each year.

References

1. Calne RY, White DJG, Thiru S, et al: Cyclosporin A in patients receiving renal allografts from cadaver donors. Lancet 2:1323, 1978.

2. Canadian Multicentre Trial Study Group: Cyclosporin in cadaveric renal transplantation: one-year follow-up of a multicentre trial. Lancet 2:986, 1983.

3. Starzl TE, Iwatsuki S, Van Thiel DH, et al: Report of Colorado and PIttsburgh liver transplantation studies. Transplant Proc 15:2582, 1983.

4. Oyer PE, Stinson EB, Jameson SA, et al: Cyclosporine in cardiac transplantation: a 2 1/2 year follow-up. Transplant Proc 15:2546, 1983.

5. Nussenblat RB, Palestine AG: Cyclosporine: immunology, pharmacology and therapeutic uses. Surv Ophthalmol 31:159, 1986.

6. Amor B, Dougados M: Ciclosporin in rheumatoid arthritis. Open trials with different dosages. In Schindler R (ed): Ciclosporin in Autoimmune Diseases. Berlin, Springer-Verlag, 1985, p 283.

7. Dupre J, Stiller CR, Gent M, et al: Effects of ciclosporin on insulin secretion in recent onset type 1 diabetes mellitus. In Schindler R (ed): Ciclosporin in Autoimmune Diseases. Berlin, Springer-Verlag, 1985, p 120.

8. Kappos L, Patzold U, Dommasch D, et al: Cyclosporine versus azathioprine in the long-term treatment of multiple sclerosis—results of the German multicenter study. Ann Neurol 23:56, 1988.

9. Myers B, Ross J, Newton L, et al: Cyclosporine-associated chronic nephropathy. N Engl J Med 311:699, 1984.

10. Myers BD (principal discussant, Nephrology Forum, Stanford University School of Medicine, Stanford, California): Cyclosporine nephrotoxicity. Kidney Int 30:964, 1986.

11. Rooth P, Dawidson I, Diller K, Taljedal I-B: Protection against cyclosporine-induced impairment of renal microcirculation by verapamil in mice. Transplantation 45:433, 1988.

12. Rooth P, Dawidson I, Clothier N, Diller K: In vivo fluorescence microscopy of kidney subcapsular blood flow in mice: Effects of cyclosporine A (CsA), (Nva^2)-cyclosporine (CsG) and isradipine, a new calcium antagonist. Transplantation 46:566, 1988.

13. McKenzie N, Devineni R, Vezina W, Keown P, Stiller C: The effect of cyclosporine on organ blood flow. Transplant Proc 17:1973, 1985.

14. Murray BM, Paller MS, Ferris TF: Effect of cyclosporine administration on renal hemodynamics in conscious rats. Kidney Int 28:767, 1985.

15. Murray BM, Paller MS: Beneficial effects of renal denervation and prazosin on GFR and renal blood flow after cyclosporine in rats. Clin Nephrol 25:S37, 1986.

16. Curtis JJ, Luke RG, Dubovsky E, Diethhelm AG, Whelchel JD, Jones P: Cyclosporine in therapeutic doses increases renal allograft vascular resistance. Lancet 2:477, 1986.

17. Fry WR, Dawidson I, Alway C, Rooth P: Cyclosporine A induces decreased blood flow in cadaveric kidney transplants. Transplant Proc 20:222, 1988.

18. Dawidson I, Rooth P, Fry WR, Coorpender L, Reisch J: Verapamil ameliorates acute cyclosporine A nephrotoxicity and improves immunosuppression after cadaver renal transplantation. Transplant Proc 21:1511, 1989.

18a. Dawidson I, Rooth P, Fry W, et al: Prevention of acute cyclosporine A-induced renal blood flow inhibition and improved immunosuppression with verapamil. Transplantation Oct. 1989 (in press).

19. Marbet UA, Graff U, Mihatsch MJ, Gratwohl A, Muller W, Thiel G: Renale nebenwirkungen der therapie mit cyclosporin A bei chronischer polyarthritis und nach knochenmarkstransplantation. Schweiz Med Wochenschr 110:2017, 1980.

20. Verpooten GA, Wybo I, Pattyn VM, et al: Cyclosporine nephrotoxicity: comparative cytochemical study of rat kidney and human allograft biopsies. Clin Nephrol 25:S18, 1986.

21. Mihatsch MF, Ryffel B, Hermle M, Brunner FP, Thiel G: Morphology of cyclosporine nephrotoxicity in the rat. Clin Nephrol 25:S2, 1986.

22. Sibley R, Rynasiewicz J, Ferguson R, et al: Morphology of cyclosporine nephrotoxicity and acute rejection in patients immunosuppressed with cyclosporine and prednisone. Surgery 94:225, 1983.

23. Bia MJ, Tyler KA: Effect of cyclosporine on renal ischemic injury. Transplantation 43:800, 1987.

24. Sommer B, Henry M, Ferguson R: Sequential antilymphoblast globuline and cyclosporine for renal transplantation. Transplantation 43:85, 1987.

25. Novick AC, Ho-Hsieh H, Steinmuller D, et al: Detrimental effect of cyclosporine on initial function of cadaver renal allograft following extended preservation. Transplantation 42:154, 1986.

26. Sagalowsky A, Reisman ME, Dawidson I, Toto R, Peters PC, Helderman JH: Late cyclosporine conversion carries risk of irreversible rejection. Transplant Proc 20:157, 1988.

27. Dawidson I, Berglin E, Brynger H, Reisch J: Intravascular volumes and colloid dynamics in relation to fluid management in living related kidney donors and recipients. Crit Care Med 15:631, 1987.

28. Dawidson I, Coorpender L, Drake D, et al: Intraoperative albumin improves the outcome of cadaver renal transplantation. Transplant Proc 19:4137, 1987.

29. Rooth P, Dawidson I, Diller K, Taljedal I-B: Beneficial effects of calcium antagonist pretreatment and albumin infusion on cyclosporine A-induced impairment of kidney microcirculation in mice. Transplant Proc 19:3602, 1987.

30. Dieperink H, Leyssac P, Starklint H, Jorgensen K, Kemp E: Antagonist capacities of nifedipine, captopril, phenoxybenzamine, prostacyclin and indomethacin on cyclosporin A-induced impairment of rat renal function. Eur J Clin Invest 16:540, 1986.

31. Agatstein E, Farrer J, Kaplan L, Randazzo R, Glassock R, Kaufman J: The effect of verapamil in reducing the severity of acute tubular necrosis in canine renal autotransplants. Transplantation 44:355, 1987.

32. Shapiro J, Cheung C, Itabashi A, Chan L, Schrier R: The effect of verapamil on renal function after warm and cold ischemia in the isolated perfused rat kidney. Transplantation 40:596, 1985.

33. Woolley J, Barker G, Jacobsen W, et al: Effect of the calcium entry blocker verapamil on renal ischemia. Crit Care Med 16:48, 1988.

34. Neumayer HH, Wagner K: Prevention of delayed graft function in cadaver kidney transplants by diltiazem: Outcome of two prospective, randomized clinical trials. J Cardiovas Pharmacol 10:S170, 1987.

35. Loutzenhiser R, Epstein M: Modification of the renal hemodynamic response to vaso-constrictors by calcium antagonists. Am J Nephrol 7:7, 1987.

36. Loutzenhiser RD, Epstein M: Renal hemodynamic effects of calcium antagonists. Am J Med 82:23, 1987.

37. Loutzenhiser R, Epstein M, Horton C: Modification by dihydropyridine-type calcium antagonists of the renal hemodynamic response to vasoconstrictors. J Cardiovasc Pharmacol 9:70, 1987.

38. Feehally J, Walls J, Mistry N, et al: Does nifedipine ameliorate cyclosporin A nephro-toxocity? Br Med J 295:310, 1987.

39. Pochet J, Pirson Y: Cyclosporin-diltiazem interaction. Lancet 1:979, 1986.

40. Grino JM, Sabate I, Cateslao A, Alsina J: Influence of diltiazem on cyclosporin clearance. Lancet 1:1387, 1986.

41. Bourbigot B, Guiserix J, Airiau J, Bressollette L, Morin JF, Cledes J: Nicardipine increases cyclosporin blood levels. Lancet 21:1447, 1986.

42. Lindholm A, Henricsson S: Verapamil inhibits cyclosporin metabolism. Lancet 1:1262, 1987.

43. Renton KW: Inhibition of hepatic microsomal drug metabolism by the calcium channel blockers diltiazem and verapamil. Biochem Pharmacol 34:2549, 1985.

44. Wagner K, Philipp Th, Heinemeyer G, Roots I, Brockmuller F, Neumayer HH: Inter-action of calcium antagonists and ciclosporin. Transplant Proc 1989 (in press).

45. Lichtman AH, Segel GB, Lichtman MA: The role of calcium in lymphocyte proliferation. Blood 61:413, 1983.

46. Bachvaroff RJ, Miller F, Rapaport FI: The role of calcium in the regulation of human lymphoctye activation. Cell Immunol 85:135, 1984.

47. McMillen MA, Lewis T, Jaffe BM, Wait RB: Verapamil inhibition of lymphocyte proliferation and function in vitro. J Surg Res 39:76, 1985.

48. McMillen MA, Tesi RJ, Baumgarten WB, Jaffe BM, Wait RB: Potentiation of cyclosporine by verapamil in vitro. Transplantation 40:444, 1985.

49. Colombani PM, Bright EC, Monastyrskyj O, Hess AD: Subcellular action of cyclosporine: Interaction between CsA and calmodulin antagonists. Transplant Proc 19:1171, 1987.

50. LeGrue SJ, Munn CG: Comparison of the immunosuppressive effects of cyclosporine, lipid-soluble anesthetics, and calmodulin antagonists. Transplantation 42:679, 1986.

51. McMillen MA, Baumgarten WK, Schaefer HC, et al: The effect of verapamil on cellular uptake, organ distribution, and pharmacology of cyclosporine. Transplantation 44:395, 1987.

52. Iyer AP, Pishak SA, Sniezak MJ, Mastro AM: Visualization of protein kinases in lymphocytes stimulated to proliferate with concanavalin A or inhibited with a phorbol ester. Biochem Biophys Res Commun 121:392, 1984.

53. Tesi RF, Hong J, Butt KMH, Jaffe BM, McMillen MA: In vivo potentiation of cyclosporine immunosuppression by calcium antagonists. Transplant Proc 19:1382, 1987.

Garry P. Reams, M.D.
John H. Bauer, M.D.

15

Acute and Chronic Effects of Calcium Antagonists on the Essential Hypertensive Kidney

A large number of calcium entry blocking drugs are currently undergoing clinical investigation. They are a chemically heterogeneous group of drugs, sharing a common antihypertensive mechanism of action: interference with entry of calcium into smooth muscle cells of resistance arterioles through voltage (potential) dependent channels. Systemic vascular resistance is reduced; heart rate and cardiac output are maintained or increased. There are three currently available subclasses of calcium antagonists. This chapter focuses on the renal function effects of the benzothiazepine derivative, diltiazem; the diphenylalkylamine derivative, verapamil; and the dihydropyridine derivatives: amlodipine, felodipine, isradipine, nicardipine, nifedipine, and nitrendipine. Each of these drugs is discussed in terms of its acute (following intravenous or initial oral dosing) and chronic (following oral dosing for days to months) effects on renal function, specifically glomerular filtration rate, effective renal plasma flow/renal blood flow, renal vascular resistance, and urinary protein excretion.

Benzothiazepine Derivative

Diltiazem. The acute intravenous administration of diltiazem to patients with essential hypertension has no significant effect on either glomerular filtration rate or effective renal plasma flow/renal blood flow (Table 1).[1] However, diltiazem administered into the renal artery of normotensive subjects with a family history of hypertension has been reported to increase renal blood flow 200%; in normotensive subjects without a family history of hypertension, renal blood flow was increased 100%.[2] The threshold dose of diltiazem required for a change in renal blood flow was similar for both groups.

The chronic oral administration of diltiazem to patients with primary or secondary renal disease and hypertension has been reported to increase both glomerular

TABLE 1. Acute and Chronic Renal Response to Diltiazem and Verapamil Monotherapy

Investigator (year)	Patient Number/Type	Dose; Route Administered	Duration Therapy
Benzothiazepine Derivative: Diltiazem			
Acute			
Blackshear et al. (1987)[2]	16; NT (+FH)	10-1000 ug/min; IRA	—
	36; NT (−FH)	10-1000 ug/min; IRA	—
Reams et al. (1987)[1]	18; EH	0.2-0.5 mg/kg; IV	—
Chronic			
Sakurai et al. (1972)[3]	26; RD, HTN	60-120 mg	1-4 wks
Tojo et al. (1972)[4]	9; RD, HTN	30- 90 mg	2-5 wks
Sunderrajan et al. (1986)[5]	18; EH	240-480 mg	8 wks
	10; EH[1]	240-480 mg	8 wks
	8; EH[2]	240-480 mg	8 wks
Sunderrajan et al. (1987)[6]	11; EH	240-480 mg	24 wks
	6; EH[2]	240-480 mg	24 wks
Diphenylalkylamine Derivative: Verapamil			
Acute			
Leonetti et al. (1982)[7]	8; EH	160 mg, oral	—
	8; NT	160 mg, oral	—
Chronic			
Leonetti et al. (1980)[8]	12; EH	240-480 mg	10 days
deLeeuw & Birkenhager (1984)[9]	15; EH	480 mg	10 days
Sorensen et al. (1985)[10]	11; EH	240-360 mg	6 wks
Kubo et al. (1986)[11]	9; EH	240-480 mg	1 wk
Schmieder et al. (1987)[12]	10; EH	240-480 mg	12 wks

NT = normotensive subjects
EH[1] = glomerular filtration rate > 80 ml/min/1.73 m^2
EH[2] = glomerular filtration rate ≤ 80 ml/min/1.73 m^2
NT(+FH) = normotensive subjects with a family history of hypertension
NT(−FH) = normotensive subjects without a family history of hypertension
EH = subjects with essential hypertension
RD, HTN = renal parenchymal disease with hypertension
IV = intravenous infusion
IRA = intra-renal arterial infusion

filtration rate (+5 to +62%) and effective renal plasma flow/renal blood flow (+8 to +36%).[3−6] However, patients with essential hypertension who have normal renal function have been reported to experience a modest decrease (but to within normal limits) in both glomerular filtration rate and effective renal plasma flow.[5] Regardless, there is a marked decrease in renal vascular resistance (−15 to −42%).

Diphenylalkylamine Derivative

Verapamil. The acute oral administration of verapamil has no significant effect on creatinine clearance in either normotensive or hypertensive subjects (see Table 1).[7]

TABLE 1. (Cont.)

Δ MAP (%)	Δ GFR (%)	ΔERPF/RBF (%)	ΔRVR (%)
—	—	+200 (^{133}XE)	—
—	—	+100 (^{133}XE)	—
− 4	− 1 (inulin)	0 (PAH)	—
− 5	+18 (creatinine)	+19 (^{131}I-Hippuran)	—
− 1	+ 5 (thiosulfate)	+ 8 (PAH)	—
−11*	0 (inulin)	+ 8 (PAH)	−22*
−10	−20*(inulin)	−14 (PAH)	—
−12	+48*(inulin)	+36*(PAH)	−42*
−15*	+1 (inulin)	− 4 (PAH)	−15
−14*	+62*(inulin)	+34 (PAH)	−38*
− 5	+ 3 (creatinine)	—	—
0	+ 3 (creatinine)	—	—
−14	+ 1 (creatinine)	—	—
−18*	—	− 1 (^{125}I-Hippuran)	−16*
− 8*	+ 4 (^{125}Iothalamate)	+ 1 (^{131}I-Hippuran)	—
−17*	+ 8 (inulin)	+ 3 (PAH)	−13*
−14*	+ 6 (creatinine)	+11 (^{131}I-Hippuran)	−25*

ΔMAP = percent change in mean arterial pressure
Δ GFR = percent change in glomerular filtration rate
Δ ERPF/RBF = percent change in effective renal plasma flow/renal blood flow
Δ RVR = percent change in renal vascular resistance
PAH = para-aminohippurate
^{133}XE = 133 radioxenon
* = statistically significant change

Similarly, the chronic oral administration of verapamil has no significant effect on either glomerular filtration rate (+1 to +8%) or effective renal plasma flow/renal blood flow (−1 to +11%).[8−12] However, there is a marked decrease in renal vascular resistance (−13 to −25%).

Dihydropyridine Derivatives

Amlodipine. There are no reported data on the renal effects following the acute administration of amlodipine. However, the long-term administration of amlodipine to patients with essential hypertension has been reported to increase both glomerular filtration rate (+13%) and effective renal plasma/renal blood flow (+19%), and to

TABLE 2. The Acute Renal Response to Dihydropyridine Derivative Monotherapy

Investigator (Year)	Patient Number/Type	Dose; Route Administered
Dihydropyridine Derivatives:		
Amlodipine	NO DATA AVAILABLE	
Felodipine		
Schmitz (1987)[14]	8; NT	0.15 mg/kg; oral
Hulthen and Katzman (1988)[15]	10; EH	10 mg; oral
Isradipine	NO DATA AVAILABLE	
Nicardipine		
Van Schaik (1984)[18]	10; EH	20 mg; oral
	10; NT	20 mg; oral
Van Schaik (1985)[19]	10; NT	20 mg; oral
Baba et al. (1986)[21]	7; EH	0.5 mg; IV
Chaignon et al. (1986)[20]	10; EH	30 mg; oral
Smith et al. (1987)[22]	6; EH	80 ug/kg/hr; IV
Nifedipine		
Klutsch et al. (1972)[23]	9; EH	1 mg; IV
	11; RD, HTN	1 mg; IV
Leonetti et al. (1982)[7]	8; EH	10 mg; oral
	8; NT	10 mg; oral
Yokoyama & Kaburagi (1983)[24]	12; EH	13.3 ug/min; IV
	9; RD, HTN	13.3 ug/min; IV
	14; RD, NT	13.3 ug/min; IV
	12; NT	13.3 ug/min; IV
Tsunoda et al. (1986)[25]	15; EH	20 mg; oral
Nitrendipine		
Thananopavarn et al. (1984)[28]	9; EH	20 mg; oral
Wallia et al. (1985)[29]	8; NT	5-10 mg; oral
Lupinacci et al. (1988)[30]	7; EH	10 mg; oral
	7; NT	10 mg; oral

NT = normotensive subjects
EH = subjects with essential hypertension
RD, HTN = renal parenchymal disease with hypertension
RD, NT = renal parenchymal disease, normotensive
IV = intravenous infusion

decrease renal vascular resistance (−25%) (see Table 3).[13] Urinary protein excretion is unchanged.[13]

Felodipine. The acute oral administration of felodipine has no significant effect on glomerular filtration rate in either normotensive or hypertensive subjects (Table 2).[14,15] However, effective renal plasma flow/renal blood flow has been reported to increase (+12 to +14%), and renal vascular resistance to decrease (−22%).[14,15]

The short-term oral administration of felodipine has been reported to decrease glomerular filtration rate (−1 to −13%);[16] however, longer-term therapy is associated with a mild increase in glomerular filtration rate (+5%) (Table 3).[15] Chronic oral felodipine therapy has been reported to have no effect on effective renal plasma flow/renal blood flow (see Table 3).[15]

Isradipine. There are no reported data on the renal effects following the acute administration of isradipine. However, the chronic oral administration of isradipine

TABLE 2. (Cont.)

Δ MAP (%)	Δ GFR (%)	Δ ERPF/RBF (%)	Δ RVR (%)
−14*	0 (^{125}Iothalamate)	+12 (^{131}I-Hippuran)	−22*
−14*	+ 3 (^{51}Cr-EDTA)	+14*(^{125}I-Hippuran)	—
− 5*	+ 8 (creatinine)	—	—
− 4*	+ 6 (creatinine)	—	—
− 4	+ 5 (creatinine)	—	—
−12*	+28*(thiosulfate)	+25*(PAH)	−31*
−17*	− 8 (^{125}Iothalamate)	+13*(^{131}I-Hippuran)	−25*
−25*	+ 5 (^{51}Cr-EDTA)	+15*(^{123}I-Hippuran)	−39*
−20	+24 (inulin)	+30 (PAH)	—
−20	−12 (inulin)	+ 1 (PAH)	—
−21*	+ 7 (creatinine)	—	—
0	+17 (creatinine)	—	—
0	+46*(thiosulfate)	+45*(PAH)	−27*
0	+10 (thiosulfate)	+ 6 (PAH)	+11
− 2	+13*(thiosulfate)	+12 (PAH)	−10
− 7	+ 6 (thiosulfate)	− 2 (PAH)	− 1
−18*	+12*(creatinine)	—	—
−18*	− 3 (DTPA)	+20 (^{131}I-Hippuran)	—
0	− 1 (inulin)	+ 1 (PAH)	—
—	+ 7 (inulin)	+10 (PAH)	− 9
—	+ 7 (inulin)	+ 4 (PAH)	− 5

ΔMAP = percent change in mean arterial pressure
Δ GFR = percent change in glomerular filtration rate
Δ ERPF/RBF = percent change in effective renal plasma flow/renal blood flow
Δ RVR = percent change in renal vascular resistance
PAH = para-aminohippurate
^{51}Cr-EDTA = ^{51}Cr-ethylene diamine tetraacetate
DTPA = ^{99m}Tc-ethylene triamine penta-acetic acid
* = statistically significant change

has been reported to increase both glomerular filtration rate (+ 6%) and effective renal plasma flow (+ 9%), and to decrease renal vascular resistance (−22%)(see Table 3).[17]

Nicardipine. The acute oral administration of nicardipine has no consistent effect on glomerular filtration rate in either normotensive or hypertensive subjects (−8 to + 8%).[18−20] The intravenous administration of nicardipine has been reported to increase glomerular filtration rate (+ 5 to + 28%).[21,22] Both oral (single dose) and intravenous nicardipine have been demonstrated to increase effective renal plasma flow/renal blood flow (+ 13 to + 25%), and to decrease renal vascular resistance (−25 to −39%) (see Table 2).[20−22] The short-term oral administration of nicardipine has no consistent effect on either glomerular filtration rate (−3 to + 20%)[18−22] or effective renal plasma flow/renal blood flow (0 to + 10%).[20,22] However, renal vascular resistance is decreased (−26 to −31%)(see Table 3).[20,22]

TABLE 3. The Chronic Renal Response to Dihydropyridine Derivative Monotherapy

Investigator (year)	Patient Number/Type	Dose	Duration Therapy
Dihydropyridine Derivatives:			
Amlodipine			
Reams et al. (1987)[13]	19; EH	5-10 mg	6 wks
Felodipine			
Leonetti et al. (1984)[16]	11; EH	37.5 mg	3 days
	9; EH	75 mg	3 days
	6; EH	150 mg	3 days
Hulthen and Katzman (1988)[15]	10; EH	20 mg	8 wks
Isradipine			
Krusell et al. (1987)[17]	10; EH	20–40 mg	14 wks
Nicardipine			
Van Schaik et al. (1984)[18]	10; EH	60 mg	1 wk
	10; NT	60 mg	1 wk
Van Schaik et al. (1985)[19]	10; NT	60 mg	1 wk
Chaignon et al. (1986)[20]	10; EH	90 mg	6 days
Smith et al. (1987)[22]	6; EH	90–160 mg	6 wks
Nifedipine			
Bruun et al. (1986)[26]	18; EH	40–80 mg	12 wks
Reams et al. (1988)[27]	26; EH	30–120 mg	4 wks
	18; EH(R+)	30–120 mg	4 wks
	7; EH(R−)	30–120 mg	4 wks
Nitrendipine			
Thananopavarn et al. (1984)[28]	9; EH	20–40 mg	2 wks
Simon et al. (1984)[31]	11; EH	32 mg	5 wks
Luft et al. (1985)[32]	8; EH	40 mg	8 days
	8; NT	40 mg	8 days
Pedrinelli et al. (1986)[33]	13; EH	40 mg	2 wks
Lupnacci et al. (1988)[30]	7; EH	20 mg	11 days
	7; NT	10 mg	11 days

EH = subjects with essential hypertension
EH(R+) = responders
EH(R−) = non-responders
NT = normotensive subjects

Nifedipine. The intravenous administration of nifedipine to patients with essential hypertension has been reported to increase glomerular filtration rate ($+24$ to $+46\%$) and to increase effective renal plasma flow/renal blood flow ($+30$ to $+45\%$)(see Table 2).[23-24] However, the intravenous administration of nifedipine to patients with renal disease, with or without hypertension, has a more variable effect on glomerular filtration rate (-12 to $+13\%$), although effective renal plasma flow/renal blood flow is either unchanged or increased ($+1$ to $+12\%$).[23,24] The acute oral administration of nifedipine has been reported to increase glomerular filtration rate in both normotensive and essential hypertensive patients.[7,25]

The renal response to long-term nifedipine administration is variable (see Table 3). Bruun et al.[26] have reported that nifedipine has no effect on glomerular filtration rate. However, Reams et al.[27] have reported that nifedipine increased glomerular filtration rate ($+13\%$) and effective renal plasma flow/renal blood flow ($+20\%$). Renal vascular resistance was decreased (-25%). The observed renal responses

TABLE 3. *(Cont.)*

Δ MAP (%)	Δ GFR (%)	Δ ERPF/RBF (%)	Δ RVR (%)
−12*	+13*(inulin)	+19*(PAH)	−25*
−19*	− 1 (creatinine)	—	—
−21*	− 8 (creatinine)	—	—
−23*	−13 (creatinine)	—	—
−13*	+ 5 (^{51}Cr-EDTA)	0 (^{125}I-Hippuran)	—
−14*	+ 6*(^{125}Iothalamate)	+ 9* (^{131}I-Hippuran)	−22*
− 6*	+20*(creatinine)	—	—
− 6*	0 (creatinine)	—	—
− 2*	+ 1 (creatinine)	—	—
−24	− 3 (^{125}Iothalamate)	+10 (^{131}I-Hippuran)	−31*
−22*	0 (^{51}Cr-EDTA)	0 (^{123}I-Hippuran)	−26*
−10*	− 1 (^{51}Cr-EDTA)	—	—
−12*	+13*(inulin/DTPA)	+20*(PAH)	−25*
−15*	+13 (inulin/DTPA)	+19*(PAH)	—
− 3	+13 (inulin/DTPA)	+20*(PAH)	—
−14*	+20 (DTPA)	0 (^{131}I-Hippuran)	—
−12	− 4 (creatinine)	—	—
− 1	+14 (creatinine)	—	—
+ 2	+ 1 (creatinine)	—	—
−13*	+10 (^{125}Iothalamate)	+ 5 (^{131}I-Hippuran)	−18
− 5	+ 6 (inulin)	+ 3 (PAH)	+ 3
0	+ 1 (inulin)	+10 (PAH)	− 8

ΔMAP = percent change in mean arterial pressure
Δ GFR = percent change in glomerular filtration rate
Δ ERPF/RBF = percent change in effective renal plasma flow/renal blood flow
Δ RVR = percent change in renal vascular resistance
PAH = para-aminohippurate
^{51}Cr-EDTA = ^{51}Cr-ethylene diamine tetraacetate
DTPA = ^{99m}Tc-ethylene triamine penta-acetic acid
* = statistically significant change

by Reams et al.[27] were independent of the patient's initial level of glomerular filtration rate and were independent of the patient's level of blood pressure control. These investigators also observed no significant change in urinary albumin excretion.

Nitrendipine. The acute oral administration of nitrendipine has no consistent effect on glomerular filtration rate in either normotensive or hypertensive subjects (−1 to +7%)(see Table 2).[28–30] However, effective renal plasma flow/renal blood flow has been reported to increase (+10 to +20%) in hypertensive subjects. Renal vascular resistance is decreased (−5 to −9%). The long-term administration of oral nitrendipine therapy to both normotensive and hypertensive subjects has no consistent effect on either glomerular filtration rate (−4 to −20%)[28,30–33] or effective renal plasma flow/renal blood flow (0 to +10%)(see Table 3).[28,30,33]

Conclusions

Among the calcium antagonists discussed, only the dihydropyridine derivatives (felodipine, nicardipine, nifedipine, and nitrendipine) have been demonstrated consistently to acutely increase effective renal plasma flow/renal blood flow. The acute effects of calcium antagonists on glomerular filtration rate are more variable; no consistent pattern is observed. With respect to chronic therapy, diltiazem, amlodipine, isradipine, nicardipine, nifedipine, and nitrendipine have all been reported to produce sustained increases in glomerular filtration rate and/or effective renal plasma flow/renal blood flow. The observed improvements in effective renal plasma flow and glomerular filtration rate (in the presence of a marked reduction in mean arterial pressure) may be independent of the drug's effect on systemic blood pressure.[27]

There are several potential mechanisms for the observed increases in glomerular filtration rate and/or effective renal plasma flow associated with calcium antagonist therapy. For example as detailed in Chapter 3, calcium antagonists may increase GFR by reversing the actions of angiotensin II on glomerular mesangial cells, or by attenuating norepinephrine-induced afferent vasoconstriction. Effective renal plasma flow may be increased as a consequence of the reversal by calcium antagonists of the microvascular actions of each of these vasoconstrictors. The effect of calcium entry blockers to prevent an increase in cytosol-ionized calcium would be expected to decrease the sensitivity of the renal vasculature to both angiotensin II and norepinephrine. Indeed, several investigators have demonstrated that calcium antagonists attenuate the intrarenal effects of exogenously administered angiotensin II and norepinephrine.[34,35] Calcium antagonists may also differentially effect alpha-adrenergic receptors, preferentially antagonizing post-synaptic alpha$_2$-adrenergic receptors.[34] Since in vitro studies suggest that calcium antagonists may exert a selective interference with the vasoconstrictor actions of norepinephrine on the afferent arteriole, one might speculate that alpha$_2$-adrenoceptors may mediate afferent arteriolar vasoconstriction, whereas alpha$_1$-adrenoceptors may predominate in the efferent vessel. However, evidence to date does not support the presence of a significant alpha$_2$-adrenergic component of norepinephrine-induced renal vasoconstriction.[36,37] Nevertheless, observations in hypertensive patients, that when glomerular filtration rate is increased, the filtration fraction is unchanged, suggest a differential attenuating effect of norepinephrine on the afferent (preglomerular) capillary bed, but do not exclude the possibility of a concurrent reversal of a direct angiotensin II effect on the glomerulus (mesangium) or efferent (postglomerular) capillary bed. Reversal of angiotensin II-mediated efferent arteriolar vasoconstriction might be expected to disproportionately enhance effective renal plasma flow, decreasing the filtration fraction. However, calcium antagonists generally do not alter the filtration fraction. In a preliminary study, the acute infusion of calcium antagonists was reported to reduce glomerular capillary pressure,[38] suggesting an acute action on both pre- and postglomerular resistances. However, as detailed elsewhere in this text, other micropuncture studies have revealed that glomerular capillary hypertension persists following the administration of calcium antagonists, even in the presence of a decrease in systemic blood pressure (see Chapter 8).

Calcium antagonists can be expected to assume a prominent role in the treatment of essential hypertension because of their ability to lower systemic blood pressure while preserving or improving renal perfusion and glomerular filtration. With rare exception,[39,40] they do not adversely effect renal function. Long-term clinical trials are required to determine if the observed short-term renal responses to calcium antagonism monotherapy are sustained, and/or have the therapeutic benefit to modify the natural course of essential hypertensive renal disease, and/or to attenuate the natural progression of advanced renal parenchymal disease.

References

1. Reams GP, Lau A, Messina C, Villarreal D, Bauer JH: Efficacy, electrocardiographic and renal effects of intravenous diltiazem for essential hypertension. Am J Cardiol 60:78I–84I, 1987.

2. Blackshear JL, Garnic D, Williams GH, Harrington DP, Hollenberg NK: Exaggerated renal vasodilator response to calcium entry blockade in first-degree relatives of essential hypertensive subjects. Hypertension 9:384–389, 1987.

3. Sakurai T, Kurita T, Nagamo S, Sonoda T: Antihypertensive, vasodilating and sodium diuretic actions of D-cis-isomer of benzothiazepine derivative (CRD-401). Acta Urologica Japonica 18:695–707, 1972.

4. Tojo S, Shishido H, Yamamoto S: Effects of CRD-401 on blood pressure and renal function. Jap J Clin Exp Med 49:1958–1966, 1972.

5. Sunderrajan S, Reams GP, Bauer JH: Renal effects of diltiazem in primary hypertension. Hypertension 8:238–242, 1986.

6. Sunderrajan S, Reams G, Bauer JH: Long-term renal effects on diltiazem in essential hypertension. Am Heart J 114:383–388, 1987.

7. Leonetti G, Cuspidi C, Sampieri L, Terzoli L, Zanchetti A: Comparison of cardiovascular, renal and humoral effects of acute administration of two calcium channel blockers in normotensive and hypertensive subjects. J Cardiovasc Pharmacol 4:S319–S324, 1982.

8. Leonetti G, Sala C, Bianchini C, Terzoli L, Zanchetti A: Antihypertensive and renal effects of orally administered verapamil. Eur J Clin Pharmacol 18:375–382, 1980.

9. deLeeuw PW, Birkenhager WH: Effects of verapamil in hypertensive patients. Acta Med Scand (suppl)681:125–128, 1984.

10. Sorenson SS, Thomsen O, Danilesen H, Pedersen EB: Effect of verapamil on renal plasma flow, glomerular filtration rate and plasma angiotensin II, aldosterone and arginine vasopressin in essential hypertension. Eur J Clin Pharmacol 29:257–261, 1985.

11. Kubo SH, Cody RJ, Covit AB, Feldschuh J, Laragh JH: The effects of verapamil on renal blood flow, renal function, and neurohormonal profiles in patients with moderate to severe hypertension. J Clin Hypertens 3:38S–46S, 1986.

12. Schmieder RE, Messerli FH, Garavaglia GE, Nunez BD: Cardiovascular effects of verapamil in patients with essential hypertension. Circulation 75:1030–1036, 1987.

13. Reams GP, Lau A, Hamory A, Bauer JH: Amlodipine therapy corrects renal abnormalities encountered in the hypertensive state. Am J Kid Dis 10:446–451, 1987.

14. Schmitz A: Acute renal effects of oral felodipine in normal man. Eur J Clin Pharmacol 32:17–22, 1987.

15. Hulthen UL, Katzman PL: Renal effects of acute and long-term treatment with felodipine in essential hypertension. J´Hypertens 6:231– 237, 1988.

16. Leonetti G, Gradnik R, Terzoli L, Fruscio M, Rupoli L, Zanchetti A: Felodipine, a new vasodilating drug: blood pressure, cardiac, renal, and humoral effects in hypertensive patients. J Cardiovasc Pharmacol 6:392– 398, 1984.

17. Krusell LR, Jespersen LT, Schmitz A, Thomsen K, Pedersen OL: Repetitive natriuresis and blood pressure. Hypertension 10:577–581, 1987.

18. Van Schaik BAM, Van Nistelrooy AEJ, Geyskes GG: Antihypertensive and renal effects of nicardipine. Br J Clin Pharmacol 18:57–63, 1984.

19. Van Schaik BAM, Hene RJ, Geyskes GG: Influence of nicardipine on blood pressure, renal function and plasma aldosterone in normotensive volunteers. Br J Clin Pharmacol 20:88S–94S, 1985.

20. Chaignon M, Bellet M, Lucsko M, Rapoud C, Geudon J: Acute and chronic effects of a new calcium inhibitor, nicardipine, on renal hemodynamics in hypertension. J Cardiovasc Pharmacol 8:892–897, 1986.

21. Baba T, Bolu A, Ishizaki T, Sone K, Takeke K: Renal effects of nicardipine in patients with mild-to-moderate essential hypertension. Am Heart J 111:552–557, 1986.

22. Smith SA, Rafiqi EI, Gardener EG, Young MA, Littles WA: Renal effects of nicardipine in essential hypertension: Differences between acute and chronic therapy. J Hypertens 5:693–697, 1987.

23. Klutsch VK, Schmidt P, Grosswendt J: Der enfluss von BAY a 1040 auf die Nieren-femktion des Hypertonikers. Arzneim.-Forsch. (Drug Res) 22:377–380, 1972.

24. Yokoyama S, Kuburagi T: Clinical effects of intravenous nifedipine on renal function. J Cardiovasc Pharmacol 5:67–71, 1983.

25. Tsunoda K, Ake K, Omata K, et al: Hypotensive and natriuretic effects of nifedipine in essential hypertension. J Clin Hypertens 3:263–270, 1986.

26. Bruun NE, Ibsen H, Nielsen F, Nielsen MD, Moelbak A, Hartling OJ: Lack of effect of nifedipine in counterregulatory mechanisms in essential hypertension. Hypertension 8:655–661, 1986.

27. Reams GP, Hamory A, Lau A, Bauer JH: Effect of nifedipine on renal function in patients with essential hypertension. Hypertension 11:452–456, 1988.

28. Thananopavarn C, Golub MS, Eggena P, Barrett JD, Sambhi MP: Renal effects of nitrendipine monotherapy in essential hypertension. J Cardiovasc Pharmacol 6:S1032–S1036, 1984.

29. Wallia R, Greenberg A, Puschett JB: Renal hemodynamic and tubular effects of nitrendipine. J Lab Clin Med 105:498–503, 1985.

30. Lupinacci L, Palomino C, Greenberg A, Puschett JB: Chronic effects of nitrendipine on renal hemodynamics and tubular transport. Clin Pharmacol Ther 43:6–15, 1988.

31. Simon G, Snyder DK: Altered pressor responses in long-term nitrendipine treatment. Clin Pharmacol Ther 36:315–319, 1984.

32. Luft FC, Aronoff GR, Sloan RS, Finsberg NS, Weinberger MH: Calcium channel blockade with nitrendipine. Hypertension 7:438–442, 1985.

33. Pedrinelli R, Fouad FM, Tarazi RC, Bravo EL, Textor SC: Nitrendipine, a calcium-entry blocker. Arch Intern Med 146:62–65, 1986.

34. Bauer JH, Reams GP: Short- and long-term effects of calcium entry blockers on the kidney. Am J Cardiol 59:66A–71A, 1987.

35. Romero JC, Raij L, Granger JP, Ruilope LM, Rodicio JL: Multiple effects of calcium entry blockers on renal function in hypertension. Hypertension 10:140–151, 1987.

36. Edwards RM, Trizna W: Characterization of alpha-adrenoceptors on isolated rabbit renal arterioles. Am J Physiol 254:F178–F183, 1988.

37. Wolff DW, Gesek FA, Strandhoy JW: In vivo assessment of rat renal vascular adrenoceptors. J Pharmacol Exp Ther 241:472–476, 1987.

38. Anderson S, Clarey LE, Riley SL, Troy JL: Acute infusion of calcium channel blockers (CCB) reduces glomerular capillary pressure (P_{GC}) in rats with reduced renal mass (abstract). Kid Internat 22:370A, 1988.

39. Diamond JR, Cheung JY, Fang LS: Nifedipine induced renal dysfunction. Am J Med 77:905–909, 1984.

40. TerWee PM, Rosman JB, Van der geest S: Acute renal failure due to diltiazem. Lancet 2:1337–1338, 1984.

William H. Frishman, M.D.

16

CALCIUM ANTAGONISTS IN SYSTEMIC HYPERTENSION

Calcium antagonists are a distinct group of compounds that interfere with the normal transmembrane flux of extracellular calcium ions on which vascular tissue depends for contraction or impulse generation (See Chapter 1).[1] They reduce the contractile activity of the heart and promote coronary and systemic vasodilation. These effects provide the clinical rationale for the use of calcium antagonists in the management of ischemic heart disease, hypertrophic cardiomyopathy, and certain arrhythmias.[2,3] Since systemic vasodilation can be expected to reduce elevated arterial blood pressure, interest has been focused on the use of the calcium antagonists in the medical management of systemic hypertension.[4,5] This chapter examines the role of calcium antagonists in the treatment of arterial hypertension and reviews the clinical experience to date with use of the three prototype agents: nifedipine, verapamil and diltiazem (Fig. 1).

RATIONALE FOR USE OF CALCIUM ANTAGONISTS IN HYPERTENSION

Calcium Antagonists as Vasodilators

The beneficial effects of the calcium antagonists in hypertension relate to their ability to induce systemic arterial vasodilation.[6] In isolated human blood vessels, nifedipine has been demonstrated to produce concentration-dependent relaxation of noradrenaline or adrenaline-induced constriction of arteries and veins.[7] In clinical use, the partial venodilator effects of nifedipine are usually overcome by the sympathetic reflex activity elicited by the drug, leaving arterial dilatation as the predominant vascular effect.[8] The potent β-adrenergic stimulating responses elicited by nifedipine also result in increases in heart rate and myocardial contractility.[2]

Studies of the cardiac effects of verapamil have found the drug to produce little change in heart rate or cardiac output.[2,9] Like nifedipine, the principal hypotensive

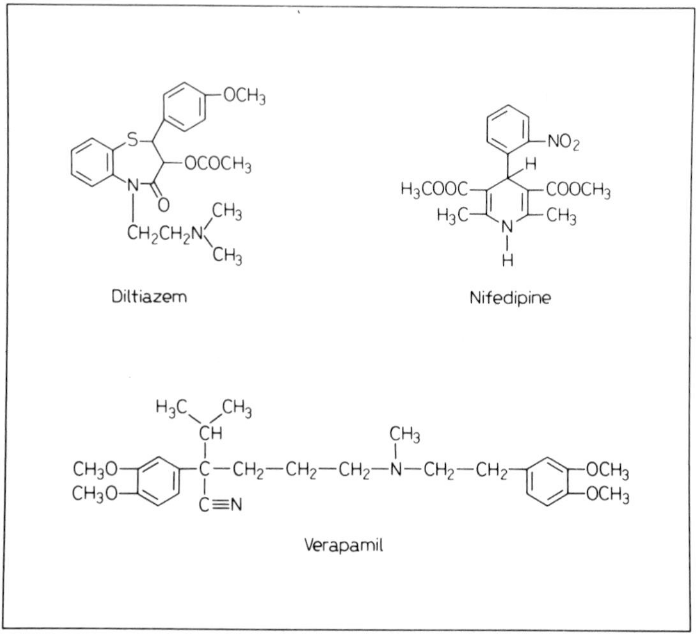

FIGURE 1. Molecular structure of the three major calcium antagonists—nifedipine (a dihydropyridine derivative), verapamil (structurally similar to papaverine), and diltiazem (a benzothiazepine derivative).

action of verapamil is mediated by peripheral vasodilation with reduction in peripheral vascular resistance. However, with verapamil, the reflex sympathetic stimulation noted with nifedipine and other vasodilators is blunted due to the drug's concomitant negative inotropic and negative chronotropic effects. Administration of diltiazem also produces little change in heart rate or cardiac output.[2,10] The comparative hemodynamic and electrophysiologic effects of the various calcium antagonists are shown in Table 1.

Experimental Use of Calcium Antagonists in Hypertensive Animals

Nifedipine has been utilized as an antihypertensive agent in rats with spontaneous hypertension, renovascular hypertension, deoxycorticosterone-induced hypertension, and chronic neurogenic hypertension.[11] Significant and dose-related decreases in blood pressure were seen in all experimental models. Nifedipine has also been compared with hydralazine in the rat model.[12] Both drugs effectively reduced blood pressure and increased heart rate, but the tachycardia was less pronounced with nifedipine than with hydralazine.

TABLE 1.   Hemodynamic and Electrophysiological Effects of the Calcium Antagonists

	Heart Rate Acute	Chronic	Conduction SA Node	Conduction AV Node	Myocardial Contractility	Peripheral Vasodilation	Cardiac Output	Coronary Blood Flow	Myocardial O$_2$ Demand
D	↓	↓	↓	↓	↓	↓	V	↑	↓
N	↑*	V*	—	—	V	↓↓	↑	↑	↓
V	↑	↓	↓	↓	↓↓	↓	V	↑	↓

* No change in heart rate occurs with nifedipine GITS, as discussed in text.
↓ = decrease; ↑ = increase; — = no change; and V = variable.

In conscious hypertensive rats, the use of diltiazem has been demonstrated to produce dose-related decreases in blood pressure and increases in heart rate;[13] the latter was attenuated by pretreatment with propranolol, suggesting that reflex sympathetic stimulation was likely the cause of diltiazem-induced tachycardia. Long-term oral administration of diltiazem to these experimental animals prevented the expected progressive increase in blood pressure typical of this breed.

In another study,[14] long-term administration of diltiazem to young, spontaneously hypertensive rats initially brought blood pressure to normal levels, but later had only weak effects in reducing blood pressure. This loss of blood pressure control may have reflected an inadequate long-term dosing regimen.

Clinical Use Of Calcium Antagonists In Systemic Hypertension

The introduction of calcium antagonists for clinical use represents an important advance in the treatment of hypertension. The calcium antagonists have been studied extensively as single agents and in combination with conventional antihypertensive agents. The following is a review of the currently available clinical studies using calcium antagonists in the treatment of hypertension.

Nifedipine

Hemodynamic Effects.   Detailed clinical investigations have documented the hemodynamic effects of nifedipine on the circulatory system in hypertensive patients. In one study,[15] a single 10 mg oral dose of nifedipine in 27 hypertensive patients reduced mean arterial pressure by 21% from the control value, with an average fall of 28 mmHg; the hemodynamic response to nifedipine was characterized by a reduction in peripheral vascular resistance and a concomitant rise in cardiac output. After the initial hemodynamic assessment, patients were treated with nifedipine for a 3-week period; during this time, blood pressure remained well controlled with 10 mg every 6 hours for 3 weeks, and no evidence of tachyphylaxis was observed. The hemodynamic effects of nifedipine recorded after 3 weeks of treatment were similar to the responses seen during acute administration of the drug. At the end of the trial, substitution of placebo for nifedipine caused a return of arterial blood pressure to pretreatment levels within 2 days. Similar results have been reported by Murakami et al.[16]

From these studies, it would appear that the negligible effects of nifedipine on capacitance vessels do not cause venous pooling, because, although cardiac output increases, right atrial pressure usually does not change. This is consistent with the findings of Mostbeck et al.[8], who performed whole-body scanning with a gamma camera after an intravenous injection of technetium 99m-labeled human albumin and found that no shift in fluid volume from the limbs to the trunk occurred after nifedipine administration. Guazzi et al.[15] attributed the tendency of some patients to have edema after nifedipine to arteriolar vasodilatation without venous vasodilatation, effects that could increase capillary blood pressure and result in edema.

The effect of nifedipine treatment on cerebral blood flow was investigated using xenon 133 in 10 hypertensive patients randomly allocated to receive either oral nifedipine or intravenous clonidine.[17] Before treatment, global cerebral blood flow was normal in all 10 patients tested. Oral nifedipine and intravenous clonidine were equally effective in lowering blood pressure, but significantly different changes in cerebral blood flow were observed between the two groups. Cerebral blood flow increased in four of the five patients treated with nifedipine; the fifth patient showed a slight decrease. This observation is consistent with findings of animal experiments that have demonstrated a selective increase in cardiac and cerebral blood flow after vasodilatation with nifedipine.[18] Intravenous administration of clonidine significantly reduced cerebral blood flow by as much as 28%. The decline noted with clonidine is probably related to a decrease in cardiac output and a slight concomitant increase in peripheral vascular resistance.[19]

Although much attention has been devoted to characterization of the ability of calcium antagonists to improve perfusion of the ischemic heart and augment cerebral blood flow, only recently has attention begun to focus on their salutary renal effects.[20] These striking effects are detailed elsewhere in this volume.

Effects on Plasma Renin Activity.   There is no consensus as to the effect of nifedipine on plasma renin activity.[21-25] In a study by Pederson et al.,[22] plasma renin activity increased after short-term administration of nifedipine, the most marked increases being seen in those patients with the highest plasma renin activities prior to treatment. However, long-term administration of nifedipine for 6 weeks produced no humoral changes. Thibonnier et al.[23] were unable to demonstrate an alteration of plasma renin activity after short-term administration of nifedipine. Olivari et al.[24] observed no change in plasma renin activity after 3 weeks of drug administration. Clearly, methodologic differences (e.g., the times at which plasma renin activity was measured, the assay system employed, the baseline renin level of the subjects, and the size of the study group) may explain much of the discrepant data, and further research should help resolve these questions. Insofar as calcium is important for the proper functioning of the feedback loop of the macula densa, which mediates renin release, calcium antagonists may inhibit this humoral loop and thereby inhibit renin release, depite significant vasodilation and reduction of systemic arterial pressure.[24,26]

Monotherapy.   Nifedipine monotherapy in the treatment of systemic hypertension has been actively investigated.[4,27] Beer et al.[5] evaluated the short-term use of nifedipine in blood pressure control in 43 patients with either moderate or severe hypertension. In the severely hypertensive patients, single 20 mg sublingual doses of nifedipine led to reductions in systolic and diastolic blood pressures of 44 and 31 mmHg, respectively. In patients with moderate hypertension, 10 mg of nifedipine was administered sublingually; the average systolic blood pressure reduction was 32 mmHg, whereas diastolic blood pressure fell 21 mmHg. Forty-two of the 43 patients responded favorably to a single sublingual dose. While an insignificant rise in heart rate occurred with a 10 mg sublingual dose, the heart rate rose an average of 13 beats/min in response to the 20 mg dose. Guazzi et al.[28] treated 26 patients with severe essential hypertension with 10 mg of nifedipine, administered either orally or sublingually. Maximum mean arterial pressure reduction was 36 mmHg 30 min after drug administration. Mean arterial pressure was 19.5% less than the control value 120 min after nifedipine was given. Side effects occurred in several patients; headache, palpitations with dysrhythmia, and burning leg and facial paresthesias were most common.

In a double-blind, crossover study, the antihypertensive effects of nifedipine (20 mg slow-release twice daily*) were compared with verapamil (160 mg three times daily.)[29] Although more side effects were reported with nifedipine, both agents provided antihypertensive efficacy. In a similar study, nifedipine and diltiazem used as antihypertenstive agents were both shown to be effective in lowering blood pressure.[30] Twenty-four–hour ambulatory blood pressure monitoring has confirmed that nifedipine was effective consistently in ambulatory patients, and that in the long-term follow up of these patients, drug action was sustained.[31]

Combination Therapy. Because reflex activation of the sympathetic nervous system is responsible for many of the drug's adverse effects, conventional nifedipine has been used together with antihypertensive drugs that attenuate adrenergic responses.

Guazzi et al.[15] administered nifedipine alone (10 mg orally, four times daily) and then together with methyldopa (250 mg orally four times/daily) to 23 patients with essential hypertension whose diastolic blood pressures exceeded 120 mmHg. Blood pressure decreased from 210/126 to 170/101 mmHg on nifedipine alone, and to 145/87 mmHg with nifedipine plus methyldopa. During combined therapy, systemic vascular resistance and heart rate were significantly reduced; cardiac index rose modestly, while pulmonary artery and pulmonary capillary wedge pressures declined. Of 23 patients who entered the study, 18 were continued on combined treatment for 1 year. Although clinical data were not reported, titration of the doses of both drugs was sufficient to maintain diastolic blood pressures between 84 and 100 mmHg. Aoki et al.[32] reported the first study, which evaluated nifedipine combined with propranolol. In 24 patients with an average blood pressure of 176/109 mmHg, propranolol potentiated the hypotensive effects of sublingual nifedipine, while suppressing nifedipine-induced tachycardia and abolishing nifedipine-related side-effects. Similar findings were observed by other investigators who combined nifedipine with β-blockers.[33–36]

Nifedipine has been combined with many other types of antihypertensive drugs as well.[37,38] In a study of 14 patients with severe systemic hypertension, nifedipine was combined with the angiotensin converting enzyme (ACE) inhibitor captopril.[38] The antihypertensive response of the combination was synergistic so that blood pressure was controlled.

*Preparation not available in the U.S.

Studies have shown nifedipine to be effective when other third-line agents, such as hydralazine, captopril and minoxidil, have proven ineffective or produced troublesome side effects. [39–42]

Controlled-release Nifedipine (The Osmotic Pump).   Recently, a new controlled-release drug-delivery system was developed by Alza Corporation, which allows nifedipine to be used once daily in hypertension or angina. [43,44] This drug-delivery system is an osmotic pump (Fig. 2) that allows nifedipine to be released over 18–36 hr without the abrupt plasma peaks of drugs usually associated with adverse reactions (Fig. 3). [43,44] Studies suggest that this new preparation, nifedipine GITS, is effective in reducing elevated blood pressure. [45] At the same time, nifedipine GITS is well tolerated, even at high doses. [45] There is a low incidence of vasodilatory side effects. Finally, in comparison to sustained-release propranolol (Inderal LA) in patients receiving diuretics, nifedipine GITS appears to be more effective and well tolerated. [45]

Hypertensive Patients with Angina Pectoris.   Nifedipine monotherapy has been used successfully in patients with hypertension and concomitant angina pectoris. [50] In a recent double-blind, crossover trial in 10 patients with angina and hypertension, [51] nifedipine was shown to be as effective as diltiazem in relieving anginal symptoms and reducing nitroglycerin consumption. The drugs also caused increases in excercise tolerance while reducing elevated systemic blood pressure.

Verapamil

Hemodynamic Effects.   Like nifedipine, verapamil produces significant decreases in arterial blood pressure because of its ability to reduce systemic vascular resistance. The

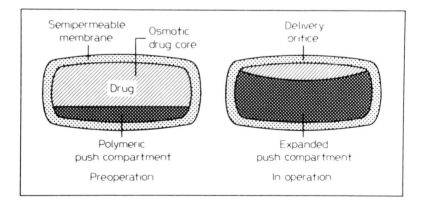

FIGURE 2.   The GITS system is a bilayer tablet surrounded by a semipermeable membrane. One layer contains the drug and the other osmotic excepients. A precisely measured hole is drilled by laser in the membrane above the drug compartment. When the tablet is swallowed, fluid from the gastrointestinal tract enters both layers. The drug is put into suspension and the osmotic excepients expand, pushing the drug out the laser-drilled hole and releasing the drug at a fairly constant rate. Figure provided by Felix Theeuwes, DSc.

expected activation of the sympathetic nervous system occurs, but its effects on the myocardium and sinus node are attenuated by verapamil's direct negative inotropic and chronotropic effects. The observed hemodynamic effects of verapamil are the net result of these two opposing forces; hence, it is not surprising that the drug's effects on cardiac output and heart rate have been reported to vary widely.[2,9,42,51,52] After verapamil, heart rate may increase, not change, or decline; similarly, cardiac output may increase, remain the same, or decrease. Nevertheless, most investigators agree that verapamil must be used cautiously in patients with heart failure.[2,42,51-53] The vasodilating capacity of the drug cannot always be relied on to overcome its negative inotropic effects.

Monotherapy. A number of studies have investigated the acute and long-term hypotensive effects of verapamil in hypertensive patients.[54-61] Muiesan et al.[54] evaluated the antihypertensive effects of verapamil in 28 patients with mild to moderate hypertension. Verapamil (160 mg orally) reduced blood pressure within 1 hr, with a peak effect at 1.5 to 2.0 hr, and a duration of action of 4 hours; heart rate and plasma renin activity were unaltered. Twelve patients received verapamil 80 mg three times daily for 8 days; the mean reduction in supine systolic and diastolic pressures was 23 and 15 mmHg, respectively; heart rate, plasma renin activity, plasma and urinary catecholamines, plasma and urinary aldosterone, and plasma volumes were not

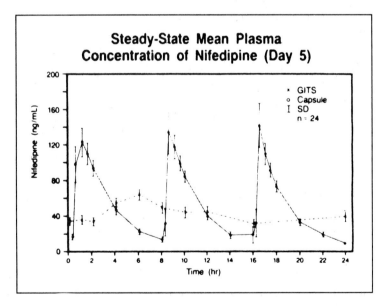

FIGURE 3. Nifedipine GITS provides—in a single dose—a relatively constant delivery of drug over a 24-hour period with minimal fluctuation in peak plasma concentrations. This figure demonstrates that nifedipine capsules may exert a bolus effect immediately after ingestion, although the range of fluctuation is still quite small (between zero and 200 ng/mL), while nifedipine GITS provides a more even delivery of medication with a highter C_{min} and lower C_{max}. The total daily dose of medication in these patients was 90 mg for both formulations of nifedipine. Figure provided by Felix Theeuwes, DSc.

significantly affected. Six hypertensive patients who received verapamil 80 mg three times daily for 2 to 3 months experienced a sustained reduction in mean supine blood pressure without significant changes in heart rate, plasma renin activity, or plasma catecholamines. Gould et al.[55] evaluated the blood pressure response in 16 hypertensive patients analyzed by intraarterial ambulatory blood pressure monitoring after at least 6 weeks of verapamil 120 to 160 mg three times daily. The drug produced a consistent reduction of blood pressure over 24 hr. Mean daytime intraarterial ambulatory blood pressure was reduced from 180/95 to 158/79 mmHg; at night, mean intraarterial supine blood pressure fell from 173/88 to 146/71 mmHg. Verapamil also caused an overall reduction in blood pressure with dynamic and isometric exercise. Side effects included mild constipation and epigastric pain.

Twelve hospitalized patients with mild to moderate hypertension were given verapamil 80 to 160 mg in three divided doses over 10 days.[56] Supine systolic pressure decreased from 177 to 150 mmHg, and diastolic pressure decreased from 111 to 96 mmHg. The antihypertensive effect was dose-dependent and remained constant throughout the day. Heart rate did not change significantly. In addition, plasma renin activity did not increase, there was no retention of salt and water, and creatinine clearance was unchanged. Side effects consisted of facial flushing in two patients, and Mobitz 1 atrioventricular block in one patient. Frishman et al.[57] found verapamil (320 mg/day) given in two divided doses also to be safe and effective in the treatment of essential hypertension. A trough verapamil plasma level of ›80 ng/ml was associated with a good hypotensive response, as patients with levels above this number had sitting blood pressure reductions from 153/104 to 137/88.

Lewis et al.[58] investigated the hypotensive effects of oral verapamil in 48 patients with hypertension; 26 had previously received no therapy and 22 had been treated with β-blockers or methyldopa, both of which were discontinued just prior to the trial; thiazide diuretics were continued in the 25 patients who were receiving this medication. Verapamil was administered in doses of 80 to 240 mg three times daily. In the 26 patients on no previous blood pressure therapy, verapamil reduced supine systolic pressure by an average of 37 mmHg and reduced supine diastolic pressure by an average of 27 mmHg. There was no significant change in heart rate. The patients who previously received β-blockers and methyldopa were better controlled when verapamil was substituted for the original drug. Side effects with verapamil included constipation and mild flushing. In another study, verapamil administered at a dose of 120 mg three times daily for 3 weeks, and then 160 mg three times daily for 3 more weeks, was compared to propranolol given at a dose of 60 mg three times daily for 3 weeks and then 80 mg three times daily for 3 more weeks.[59] Verapamil decreased mean supine blood pressure from 179/104 to 148/84 mmHg without significantly affecting heart rate; this response was superior to propranolol in the doses used. In addition, verapamil was well tolerated with minimal side effects. In a more recent study,[60] the levels of blood pressure reductions after chronic therapy with propranolol (40–240 mg twice daily) and verapamil (120–240 mg twice daily) were compared. Both drugs were shown to produce a uniform and comparable reduction in blood pressure throughout the whole day, together with a reduction in heart rate, which was greater with propranolol. Both drugs were equally well tolerated without patient withdrawals being observed.

The antihypertensive efficacy of verapamil was evaluated in 43 patients with essential hypertension in a study that also examined relationships between age and pretreatment renin and blood pressure, and compared intraindividually the responses with those obtained using β-blockers (n = 29) and diuretic therapy (n = 18).[61] Verapamil produced a decrease in mean blood pressure that was directly related to the patient's age and pretreatment blood pressure, but inversely to pretreatment renin. Although there was no difference in overall pressure response between verapamil, β-blocker, and diuretic therapy, the pressure responses with diuretics paralleled those obtained with verapamil, whereas, in contrast, responses with β-blockers correlated indirectly with the patient's age and directly with pretreatment renin. The authors proposed use of verapamil as the first choice for the older and low-renin patients in place of a diuretic agent and a β-blocker as the first-line drug for the younger and high-renin patients.

In a large, double-blind trial, verapamil (80, 120, 160 mg three times daily) was compared to propranolol (40, 80, 120 mg three times daily). Verapamil lowered blood pressure more effectively than propranolol in both black and white patients.[62,63] Verapamil was equally effective in both black and white patients, whereas propranolol was most effective in white patients.[62,63]

Combination Therapy. Lewis[58] evaluated 75 patients who were treated for hypertension with verapamil over 1 year. Most of these patients were also on a thiazide diuretic, and some were on methyldopa or clonidine. Fourteen patients stopped the drug because of side effects (most commonly constipation), poor control of blood pressure, or noncompliance. The addition of verapamil caused a 25 to 30 mmHg decline in diastolic blood pressure. The decrease in blood pressure after 1 month remained at the same level for 12 months.

Combination verapamil–β-Blocker therapy for the treatment of hypertension has generally been avoided because of the common negative inotropic and chronotropic actions of these drugs, and the availability of other antihypertensive agents. Studies evaluating combination verapamil-propranolol therapy in patients with angina pectoris have found the two drugs used together to have potent hypotensive effects.[64] The concomitant use of these two drugs for blood pressure control requires further clarification.

Sustained-release Verapamil. A new sustained-release formulation of verapamil for the treatment of hypertension is available. Midtbo et al.[65] evaluated 24 patients with mild to moderate systemic hypertension using sustained-release (240 mg tablet). Frishman et al. compared sustained-release verapamil twice daily to instant-release verapamil (160 mg thrice daily).[66] Both formulations were effective in reducing blood pressure. Zachariah et al.,[67] using ambulatory blood pressure monitoring, demonstrated that sustained-release verapamil might even be useful once daily.

Hypertensive Crisis. Several hundred patients have been treated with intravenous verapamil for hypertensive emergencies, with most of the experience being reported from Europe and Brazil.[47,68,69] In one study of 47 patients with renovascular hypertension, verapamil 5 mg administered intravenously caused a 20 to 25% fall in systolic and diastolic pressures within 1 min.[68] In another study, 20 children with severe hypertension accompanying renovascular disease or chronic renal failure were treated with verapamil.[69] A single intravenous injection of 0.1 mg/kg was followed by a 25%

decrease in systolic blood pressure; maximal effects were observed at 30 min. A continuous intravenous infusion was used successfully for prolonged hypertensive crises.

Hypotension has been reported rarely (eight patients of approximately 400);[47] these few instances were in cases in which a large dose (up to 50 mg) of verapamil had been infused over several hours. The effect was quickly reversed by halting the infusion.

Hypertensive Patients with Angina Pectoris. Frishman et al.[70] compared oral propranolol and verapamil in patients with hypertension and angina pectoris in a placebo-controlled, double-blind, randomized, crossover trial involving 12 patients with stable angina pectoris and mild to moderate hypertension. Doses of propranolol were titrated from 60 to 320 mg/day and doses of verapamil were titrated from 240 to 480 mg/day. No significant differences in effects on angina or on total exercise work were found between the two drugs. Similarly, both drugs reduced supine and standing systolic and diastolic blood pressure at rest and with exercise. Verapamil, however, caused a significantly greater fall in standing diastolic pressure compared with propranolol. Five patients were maintained on verapamil 480 mg/day for 1 year with good long-term antianginal and antihypertensive effects.

Diltiazem

Hemodynamic Effects. In 20 patients with coronary artery disease or hypertension who underwent cardiac catheterization, diltiazem 60 mg orally decreased systolic blood pressure, heart rate, cardiac index, and peripheral resistance. [71] Similar results were seen in a long-term study using 90 mg of the drug orally three times daily.[72] In an experimental study, the effects of diltiazem on renal blood flow and renal function were observed in anesthetized dogs.[73] Infusion of diltiazem into the renal artery increased renal blood flow. In addition, diltiazem induced a natriuresis that persisted even when renal blood flow was held constant. The clinical implications of this finding in hypertensive patients are not known.

Clinical Studies. Maeda et al.[74] studied the hypotensive effect of diltiazem in 28 patients with mild, moderate, and severe essential hypertension. Two treatment protocols were used; one group received only diltiazem 180 mg orally per day, and a second group received diltiazem in combination with a thiazide diuretic. Diltiazem alone reduced systolic and diastolic pressures in 89 and 67% of the patients, respectively. This effect was seen after the first week of therapy and became more pronounced after 6 to 8 weeks of treatment. The combination of diltiazem and diuretic was effective in all patients, including those who did not respond to diltiazem alone. The maximum hypotensive effect of diltiazem after a single oral dose occurred at 3 to 4 hours. There was a gradual rise in blood pressure after this period, though the duration of effect was not determined. Only two patients experienced side effects; one had dizziness and the other "gastric fullness. " In another study,[75] 14 patients with mild or moderate hypertension were treated with diltiazem, 180 to 360 mg daily, in divided doses for 2 months. The drug reduced sitting systolic blood pressure by a mean of 18 mmHg and diastolic blood pressure by 16 mg. All but one patient had at least a 10 mmHg reduction in diastolic pressure, to a value less than 90 mmHg. In these patients, the blood presure reduction with diltiazem was similar to that with diuretics. Although plasma norepinephrine was higher after even 2 months, heart rate was unaffected. There was a low incidence of side effects.

The safety and efficacy of sustained-release diltiazem (120, 180 mg tablets) used twice daily were compared to that of hydrochlorothiazide (25, 50 mg tablets) administered twice daily in 207 patients with mild-to-moderate hypertension in a placebo run-in, randomized, double-blind, parallel titration study.[76] Patients whose conditions were not well controlled on either drug alone received combination therapy. Both drugs were shown to be effective in reducing systolic and diastolic blood pressures for up to 6 months and were equally effective in black patients and the elderly. The combination of diltiazem and hydrochlorothiazide was found to be more effective than either drug used alone. Side effects were minimal with both drugs; however, more patients developed hypokalemia with hydrochlorothiazide and combination therapy than with diltiazem alone.

Hypertensive Crisis. There is very limited experience with diltiazem in the treatment of severe hypertension or hypertensive crisis.[47] In one study[77] involving only five patients, a moderate response was demonstrated. Intravenously administered diltiazem caused a reduction of blood pressure from 225/125 mmHg to approximately 175/100 mmHg in 35 to 40 min. In this study, patients were treated with an escalating dose schedule starting at 5mg, increasing to 10mg at 30 min, and further increasing to 20 mg at 40 min. The hypotensive effect persisted for approximately 3 hours. There were no major effects on heart rate and no side effects were reported.

Hypertensive Patients with Angina Pectoris. As mentioned earlier, Frishman et al.[50] compared oral nifedipine to diltiazem in patients with concomitant systemic hypertension and angina pectoris. The drugs were equally effective in reducing angina attacks, improving exercise tolerance, and reducing blood pressure. Diltiazem, however, was associated with fewer adverse reactions.

TABLE 2. Results of Clinical Studies Evaluating the Effects of Calcium Antagonists on Left Ventricular Hypertrophy Regression

Study	Drug	No. Pts.	Follow-up Time	Results*
Ferrara et al.[80]	Nitrendipine	20	8 wks	LVM 3.6% (cross-sectional area 2%)
Muiesan et al.[81]	Verapamil	7	8 mos	LVM 17%
Muiesan et al.[81]	Nifedipine	7	3 mos	LVM 13.4%
DeSimone et al.[82]	Nifedipine	20	2 mos	No regression
Strauer et al.[83]	Nifedipine	12	3.9 mos (mean)	LVM 10.5% PWT 3.6% LVST 15.1%
Amodeo et al.[84]	Diltiazem	10	4 wks	LVM 10.3%

*LVM = left ventricular mass; PWT = posterior wall thickness; LVST = left ventricular septal wall thickness.

Calcium Antagonists and Left Ventricular Hypertrophy

Left ventricular hypertrophy is a common complication of longstanding systemic hypertension. Left ventricular hypertrophy is not just an adaptive process to normalize ventricular wall stress but is a pathological entity that increases the risk of sudden death, myocardial ischemia, arrhythmia, and congestive heart failure in hypertensive patients.[78] Left ventricular hypertrophy has been shown to regress with various antihypertensive drugs, with a parallel reduction in blood pressure.[78] Various calcium antagonists can reduce left ventricular hypertrophy in hypertensive patients, while at the same time suppressing ventricular ectopy, improving ventricular compliance, and alleviating myocardial ischemia.[78,79] Table 2 summarizes the results of some echocardiographic studies evaluating the effects of various calcium antagonists on left ventricular hypertrophy regression.[80-84]

New Calcium Antagonists

Although not discussed in detail in this chapter, there are other calcium antagonists that are being used in hypertension. Gallopamil, which has structural similarities to verapamil, is now being studied in hypertensive patients. Three long-acting dihydropyridine compounds—amlodipine, isradipine, and nitrendipine—appear to be useful as once- or twice-daily antihypertensive drugs. Shorter acting dihydropyridine compounds— nicardipine (which is now available for clinical use) and nivaldipine— also appear useful in systemic hypertension.

Conclusion

Scientific rationale and clinical investigation suggest a potentially important role for calcium antagonists in the treatment of systemic hypertension, as monotherapy and in combination with other antihypertensive drugs. The calcium antagonists offer many advantages over the currently available armamentarium for the treatment of systemic hypertension, although they are not without their disadvantages (Table 3).[85-90] Aside

---

TABLE 3. Calcium Antagonists in the Treatment of Systemic Hypertension*

Advantages
1. No detrimental effects on lipid profile and glucoregulatory hormones.
2. No hypokalemic effects.
3. Safe in patients with bronchospasm, peripheral vascular disease, and renal dysfunction.
4. Low incidence of depression and sexual dysfunction.
5. Effective in treating co-existing angina pectoris and/or arrhythmias.
6. Effective in black and white patients.
7. Effective in young and old patients.
8. Possible antiatherogenic effects.

Disadvantages
1. Can exacerbate congestive heart failure.
2. Can adversely affect atrioventricular and sinus node function.

---

*Adapted from references 85–90.

from a favorable side-effect profile, they have been shown to exert beneficial effects on several important target organs — the heart and the cerebral circulation. As detailed elsewhere in this book, calcium antagonists exert salutary effects on renal perfusion and electrolyte excretion, further commending this class of drug for the treatment of hypertension. They may also have antiatherogenic effects.[90] The true place of these drugs in the treatment of hypertension will ultimately be defined through further clinical research and by their widespread use in clinical practice.

References

1. Fleckenstein A, Tritthart H, Fleckenstein B, Herbst A, Grun G: A new group of compatible Ca^{++} antagonists (iproveratril, D600, prenylamine) with highly potent inhibitory effects on excitation-contraction coupling in mammalian myocardium. Fluegers Arch 307:25–32, 1969.
2. Stone PH, Antman EM, Mueller JE, Braunwald E: Calcium channel blocking agents in the treatment of cardiovascular disorders. Part II: Hemodynamic effects and clinical applications. Ann Intern Med 93:886–904, 1980.
3. Krikler DM, Rowland E: Critical value of calcium antagonists in treatment of cardiovascular disorders. J Am Coll Cardiol 1:355–364, 1983.
4. Frishman WH, Stroh JA, Greenberg SM, Suarez T, Karp A, Peled HB: Calcium-channel blockers in systemic hypertension. Curr Probl Cardiol 12:287–346, 1987.
5. Beer N, Gallegos I, Cohen A, Klein N, Sonnenblick E, Frishman W: Efficacy of sublingual nifedipine in the acute treatment of systemic hypertension. Chest 79:571–574, 1981.
6. Frishman WH, Charlap S, Michelson EL: Calcium-channel blockers in systemic hypertension. Am J Cardiol 58:157–160, 1986.
7. Mikkelsen K, Andersson KE, Pedersen OL: The effect of nifedipine on isolated human peripheral vessels. Acta Pharmacol Toxicol 43:291–298, 1978.
8. Mostbeck A, Partsch H, Peschl L: Investigations on peripheral blood distribution. Third international Adalat Symposium, 1976. Amsterdam Excerpta Medica, 1976, pp 91–97.
9. Ferlinz J: Effects of verapamil on normal and abnormal ventricular functions in patients with ischemic heart disease. In Zanchetti, Krikler (eds): Calcium Antagonism in Cardiovascular Therapy: Experience with Verapamil. Amsterdam, Excerpta Medica, 1981, pp 92–105.
10. Bourassa MG, Cote P, Theroux P, Tubau JF, Genain C, Waters DD: Hemodynamics and coronary flow following diltiazem administration in anesthetized dogs and in humans. Chest 78(suppl 1):225–227, 1980.
11. Iriuchijima J: Effect of calcium antagonist, nifedipine, on blood pressure of various hypertensive rats. Hiroshima J Med Sci 29:15–19, 1980.
12. Kubo T, Fujie K, Yamashita M, Misu Y: Antihypertensive effects of nifedipine on conscious normotensive and hypertensive rats. J Pharmacobiodyn 4:294–300, 1981.
13. Sato M, Murata S, Narita H, Tomita M, Yamashita K, Yamaguchi I: Hypotensive effects of diltiazem hydrochloride in the normotensive, spontaneously hypertensive and renal hypertensive rats (authors translation of abstract). Nippon Yakurigaku Zasshi 75:99–106, 1979.
14. Osada T, Kajiwara N, Kobayashi Y, et al: The inhibition of hypertension and the histological changes in SHR treated with diltiazem. Jpn Heart J 20:745, 1979.
15. Guazzi MD, Fiorentini C, Olivari MT, Bartorelli A, Necchi G, Polese A: Short and long-term efficacy of a calcium antagonist (nifedipine) combined with methyldopa in the treatment of severe hypertension. Circulation 61:913–919, 1980.
16. Murakami M, Murakami E, Takekoshi N, et al: Antihypertensive effect of 4(-2-nitrophenyl)-2, 6-dimethyl-1, 4-dihydropyridine-3, 5-dicarbonic acid dimethylester (nifedipine, Bay-a 1040), a new coronary vasodilator. Jpn Heart J 13:128–135, 1972.

17. Bertel O, Conen D, Radu EW, Muller J, Lang C, Dubach UC: Nifedipine in hypertensive emergencies. Br Med J 286:19–21, 1983.

18. Aboul-Khair M, Wicker P, Tarazi RC: Differences between the effects of hydralazine and a calcium antagonist (Baye 5009) on cerebral, renal and coronary blood flow. (abstract) Clin Res 29:704A, 1981.

19. Lowenstein J: Clonidine. Ann Intern Med 92:74–77, 1980.

20. Loutzenhiser RD, Epstein M: Renal hemodynamic effects of calcium antagonists. J Cardiovasc Pharmacol 12(suppl VI):S48–52, 1988.

21. Bartorelli C, Magrini T, Moruzzi P, et al: Haemodynamic effects of a calcium antagonistic agent (nifedipine) in hypertension. Therapeutic implications. Clin Sci Molec Med 55(suppl 4):291S–292S, 1978.

22. Pedersen OL, Mikkelsen E, Christensen NJ, Kornerup HJ, Pedersen EB: Effect of nifedipine on plasma renin, aldosterone and catecholamines in arterial hypertension. Eur J Clin Pharmacol 15:235–240, 1979.

23. Thibonnier M, Bonnet F, Corvol P: Antihypertensive effect of fractionated sublingual administration of nifedipine in moderate essential hypertension. Eur J Clin Pharmacol 17:161–164, 1980.

24. Olivari MT, Bartorelli C, Polese A, Fiorentini C, Moruzzi P, Guazzi MD: Treatment of hypertension with nifedipine, a calcium antagonistic agent. Circulation 59:1056–1062, 1979.

25. Aoki K, Yoshida T, Kato S, et al: Hypotensive action and increased plasma renin activity by calcium antagonist (nifedipine) in hypertensive patients. Jpn Heart J 17:479–484, 1976.

26. Gutsche HU, Muller-Suur R, Schurek JH: Ca^{++}-antagonist prevents feedback induced SN-GFR decrease in rat kidney. Kidney Int 8:(suppl 4-5)477, 1975.

27. Ferlinz J: Nifedipine in myocardial ischemia, systemic hypertension, and other cardiovascular disorders. Ann Intern Med 105:714–29, 1986.

28. Guazzi M, Oliveri MT, Polese A, Fiorentini C, Magrini R, Moruzzi P: Nifedipine, a new antihypertensive with rapid action. Clin Pharmacol Ther 22:528–31, 1977.

29. Midtbo K, Hals O, van der Meer: Verapamil compared with nifedipine in the treatment of essential hypertension. J Cardiovasc Pharmacol 4(suppl 3):S363–368, 1982.

30. Klein W, Brandt D, Vrecko K, Harringer M: Role of calcium antagonists in the treatment of essential hypertension. Circ Res 52(I):174–181, 1983.

31. Hornung RS, Gould BA, Jones RI, Sonecha TN, Raftery EB: Nifedipine tablets for systemic hypertension: a study using continuous ambulatory intraarterial recording: Am J Cardiol 51:1323–1327, 1983.

32. Aoki K, Kondo S, Mochizaki A, et al: Antihypertensive effect of cardiovascular Ca^{++} antagonist in hypertensive patients in the absence and presence of beta-adrenergic blockade. Am Heart J 96:218–226, 1978.

33. Husted SE, Kraemer H, Christensen CK, Pedersen OL: Long-term therapy of arterial hypertension with nifedipine given alone or in combination with β-adrenoceptor blocking agents. Eur J Clin Harmacol 22:101–103, 1982.

34. Opie LH, Jee L, White D: Antihypertensive effects of nifedipine combined with cardioselective beta-adrenergic receptor antagonism by atenolol. Am Heart J 104:606–612, 1982.

35. Yagil Y, Kobrin I, Stessman J, Ghanem J, Leibel B, Ben-Ishay D: Effectiveness of combined nifedipine and propranolol treatment in hypertension. Hypertension 5(II):113–117, 1983.

36. Ekelund LG, Ekelund C, Rossner S: Antihypertensive effects at rest and during exercise of a calcium blocker, nifedipine, alone and in combination with metoprolol. Acta Med Scand 212:71–75, 1982.

37. Hallin L, Andren L, Hansson L: Controlled trial of nifedipine and bendroflumethiazide in hypertension. J Cardiovasc Pharmacol 5:1083–1085, 1983.

38. Guazzi MD, DeCesare N, Galli C, et al: Calcium channel blockade with nifedipine and angiotensin converting enzyme inhibition with captopril in the therapy of patients with severe primary hypertension. Circulation 70:279–284, 1984.

39. Evans MG Jr, Olanoff LS, Hurwitz G, Cowart TD, Conradi EC: Use of nifedipine as an adjunct to current hypertensive therapy. Arch Intern Med 144:985–987, 1984.

40. Murphy MB, Scriven AJI, Dollery CT: Efficacy of nifedipine as a step 3 antihypertensive drug. Hypertension 5II:118–121, 1983.

41. Murphy MB, Bulpitt CJ, Dollery CT: Role of nifedipine in the treatment of resistant hypertension: comparison with hydralazine in hospital outpatients. Am J Med 77(suppl 2B):16–21, 1984.

42. Spivack C, Ocken S, Frishman WH: Calcium antagonists: clinical use in the treatment of systemic hypertension. Drugs 25:154–177, 1983.

43. Eckenhoff B, Theeuwes F, Urquart J: Osmotically actuated dosage forms for rate controlled drug delivery. Pharm Tech 5:35–44, 1981.

44. Frishman WH, Sherman D, Feinfeld DA: Innovative drug delivery systems in cardiovascular medicine: nifedipine GITS and clonidine TTS. Cardiol Clinics 5:703–16, 1987.

45. Frishman, W: Clinical utilization of nifedipine GITS in treating hypertension. Am J Cardiol 1989 (in press).

46. Ellrodt AG, Ault M, Riedinger MS, Murata GH: Efficacy of sublingual nifedipine in hypertensive emergencies. Am J Med 79:19–25, 1985.

47. Frishman WH, Weinberg P, Peled HB, Kimmel B, Charlap S, Beer N: Calcium-entry blockers for the treatment of severe hypertension and hypertensive crisis. Am J Med 77:35–45, 1984.

48. Frishman WH: Calcium-channel blockers for hypertensive emergencies. J Clin Hypertens 3 (suppl):55S–61S, 1986.

49. Jee LD, Opie LH: Acute hypotensive response to nifedipine added to prazosin in treatment of hypertension. Br Med J 287:1514, 1983.

50. Frishman WH, Charlap S: Calcium-channel blockers for combined systolic hypertension and myocardial ischemia. Circulation 75:154–162, 1988.

51. Frishman WH, Sonnenblick EH: The calcium antagonists. In Hurst JW (ed): The Heart, New York, McGraw-Hill, 1986, 1624–1639.

52. Singh B, Roche A: Effects of intravenous verapamil on hemodynamics in patients with heart disease. Am Heart J 94:593–599, 1977.

53. Charlap S, Kimmel B, Frishman WH: Calcium-channel blockers in heart failure. In Julian DG, Wenger NK (eds): Cardiology, Vol IV, Heart Failure. London, Butterworths, 1986, 179–197.

54. Muiesan G, Agabiti-Rosei E, Alicandri C, et al: Influence of verapamil on catecholamines, renin, and aldosterone in essential hypertensive patients. In Verapamil. Zanchetti and Krikler (eds), Calcium Antagonism in Cardiovascular Therapy: Experience with Verapamil Amsterdam, Excerpta Medica, 1981, pp 238–249.

55. Gould BA, Mann S, Kieso H, Subramanian VB, Raftery EB: The 24 hour ambulatory blood pressure profile with verapamil. Circulation 65:22–24, 1982.

56. Leonetti G, Sala C, Bianchini C, Terzoli L, Zanchetti A: Antihypertensive and renal effect of orally administered verapamil. Eur J Clin Pharmacol 18:375–382, 1980.

57. Frishman W, Charlap S, Kimmel B, et al: Twice-daily oral verapamil in essential hypertension. Arch Intern Med 146:561–565, 1986.

58. Lewis GR, Morley KD, Lewis BM, Bones PJ: The treatment of hypertension with verapamil. NZ Med J 87:351–354, 1978.

59. Leonetti G, Pasoti C, Ferrari GP, Zanchetti A: Double-blind comparison of the antihypertensive effects of verapamil and propranolol. In Zanchetti and Krikler (eds): Calcium Antagonism in Cardiovascular Therapy: Experience with Verapamil, Amsterdam, Excerpta Medica, 1981, pp 260–267.

60. Hornung RS, Jones RI, Gould BA, Sonecha T, Raftery EB: Propranolol versus verapamil for the treatment of essential hypertension. Am Heart J 108:554–560, 1984.

61. Buhler FR, Hulthen UL, Kiowski W, Muller FB, Bolli P: The place of the calcium antagonist verapamil in antihypertensive therapy. J Cardiovasc Pharmacol 4 (suppl):350–357, 1982.

62. Cubeddu LX: Racial differences in response to antihypertensive drugs: a focus on verapamil. J Clin Hypertens 3 (suppl): 55S–61S, 1986.

63. Cubeddu LX, Aranda J, Singh B, et al: A comparison of verapamil and propranolol for the initial treatment of hypertension. JAMA 256:2214–2221, 1986.

64. Packer M, Leon MB, Bonow RO, Kieval S, Rosing DR, Subramanian VB: Hemodynamic and clinical effects of combined therapy with verapamil and propranolol in ischemic heart disease. Am J Cardiol 50:903–912, 1982.

65. Midtbo KA, Hals O, Lauve O: A new sustained-release formulation of verapamil in the treatment of hypertension. J Clin Hypertens 3:(suppl) 125S–132S, 1986.

66. Frishman WH, Eisen G, Charlap S, Strom JA: Long-term safety and efficacy comparison of immediate-release and sustained-release oral verapamil in systemic hypertension. J Clin Hypertens 3:605–609, 1987.

67. Zachariah PK, Sheps SG, Schriger A: Efficacy of sustained-release verapamil: automatic ambulatory blood pressure monitoring. J Clin Hypertens 3:(suppl)133S–142S, 1986.

68. Brittinger WD, Schwarzbeck A, Wittenmeier KW, et al: Klinish-experimentelle untersuchungen ubere die blutdruckenende wirkung von verapamil. Dtsch Med Wochenschr 95:1871–1877, 1970.

69. Scharer K, Atlas H, Bein G: The treatment of renal hypertension with verapamil in childhood. Monatsschr Kinderheilkd 125:706–712, 1977.

70. Frishman WH, Klein NA, Klein P, et al: A comparison of oral propranolol and verapamil in patients with hypertension and angina pectoris: A placebo-controlled double-blind randomized crossover trial. Am J Cardiol 50:1164–1172, 1982.

71. Kinoshita M, Motomura M, Kusukawa R, Kawakita S: Comparison of hemodynamic effects between β-blocking agents and a new antianginal agent, diltiazem hydrochloride. Jpn Circ J 43:587–598, 1979.

72. Kusukawa R, Kinoshita M, Shimono Y, Tomonaga G, Hosino T: Hemodynamic effects of a new anti-anginal drug, diltiazem hydrochloride. Arzneim Forsch 27:878–887, 1977.

73. Yagamuchi I, Ikezawa K, Takada T, Kiyomoto A: Studies on a new 1,5- benzothiazepine derivative (CRD-401). VI: Effects on renal blood flow and renal function. Jpn J Pharmacol 24:511–512, 1974.

74. Maeda K, Takasugi T, Tsukano Y, Tanaka Y, Shiota K: Clinical study on the hypotensive effect of diltiazem hydrochloride. Int J Clin Pharmacol Ther Toxicol 19:47–55, 1981.

75. Inouye IK, Massie BM, Benowitz N, Simpson P, Loge D: Antihypertensive therapy with diltiazem and comparison with hydrochlorothiazide. Am J Cardiol 53:1588–1592, 1984.

76. Frishman WH, Zawada ET, Smith LK, et al: Comparison of hydrochlorothiazide and sustained-release diltiazem for mild to moderate hypertension. Am J Cardiol 59:615–623, 1987.

77. Rosenthal J: Die behandlung der hypertensiven kuise mit diltiazem. In Bender F, Greef K (eds): Calcium Antagonisen zur Behandlung der Angina Pectoris, Hypertonie and Arrhythmie. First Dilzen Symposium, Copenhagen 1981. Amsterdam, Excerpta Medica, 1982, pp 227–234.

78. Hachamovitch R, Sonnenblick EH, Strom JA, Frishman WH: Left ventricular hypertrophy in hypertension and the effects of antihypertensive drug therapy. Curr Probl Cardiol 13:371–421, 1988.

79. Messerli F: Effects of calcium channel blockade on cardiac repercussions of long-standing hypertension. J Cardsiovasc Pharmacol 12(suppl VI):S44–S47, 1988.

80. Ferrara LA, Fasano ML, Simone G, et al: Antihypertensive and cardiovascular effects of nitrendipine: a controlled study vs placebo. Lancet ii:850, 1977.

81. Muiesan G, Agabiti-Rosei E, Romanelli G, et al: Adrenergic activity and left ventricular function during treatment of essential hypertension with calcium antagonists.. Am J Cardiol 57:44D–49D, 1986.

82. DeSimone G, Ferrara LA, et al: Effect of slow release nifedipine on left ventricular mass and systolic function in mild or moderate hypertension. Curr Ther Res 36:537–544, 1984.

83. Strauer BE, Atef Mahmoud M, Bayer F, et al: Reversal of left ventricular hypertrophy and improvement of cardiac function in man by nifedipine. Eur Heart J 5(suppl F):53, 1984.

84. Amodeo C, Kobrin I, Ventura HO, et al: Hemodynamic effects of diltiazem in hypertension (abstr). Circulation(suppl III): III–12, 1985.

85. Lewis GRJ, Stewart DJ, Lewis BM, Bones PJ, Morley KD, Janus ED: The antihypertensive effect of oral verapamil — acute and long-term administration and its effects on the high density lipo-protein values in plasma. In Zanchetti and Krikler (eds): Calcium Antagonism in Cardiovascular Therapy: Experience with Verapamil. Amsterdam, Excerpta Medica, 1981, pp 270–277.

86. Klein WW: Treatment of hypertension with calcium channel blockers: European Data. Am J Med 77:143–146, 1984.

87. Shamoon HH, Baylor P, Kambosos D, Charlap S, Plawes S, Frishman WF: Influence of oral verapamil on glucoregulatory hormones in man. J Clin Endocrinol Metab 60:536–541, 1985.

88. Moreira J, Barata JD, Olias J: Antihypertensive action of calcium blockade in hypertensive patients with chronic renal disease. Nephron 41:314–319, 1985.

89. Schoen RE, Frishman WH, Shamoon H: Hormonal and metabolic effects of calcium-channel antagonists in man. Am J Med 84:492–504, 1988.

90. Weinstein DB: The antiatherogenic potential of calcium antagonists. J Cardiovasc Pharmacol 12(suppl IV):S29–35, 1988.

Murray Epstein, M.D.
Rodger Loutzenhiser, Ph.D.

17

Potential Applicability of Calcium Antagonists as Renal Protective Agents

With the pharmacologic effects of the calcium antagonists on renal hemodynamics in mind,[1-3] it is tempting to consider the clinical relevance of these recently delineated renal hemodynamic effects. Of particular interest are the attributes that commend their use in hypertension and their potential future applications in clinical medicine (Table 1).

Applicability of Calcium Antagonists to the Management of Hypertension

The salutary effects of calcium antagonists on renal hemodynamics suggest that they are particularly well-suited for the management of hypertension. Drugs such as hydralazine, which directly reduce peripheral vascular resistance (PVR), have been used in antihypertensive therapy for many years. Nevertheless, the effectiveness of these agents often is limited by the reactive stimulation of renal and hormonal responses that counteract their antihypertensive actions (Fig. 1).[4,5] These responses tend to produce tolerance to the vasodilatory action of hydralazine as well as volume expansion-induced pseudotolerance to its antihypertensive effects.

In contrast to nonspecific vasodilators such as hydralazine, calcium antagonists attenuate the expected adaptive changes in PVR, heart rate, cardiac output, and extracellular fluid volume that would otherwise lead to a reduction in the initial blood pressure-lowering response (Fig. 2). Calcium antagonists interfere with angiotensin II (ANG II) and alpha adrenergic-mediated vasoconstriction. An intriguing possibility is that calcium antagonists might countervail the sodium-retaining effects of decreased renal perfusion[6,7] and possibly of decreased levels of natriuretic hormones (as indicated by the symbol ‖ in Figure 2).

Aside from their role in treating hypertension, calcium antagonists, because of their favorable effects on renal hemodynamics, may have a future role in managing certain types of acute renal insufficiency.

TABLE 1. Future Applications of Calcium Antagonists in Clinical Medicine

1. Amelioration of renal insufficiency from:
   a. Radiocontrast agents
   b. Aminoglycoside nephrotoxicity
   c. Chemotherapy
2. Organ preservation during harvesting of kidneys for transplantation.

Prophylaxis Against Acute Renal Insufficiency

Possible future applications of calcium antagonists include the utilization of their ability to augment renal perfusion in clinical settings in which renal hemodynamics are compromised. Before considering such applications, it is relevant to review the effects of calcium antagonists in experimental models of acute renal failure (ARF).

Experimental Acute Renal Failure

The role of calcium antagonists as protective agents against ARF has been assessed in a number of experimental models, including glycerol-induced ARF, gentamicin-induced renal failure, and ischemia induced by vascular clamping. Lee et al.[8] studied the effects of the calcium antagonist diltiazem on the natural history of glycerol-induced ARF in rats. Animals pretreated with diltiazem for 3 days prior to the administration of glycerol developed a less severe renal failure syndrome. Treatment decreased the extent of tubular cell necrosis and was associated with a more rapid histologic and functional recovery.

Compensatory Responses to Vasodilation

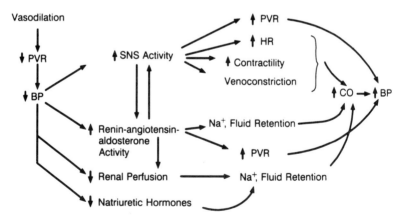

FIGURE 1. A schematic diagram summarizing the mechanisms whereby vasodilation induced by nonspecific vasodilators such as hydralazine tends to induce reactive stimulation of renal and hormonal responses that counteract their antihypertensive actions. Reproduced with permission from Epstein and Oster, 1988.

Another experimental model that has been studied by several investigators is gentamicin nephrotoxicity. In experimental aminoglycoside-induced ARF, binding of the agent to the luminal brush border membrane of the proximal tubule has been postulated to result in alteration of the composition of membrane phospholipid, increased permeability to calcium, and subsequent impairment of mitochondrial function.[9] Because of such increased permeability to calcium, calcium antagonists might be expected to preserve cellular integrity and protect against aminoglycoside-induced nephrotoxicity, as recently suggested by Eliahou et al.[10] Lee et al.[11,12] evaluated the protective effect of a calcium antagonist on gentamicin nephrotoxicity in the rat. Administration of gentamicin for 12 days caused a substantial decrease in both glomerular filtration rate (GFR) and renal plasma flow. Concurrent treatment with the calcium antagonist nitrendipine promoted a significant increase in GFR but did not measurably influence renal blood flow. Urinary excretion of N-acetyl-glucosaminidase (NAG) and beta-glucosidase was measured to assess direct tubular cell toxicity resulting from administration of aminoglycoside. There was a progressive rise in the excretion of both enzymes beginning on day 3 and continuing throughout the study. The administration of nitrendipine in conjunction with gentamicin almost completely abrogated the increased enzymuria. Although recognizing the obvious limitations of an isolated study in an animal model, the authors recommended that additional studies be carried out to evaluate the possible protective role of calcium antagonists in the setting of aminoglycocide nephrotoxicity.

Recently, Watson et al.[13] investigated the effects of verapamil on the development of renal insufficiency and calcium accumulation in renal tissue following administration of aminoglycoside. Sprague-Dawley rats were given gentamicin (120 mg/kg body weight/day) by daily subcutaneous injection for either 6 or 9 days. Subgroups of

Modulation by Calcium Antagonists of Compensatory Responses to Vasodilation

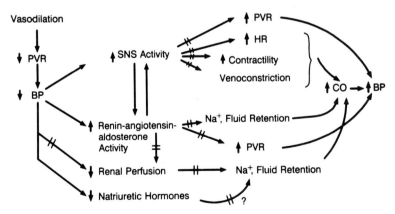

FIGURE 2. A summary of the mechanisms whereby calcium antagonists attenuate the expected adaptive changes in peripheral vascular resistance (PVR), heart rate, cardiac output, and extracellular fluid volume that would otherwise eventually lead to a reduction in the initial blood pressure-lowering response. ‖ symbols indicate countervailing mechanisms that are attenuated by calcium antagonists. Reproduced with permission from Epstein and Oster, 1988.

these animals received verapamil that was added to the drinking water at a concentration of 10 mg/dl commencing 2 days prior to the start of gentamicin administration. Control groups were treated with sham injections of dextrose/water for 6 or 9 days, and two of these groups had verapamil added to their drinking water. These investigators reported that the degree of functional damage and accumulation of cortical tissue calcium after 6 or 9 days of administration of gentamicin (120 mg/kg body weight/day) was not significantly different in rats whose drinking water contained verapamil (10 mg/100 ml) from those of control animals. The accumulation of tissue calcium correlated with the degree of reduction of creatinine clearance and probably reflected the extent of lethal tubular cell injury.

Although data in man are lacking, studies from some (but not all) investigations in animal models suggest that future clinical trials may be considered to assess the possibility that calcium antagonists are protective against aminoglycoside nephrotoxicity (this topic is considered in greater detail in Chapter 10).

Models of Postischemic Acute Renal Failure

Another experimental model that has attracted investigative attention is that of postischemic ARF induced by vascular clamping. The available data are conflicting with respect to the effects of calcium antagonists in this setting. Malis et al.[14] did not observe a protective effect with verapamil treatment, whereas in the same species, Goldfarb et al.[15] showed that verapamil had a protective influence on ARF. These differences might be explained by the use of varying doses of calcium antagonists, different preischemic infusion periods (some of which lasted only 20 minutes),[13] and various periods of postischemic infusion (some lasting only 15 minutes).[14] In none of these experiments was the long-term application of calcium antagonists evaluated.

Recently Hertle and Garthoff[16] have examined the effects of nisoldipine on renal function following contralateral nephrectomy and, subsequently, 60 minutes of normothermic ischemia. Nisoldipine (300 ppm) was incorporated into a standard diet as well as being administered 1 hour prior to ischemia (10 mg/kg orally). The investigators assessed the effects of nisoldipine on survival, serum urea, serum creatinine, urine volume and creatinine clearance. Treatment with nisoldipine resulted in the survival of all animals (compared to 67% in the untreated group) and improved immediate and long-term renal function (14 days). In contrast, nisoldipine was not effective when administered only in the postischemic period.

Most investigations of the effects of calcium antagonists on experimental ARF have been carried out in the anesthetized dog or rat. In order to circumvent the confounding influence of anesthesia, Wagner et al.[17] investigated the effects of therapy with calcium antagonists in a model of postischemic ARF in conscious dogs monitored by an implanted electromagnetic flow probe. Acute renal failure was induced by inflating a cuff that was placed around the left renal artery in 18 conscious, previously uninephrectomized, dogs. The animals were divided into three groups: Group A constituted the control group, receiving solely 0.9% NaCl; Group B received intra-aortic diltiazem (5 μg/min/kg) beginning at the end of the ischemic period until the 7th day after ischemia; and Group C received diltiazem from the 3rd day prior to induction of ischemia until the 7th day after ischemia. Renal blood flow and GFR were determined on the day before induction of ischemia and on days 1, 3, and 7 following ischemia. When diltiazem was administered before and after ischemia, both GFR and renal blood flow were preserved. In contrast, when diltiazem was administered only following induction of ischemia (Group B), there was an improvement in renal blood flow but no significant effect on GFR. The authors attributed the protective effect of diltiazem to a reversal of the vasoconstriction as well as a protective effect of calcium antagonists on the ischemic tubular cell.

Protection Against Radiocontrast-induced Acute Renal Failure

Several lines of evidence have demonstrated that the intrarenal administration of radiocontrast medium results in a prolonged vasoconstrictive response and reduction in GFR.[18-22] Bakris and Burnett[22] have investigated the effects of calcium entry modulation on the renal hemodynamic response to radiocontrast agents. They demonstrated that injection of radiocontrast solution (diatrizoate meglumine) in anesthetized dogs reduced mean GFR by 42% (Fig. 3). In contrast, this decrement was attenuated by the infusion of either verapamil (50 μg/min), or diltiazem (40 μg/min). Similarly, chelation with ethyleneglycoltetraacetic acid (EGTA) (10 μmoles/min) attenuated the renal vasoconstriction. These hemodynamic responses were achieved at intrarenal doses that did not alter systemic arterial pressure or baseline renal blood flow (RBF). They concluded that calcium antagonism with several different agents, or chelation of calcium with EGTA, attenuates both the magnitude and duration of radiocontrast-mediated intrarenal vasoconstriction. These studies suggest that calcium entry constitutes an important mediator in the vasoconstrictive phase that attends administration of radiocontrast medium.

Recently, Oliet et al.[23] have extended these observations to humans. In a preliminary communication,[23] they reported the results of a small randomized double-blind study of the protective effect of nifedipine in patients undergoing renal arteriography. Patients treated with placebo manifested a blunted natriuresis and diuresis and an increase in excretion of NAG. In contrast, patients treated with nifedipine sublingually did not develop these renal functional alterations.[23] The authors interpreted their data as suggesting that a calcium antagonist may ameliorate renal damage associated with radiocontrast agents. Additional studies will be necessary to delineate the possible protective role of calcium antagonists in this clinical setting.

Cacoub et al.[24] have recently reported in preliminary form the results of a retrospective study in assessing the protective effects of nifedipine against radiocontrast-induced ARF in patients with pre-existing chronic renal failure. The investigators retrospectively analyzed the clinical course of 26 patients with mild-to-moderate chronic renal failure (creatinine clearance [C_{Cr}] ranging from 20 to 60 ml/min) who received radiocontrast agents intravenously. Acute renal failure was defined as an increase of at least 20% of the baseline serum creatinine value during the 5-day period following radiocontrast administration. The patients were divided into two groups according to whether or not they were treated with nifedipine before and after the radiocontrast procedure. The indication for treatment in all patients was hypertension, and daily mean dosage of nifedipine was 40 mg. The groups were matched for type and quantity of radiocontrast agent injected. Four of eleven (36%) patients who were treated with nifedipine developed ARF, versus 38% (6/16) of those who did not receive this drug. Based on this abbreviated, retrospective study, the authors suggested that calcium antagonists do not protect against radiocontrast-induced ARF in the setting of chronic renal insufficiency. The authors were careful to note, however,

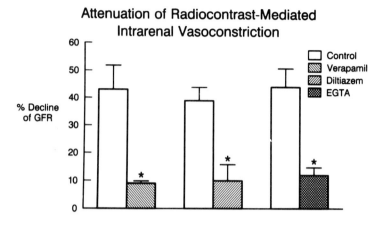

FIGURE 3. Effects of calcium entry modulation on glomerular filtration rate (GFR) in anesthetized dogs receiving radiocontrast solution (diatrizoate meglumine). Injection of radiocontrast reduced mean GFR by 42%. This decrement was attenuated by infusion of verapamil, diltiazem, or EGTA. Redrawn from data of Bakris and Burnett.[22]

that careful prospective studies are required to resolve this important issue. In summary, preliminary observations suggest that calcium antagonists may be protective against the development of acute renal insufficiency in patients receiving radiocontrast agents. Controlled, prospective, randomized trials are warranted to substantiate whether this obtains in a clinical setting.

Role in Transplant-associated Acute Renal Failure

It has been proposed that the prophylactic administration of calcium antagonists to donor kidneys might serve to ameliorate post-transplantation renal insufficiency. Since the human kidney cannot sustain warm ischemic periods greater than 30–60 minutes without resulting in irreversible renal injury, renal hypothermia has been used widely to decrease the metabolic demands of the tissue and diminish renal injury. Harvested human cadaver kidneys, flushed with a cold physiologic solution mimicking intracellular fluid, can be stored for up to 72 hours with good functional result. Despite this attempt to minimize renal ischemia by hypothermia, up to 60% of cold-stored cadaver kidneys undergo a period of reversible acute tubular necrosis (ATN) after transplantation. Recently, a number of investigations have been undertaken to study enhancement of hypothermic protection with the addition of calcium antagonists.

Agatstein et al.[25] studied the ability of calcium antagonists to decrease the severity of ATN after 24-hour cold storage, and autotransplantation was studied in a randomized, paired study of 12 dogs. Experimental animals pretreated with intraarterial verapamil and flushing of the harvested kidney with cold intracellular solution containing verapamil demonstrated significantly greater renal function preservation (p < 0.05) over their matched controls. Golueke et al.[26] have recently purported findings that are not in accord with the above studies. The latter authors investigated the ability of verapamil to decrease the severity of postischemic renal failure induced by 5 minutes of warm ischemia and 48-hour storage in autotransplanted, contralaterally nephrectomized dogs. They reported that verapamil, when either added to the flush and preservation fluid or infused regionally into the autotransplanted kidney or both, did not significantly alter posttransplant function or animal survival.

Recent reports of the efficacy of calcium antagonists in humans confirm earlier suggestions of their applicability in clinical transplantation. Duggan et al.[27] investigated the protective effects of the calcium antagonist verapamil in the setting of cadaveric renal transplantation. Twenty patients in whom brain death had been confirmed were randomly allocated to either a control group or a treatment group (administration of verapamil 20 mg intravenously in addition to the standard regimen). Thirty-nine of the 40 perfused kidneys were subsequently transplanted. The investigators reported that recipients of kidneys treated with verapamil had a twofold greater urine output on day 1 compared to the control group. Serum creatinine on day 1 was also significantly lower in the verapamil-treated group ($p < 0.05$). These initial differences, however, were not maintained; by day 7, urine output and serum creatinine were similar in both groups, and the overall requirement for dialysis in the initial posttransplant week was similar for both groups. Based on the differences on posttransplant day 1, the authors interpreted their findings as suggesting that verapamil ameliorates postischemic ARF.[27]

In a prospective randomized trial, Wagner et al.[28] evaluated the influence of diltiazem on the development of ATN in cadaveric kidney transplantation. In this initial study, cadaver kidneys were procured from heart-beating donors locally harvested at the study center. Diltiazem was added to Eurocollin solution (20 mg/L) at donor nephrectomy. The graft recipient received a preoperative bolus injection of diltiazem (0.28 mg/kg) which was followed by an infusion of diltiazem (0.002 mg/min/kg) for 2 days. Thereafter, diltiazem was administered orally. In the control group (n = 22), 9 patients (41%) developed ATN compared with 2 patients (10%) in the diltiazem group ($p < 0.05$) (Fig. 4). In the control group, 3.5 ± 0.4 hemodialysis per patient were necessary compared with 0.6 ± 0.2 in the diltiazem group ($p < 0.005$).

Subsequently, Neumayer and Wagner[29] carried out an additional study to ascertain the importance of donor pretreatment. They investigated the effects of treatment with calcium antagonists in a group of transplant kidneys procured from distant transplant centers through a sharing agreement. In contrast to the salutary effects of combined treatment of both donor and recipient (Study 1), the authors concluded that posttransplant treatment of the recipient alone with calcium antagonists was less effective in protecting against post-graft failure.

The protective effects of calcium antagonists in renal transplantation in humans have been confirmed by Frei et al.[30] They randomized 126 recipients of cadaver kidneys to either a control group (n = 62) or a group receiving a kidney graft pretreated with diltiazem (n = 64). Grafts were reperfused immediately prior to transplantation either with or without diltiazem 100 mg/L. They observed that the diltiazem-treated group required dialysis less frequently during the initial week following transplantation (14%) than did the control group (36%). More recently, Neumayer et al.[31] have investigated the effects of treating solely the donor kidney on prevention of posttransplant ARF. They utilized locally harvested kidneys in which reperfusion was not performed. The group with addition of diltiazem (20 mg/L) to the Eurocollins solution (n = 16) was compared with an untreated

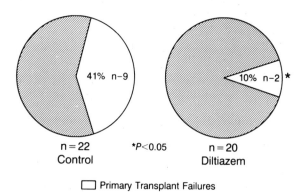

FIGURE 4. Effects of calcium antagonist administration on subsequent development of post-transplant acute renal insufficiency in 42 transplant recipients. Nine of 22 patients who did not receive diltiazem developed renal insufficiency (left panel). In contrast, only 2 of 20 patients treated with diltiazem developed renal insufficiency (right panel). Redrawn from data of Neumayer and Wagner.[29]

control group (n = 19). Glomerular filtration rate and RPF were measured on days 1, 4, and 7 after transplantation utilizing inulin and para-aminohippurate (PAH) clearances. In the control group, 11 of 19 patients (58%) developed posttransplant ARF, whereas only 3 of 16 patients treated (19%) developed delayed graft function. Of interest, pretreatment with the prostacyclin analogue iloprost induced similar protective effects. The investigators concluded that pretreatment of the donor kidney with diltiazem is protective against the development of ARF.

Finally, as detailed elsewhere in this book, Dawidson and Rooth have demonstrated that verapamil and isradipine are also protective in the setting of cadaveric renal transplantation (see Chapter 14).

Collectively, these observations indicate that calcium antagonists have a role in ameliorating the course of acute renal insufficiency following cadaveric transplantation. Whether pretreatment of the donor kidney suffices to exert a protective effect remains to be defined by future prospective studies.

Protection Against Cyclosporine Nephrotoxicity

Cyclosporine A (CyA) is now established as the immunosuppressant of choice in human organ transplantation because it improves graft survival and is not associated with myelosuppression. It is also used as a prophylaxis against graft-versus-host disease in bone marrow transplant recipients. In the future, it may also be used for the treatment of several autoimmune diseases, including diabetes mellitus. Nevertheless, abundant evidence has accumulated indicating that CyA therapy can lead to a wide spectrum of nephrotoxicity.[32] This nephrotoxicity remains the major hurdle in the wider application of this important drug.

Despite much study, the mechanism by which cyclosporine injures the kidney remains incompletely defined. The nephrotoxicity of CyA was initially considered to be primarily a tubulotoxic effect, but a number of recent studies suggest an important hemodynamic component. Thus, clinical studies suggest that nephrotoxicity is associated with renal vasoconstriction, with rapid improvement in renal function when CyA dosage is reduced.[32] In renal allograft recipients converted from CyA to azathioprine, RBF (assessed by the clearance of I[131] orthoiodohippurate) increased, suggesting that a CyA-associated rise in renal vascular resistance was reversible even after 12 months of therapy.[33] Finally, cardiac allograft recipients receiving CyA have a twofold elevation in renal vascular resistance when compared with those receiving azathioprine.[34]

Sabbatini et al.[35] investigated the effects of cyclosporine on glomerular dynamics. They compared cyclosporine with placebo in a randomized, double-blind study performed in Munich-Wistar rats by micropuncture techniques. The cyclosporine group received cyclosporine, 20mg/kg of body weight dissolved in saline, in 1 hour, whereas the control group received an equivalent amount of saline without drug. Total kidney GFR and single-nephron GFR were significantly decreased in the CyA group. Afferent arteriolar blood flow was greatly depressed in the CyA group. This fall was accounted for by a marked increase in both afferent and efferent arteriolar resistance. Single nephron filtration fraction was unchanged. These results show that acute CyA nephrotoxicity is associated with a functional modification of glomerular dynamics.

Recently, attention has focused on the possible role of calcium antagonists in protecting against cyclosporine nephrotoxicity. With the use of intravital fluorescent microscopy to monitor the linear velocity of blood cells as an estimate of subcapsular blood flow in mice, Dawidson and Rooth (see Chapter 14), have demonstrated that cyclosporine markedly decreases subcapsular blood flow. Pretreatment with verapamil (0.3–0.4 mg/kg) or dihydropyridine (isradipine) prevented cyclosporine-induced impairment of blood flow.[36] In contrast, pretreatment with the alpha-blocking agent phentolamine did not prevent these effects.

Dieperink et al.[37] have extended these findings. They investigated the protective effects of nifedipine as well as other vasoactive agents in ameliorating CyA nephrotoxicity in the rat. Based on their earlier observations, they proposed that net ultrafiltration pressure is reduced by the effects of CyA on afferent arteriolar resistance and/or on the filtration coefficient (K_f). They observed that concomitant treatment with nifedipine improved GFR as compared with placebo-treated controls. In contrast, other vasoactive agents, including captopril, phenoxybenzamine, and prostacyclin, failed to provide protection. Based on their findings, the authors postulated that the beneficial effects of nifedipine were most likely mediated by preglomerular vasodilation.

The mechanisms whereby CyA mediates renal vasoconstriction are incompletely defined. Recent attention has focused on the role of the renin-angiontensin system and eicosanoid synthesis. It has been suggested that enhanced TXA_2 production may mediate this vasoconstriction. As detailed elsewhere in this book (see Chapter 3), TXA_2 has powerful actions on renal vascular smooth muscle, promoting vasoconstriction, and affects mesangial function. Duarte[38] was the first to suggest a potential role for TXA_2 in CyA nephrotoxicity in promoting vasoconstriction and microthrombosis. Several studies have been published supporting this view.[39,40] As an example, Kawaguchi et al.[39] noted a gradual rise in urinary excretion of TXB_2 in Fischer rats given 15 mg/kg of CyA, reaching a plateau excretion rate in 1 week. In a second set of experiments this excretion pattern was seen at a lower dose of CyA (1.5 mg/kg).[41] A close correlation was observed between plasma CyA levels and urinary TXB_2 excretion which rose above baseline during allograft rejection.

In light of several studies from our laboratory demonstrating that calcium antagonists reverse thromboxane-mediated afferent arteriolar vasoconstriction,[42,43] our findings provide a scientific framework for anticipating a protective effect of calcium antagonists on CyA-induced renal vasoconstriction (see Chapter 3).

Sumpio et al.[44] have assessed the protective role of calcium antagonists in a model of cyclosporine nephrotoxicity. Utilizing the isolated perfused rat kidney model (see Chapter 3), they demonstrated that the addition of cyclosporine (500 ng/ml) to the perfusate induced a marked reduction of GFR, urine output, and renal perfusate flow. Pretreatment with verapamil (1 μg/ml added 10 minutes before CyA) markedly improved GFR and renal perfusate flow. Of interest, pretreatment with a combination of verapamil and adenosine triphosphate/magnesium chloride (ATP-$MgCl_2$) pretreatment returned GFR to control values and significantly improved renal perfusate flow and urinary output.

The above-mentioned observations suggest that calcium antagonists might be useful in ameliorating cyclosporine nephrotoxicity in humans. The reader is referred to Chapter 14 for more comprehensive discussion of this topic.

Cyclosporine-Calcium Antagonist Clinical Interactions. The administration of calcium antagonists in the setting of concomitant cyclosporine therapy has additional important clinical implications. During the course of a controlled trial of the effect of calcium antagonists in preventing renal insufficiency during cadaveric transplantation, Wagner and Neumayer observed an increase in cyclosporine blood trough levels.[45] More recently, Brockmoller et al.[46] observed that blood levels of cyclosporine were significantly higher in transplant recipients treated with diltiazem than in a corresponding control group. Although the mechanisms have not been established, the authors speculated that concomitant administration of diltiazem and cyclosporine might have inhibited the degradation of cyclosporine in the liver. Of interest, despite the higher blood levels of cyclosporine, the diltiazem-treated group did not manifest cyclosporine nephrotoxicity, and indeed, RBF tended to be higher in this group. In contrast, Poochet and Pirson[47] and Grino et al.[48] reported a reversible deterioration of renal function due to increased cyclosporine levels during concomitant treatment with diltiazem.

Although the mechanism(s) whereby cyclosporine nephrotoxicity did not occur despite the higher cyclosporine levels have not been elucidated, the clinical implications are apparent. It is clear that in the setting of concomitant administration of diltiazem and cyclosporine, appropriate levels of cyclosporine can be obtained with a reduction in the usual dosage. Additional studies are required to elucidate the mechanisms that mediate this interesting interaction.

Protection Against Cisplatin-Induced Nephrotoxicity

Cisplatin is an antineoplastic agent frequently used in the treatment of a variety of tumors, with specific efficacy in patients with disseminated testicular and ovarian cancer.[49,50] Although there are several well-established side effects of cisplatin, the dose-limiting adverse effect is nephrotoxicity. Specifically, cisplatin not infrequently produces acute renal insufficiency.[51] Offerman et al.[52] demonstrated that a regimen consisting of cisplatin in conjunction with vinblastine and bleomycin (the Einhorn regimen) acutely diminished effective renal plasma flow (ERPF) with consequent decrements in GFR (and with a resultant increase in filtration fraction). They further proposed that these hemodynamic effects were indirect and could be attributable to the actions of angiotensin II.[53,54]

Recently, Sleijfer et al.[55] assessed the efficacy of a calcium antagonist (verapamil 80 mg, t.i.d.) and cimetidine (200 mg, t.i.d.) in conjunction with administration of cisplatin. Nine patients with cancer were treated with cisplatin together with vera-pamil and cimetidine, whereas 9 additional patients were treated with cisplatin alone (controls). Glomerular filtration rate and the ERPF were determined simultaneously utilizing ^{125}I sodium-iothalamate and ^{131}I-hippurate, respectively, on the day prior to cisplatin therapy, on day 10, and finally on day 21. Patients treated with vera-pamil/cimetidine manifested a smaller decrease in ERPF when compared with the control group on day 21. Of importance, the decrease in GFR of patients receiving cisplatin was completely prevented by administration of verapamil-cimetidine.

Subsequent studies by Sleijfer et al. have not been consistent with regard to renal protection in this setting (personal communication).

Protection Against Amphotericin B Nephrotoxicity

Cheng et al.[56] reported increased afferent resistance and decreased glomerular cap-illary pressure as the primary causes of impaired glomerular function following the administration of amphotericin. Since calcium antagonists produce preferential affer-ent arteriolar vasodilation, it is of interest to consider whether they may have a protec-tive role in modulating amphotericin nephrotoxicity. Tolins and Raij[57] have recently reported that pretreatment of rats with verapamil completely inhibited amphotericin-induced renal vasoconstriction and blunted the fall in GFR during acute drug infusion. Based on these preliminary observations, additional studies are warranted to further delineate the potential protection afforded by calcium antagonists against ampho-tericin nephrotoxicity.

Role in Chronic Renal Failure

Effects in Experimental Chronic Renal Failure

Within the past several years, major investigative interest has focused on the deter-minants of the progression of chronic renal disease. Chronic renal insufficiency, once established, tends to progress to end-stage renal failure. The mechanisms underlying the progression of renal disease have remained incompletely defined. Numerous stud-ies have attempted to characterize the deleterious intrarenal processes that arise as a result of the initial insult and persist after its cause has disappeared. [58−62] In light of studies suggesting that calcium antagonists exert a protective effect in diverse models of experimental ARF, it is interesting to consider their effects in models of experi-mental chronic renal failure. Goligorsky et al.[58] have demonstrated that the chronic administration of verapamil protects against nephrocalcinosis, abnormal tubular cell Ca^{2+} kinetics, and mitochondrial and morphologic changes in tubular basement membrane in the rat 3 weeks after partial nephrectomy. At this early stage, however, changes in renal function had not yet occurred.

Subsequently, Harris et al.[59] investigated the effects of long-term administration of calcium antagonist on the progression of experimental chronic renal failure in the rat. The indices studied included the degree of renal functional deterioration, the extent of histologic damage and nephrocalcinosis, and cumulative survival. Fourteen days following staged subtotal nephrectomy, rats were paired according to renal functional impairment, mean arterial pressure (MAP), and body weight. Rats were pair-fed and received either verapamil (0.1 μg/g subcutaneously b.i.d., n = 10) or saline (n = 10) for up to 23 weeks. Members of each pair were sacrificed after the control rat developed severe uremia. At sacrifice, rats treated with verapamil had a lower serum creatinine (2.29 vs. 2.99 mg/dl; p < 0.05) and a higher creatinine clearance (318 vs. 164 μl/min; p < 0.05) than did controls. In a second experiment, survival was superior in rats treated with verapamil compared to controls from week 7 (p < 0.0025 by week 14). Serum creatinine was higher at week 10 in control rats (1.68 vs. 1.10 mg/dl; p < 0.05). Apparently, MAP was not different in the two groups. Histologic damage and nephrocalcinosis were worse, and renal calcium content was higher in controls. The authors concluded that verapamil protects against renal dysfunction, histologic damage, nephrocalcinosis, and myocardial calcification, and improves survival in the remnant model of chronic renal disease.[59]

Although Harris et al.[59] attributed the protective effects of verapamil to a reduction in the accumulation of calcium in renal tissue, their results did not exclude the possibility that verapamil also afforded protection by affecting glomerular dynamics in remnant nephrons, or that other mechanisms affected the course of progressive renal disease[60] (see Chapter 8 for a detailed discussion). Recently, these investigators extended their studies to the remnant kidney model by using micropuncture techniques to assess the effects of chronic administration of verapamil on glomerular capillary dynamics in rats with reduced renal mass.

Pelayo et al.[63] observed that verapamil did not reduce glomerular capillary hydrostatic pressure in the remnant kidneys of Munich-Wistar rats. Nevertheless, they observed an increase in the hydrostatic pressure within Bowman's space. Glomerular ultrafiltration coefficient (LpA) was significantly lower in nephrectomized rats given saline (Nx-SAL) (p < 0.005) than in either nephrectomized rats receiving verapamil (Nx-VER) or in control rats. Urinary protein excretion and the magnitude of glomerular sclerosis in Nx-SAL and Nx-VER rats were not different. These investigators concluded that chronic administration of verapamil normalizes LpA and reduces delta P by increasing P_{BS} in Nx rats, alterations that neutralize each other, leading to the constancy of single-nephron GFR. Unfortunately, some of the observations are not consistent with earlier findings from the same group (Harris et al.[59]) even though an identical experimental model was used, confounding interpretation of the data. For a detailed critique of this study, see Chapter 3.

Sterzel et al.[64] recently investigated the effects of calcium antagonists on the course of experimental chronic renal disease in rats. In one study, they examined the effects of nitrendipine in rats with two models of chronic progressive renal disease: (1) chronic antiglomerular basement membrane glomerulonephritis (AGBM-GN); and (2) nephrosclerosis in salt-sensitive Dahl rats. In the absence of calcium antagonists, the urinary excretion rate of albumin increased in AGBM-GN rats as well as in Dahl rats.[64] Similarly, clearance studies disclosed a decrease in GFR approximating 63% in the untreated animals. Nitrendipine afforded protection of renal perfusion and filtration rates, with GFR persisting at near-control levels.

Eliahou et al.[65] compared the effects of the calcium antagonist nisoldipine with those of a nonspecific vasodilator (dihydralazine) on the course of renal function in the rat remnant kidney model. They studied four groups of rats: (1) a control group that ingested normal rat chow containing 21% protein; (2) a group treated with nisoldipine, 0.3–0.6 mg/kg body weight daily in drinking water; (3) a group treated with dihydralazine 15–25 mg/kg body weight daily; and (4) a group that ingested an isocaloric low-protein (6%) diet with the same sodium content as the normal chow. They assessed the deterioration in renal function at 4-week intervals for up to 20 weeks. The severity of the chronic renal failure was assessed by light microscopy and cumulative survival. All three therapeutic regimens attenuated significantly the rise in blood pressure. Cumulative survival for the 19–20 week interval was 11% in untreated rats, 70% in nisoldipine-treated animals, and 50% in dihydralazine-treated animals. Light microscopy revealed severe sclerosis in the control group. The nisoldipine-treated rats and those on a low-protein diet had the least histologic damage, whereas the dihydralazine-treated rats had intermediate damage. The authors concluded that, although reduction of the elevated blood pressure by whatever means improves survival and delays the progression of renal failure, nisoldipine conferred a greater protective effect despite similar levels of blood pressure reduction.

The observations of Yoshioka et al.[66] are pertinent in this regard. In the course of defining the determinants of proteinuria in the Munich-Wistar rat remnant kidney model, these investigators determined glomerular microcirculatory parameters, including SNGFR, P_{GC}, Q_A, R_A, and R_E. Administration of verapamil (50 μg/kg/min) produced a marked reduction in P_{GC} from 70 $\pm$ 5 to 50 $\pm$ 3 mmHg. This reduction was attributable to a decrease in calculated afferent (R_A) and efferent (R_E) arteriolar resistances. Why the vasodilatory effects of verapamil were not preferentially afferent is not readily evident. Because all previous investigations from our laboratory have used either diltiazem or dihydropyridine calcium antagonists, it is conceivable that these ostensible differences might relate to the different agents employed. Alternatively, it is possible that the renal microcirculatory effects of calcium antagonists differs in normal or hydronephrotic kidneys as compared with remnant kidneys. Additional studies of the same calcium antagonists in different experimental models will be necessary to resolve this issue.

Recently, Jackson and Johnston[67] compared the effects of treatment with an angiotensin converting enzyme inhibitor (enalapril, 5 mg/kg/day) with those of a calcium antagonist (felodipine, 30 mg/kg/day) in Sprague Dawley rats in order to assess the effects on progression of chronic renal failure. Progressive renal failure was induced by surgical removal of the right kidney, and segmental infarction of $\frac{7}{8}$ths of the left kidney. Following subtotal nephrectomy, plasma creatinine rose from 65 $\pm$ 16 μmol/L to 173 $\pm$ 19 μmol/L (p $<$ 0.001) over a period of 6 weeks, systolic blood pressure (SBP) rose from 121 $\pm$ 2 mmHg to 176 $\pm$ 7mmHg (p $<$ 0.001) and urinary protein excretion rose from 0.6 $\pm$ 0.2 to 84 $\pm$ 22 mg/24 hours (p $<$ 0.001). Rats were treated with enalapril or felodipine from 1 week after subtotal nephrectomy, and their course was compared with that of untreated rats. Systemic blood pressure decreased to a similar degree for both types of treatment. Six weeks after surgery, plasma creatinine concentration was lower in the enalapril-treated group than in the felodipine-treated group. The latter group had plasma creatinine concentrations similar to those of the untreated rats. Urinary protein excretion was reduced to 15 $\pm$ 3 mg/24 hours (p $<$ 0.001) by treatment with enalapril, and increased to 221 $\pm$ 35 mg/24 hours after treatment with felodipine. The glomerulosclerosis index (obtained from a histologic score) was reduced by enalapril but not by felodipine. The authors interpreted these results as suggesting that angiotensin-converting enzyme inhibitors may have specific intrarenal effects that retard the deterioration of renal function that occurs when renal mass has been reduced.

In summary, several (but not all) recent studies have suggested that calcium antagonists are protective against the deterioration of renal function when renal mass has been reduced either by surgical ablation of renal tissue or by primary renal disease. The mechanisms that mediate these protective effects are multiple. Reduction of severely elevated blood pressure, by whatever means, seems to improve survival and delay the progression of renal failure. Independent of this effect, attention has focused on the ability of calcium antagonists to attenuate deposition of calcium within the renal parenchyma and on the prevention of nephrocalcinosis. Additional mechanisms include the hemodynamic effects of these agents and their ability to attenuate glomerular capillary wall tension (see Chapter 8).

Clinical Experience in Chronic Renal Failure

Despite these provocative observations, there have been relatively few attempts to extrapolate these findings to the clinical arena.

Recently, Eliahou et al.[68] assessed the effect of the calcium antagonist nisoldipine on the progression of chronic renal failure in a large group of patients. Patients with a steady decrease in renal function were randomized into two groups: (1) patients given nisoldipine (n = 17); and (2) patients given standard antihypertensive therapy without calcium antagonists, with a placebo tablet resembling the nisoldipine tablet (placebo group, n = 17). The standard antihypertensive therapy included one or a combination of the following: diuretics (chlorthalidone or furosemide) in 12, beta blockers (atenolol, oxprenolol, propranolol, or metoprolol) in 10, prazosin in 3, and hydralazine in 4 patients. The monthly progress of their renal failure was assessed by a plot of the reciprocal of serum creatinine versus time in months. Blood pressure control was similar in the nisoldipine and placebo (i.e., conventional therapy) groups. After a mean follow-up of 17.4 ± 8.2 (range, 6–30) months, the nisoldipine-treated group had a significant decrease in the slope of progression (i.e., slower rate of progression of renal failure), whereas the placebo-treated patients, after 16.9 ± 7.2 (range 6–30) months of follow-up, had no significant change in the slope. In light of the salutary effects of protein restriction, it is noteworthy that the protein intake of the two groups was similar: 0.85 ± 0.2 g/kg actual body weight in the nisoldipine-treated group and 0.88 ± 0.26 g/kg in the placebo group. The authors speculated that the beneficial effects of nisoldipine may have been mediated by the ability of this calcium antagonist to prevent calcium deposition within the kidney.[68]

Finally, because studies from several laboratories have demonstrated that calcium antagonists selectively attenuate afferent arteriolar vasoconstriction[69−72] the possibility that these agents might be detrimental merits comment. Preglomerular vascular tone is thought to act as a "buffer," protecting the glomerular structure from injury in the face of elevated systemic arterial pressure.[61] Theoretically, therefore, one might anticipate that by promoting afferent arteriolar vasodilation, calcium antagonists might exert deleterious effects by potentially exacerbating glomerular hypertension.[62,73] Such extrapolations should, however, be drawn with caution. Indeed, experimental studies have shown that in subtotal nephrectomized rats, verapamil ameliorated rather than exacerbated renal damage without concomitant changes of blood pressure.[59] Furthermore, recent studies of desoxycorticosterone-induced hypertension in rats demonstrated that nifedipine prevented glomerular injury despite persistent increases of glomerular capillary pressure.[74] Finally, Eliahou et al.[68] demonstrated that nisoldipine was more effective than other antihypertensive medications in preventing the progression of chronic renal failure in humans.

Although the mechanisms of action of calcium antagonists in these settings are not established, it is likely that the potential adverse effect of increased glomerular capillary pressure is countered by concomitant salutary effects of these agents. There are many possible mechanisms whereby calcium antagonists may be renal protective, independent of their effects on the afferent arteriole (Table 2). First, it is important to emphasize that although calcium antagonists preferentially reduce afferent arteriolar resistance, the resultant PGC depends on the net effect of their systemic and renal microvascular actions. Second, as noted elsewhere in this monograph (Chapter 8, p. 155), Dr. Dworkin has proposed that calcium antagonists might ameliorate

TABLE 2. Known and Postulated Mechanisms Mediating the Renal Protective Actions of Calcium Antagonists

1. Reduction in Systemic Blood Pressure

Although calcium antagonists preferentially reduce afferent arteriolar resistance, the resultant PGC depends on the net effect of their systemic and renal microvascular actions.

2. Reduction of Renal Hypertrophy

In renal failure, increased wall tension resulting from hypertrophy of capillaries and increased PGC may act in concert to promote progressive injury and glomerular sclerosis. Calcium antagonists might reduce injury by decreasing hypertrophy (see Chapter 8, p. 155).

3. Modulation of Mesangial Traffic of Macromolecules

Sub-pressor doses of ANG II increase the mesangial uptake of macromolecules. Lodging of various macromolecules in the mesangium may result in stimulation of local inflammatory phenomena, including mesangial cell proliferation. Calcium antagonists antagonize these effects of ANG II.[75]

4. Reduction in Metabolic Activity

Calcium antagonists might slow the progression of renal disease by diminishing the enhanced metabolic activity of remnant kidneys.[59,78]

5. Amelioration of Uremic Nephrocalcinosis

In experimental renal failure, an increase in cellular calcium influx has been suggested to promote nephrocalcinosis. Calcium antagonists might ameliorate uremic nephrocalcinosis, perhaps by correcting the abnormal calcium influx.[58]

6. May Block Pressure-induced Calcium Entry

Calcium antagonists interfere with pressure-induced afferent arteriolar vasoconstriction.[79] May imply that calcium antagonists block dihydropyridine-sensitive calcium channels that are activated by an increase in transmural pressure.

7. Decreased Free Radical Formation

Free radicals are potential mediators of renal injury. Since elevated intracellular calcium plays a permissive role in many biochemical events leading to free radical formation, calcium antagonists may attenuate this process.

glomerular injury by decreasing hypertrophy with a resultant decrease in capillary wall tension. A third possibility relates to the ability of calcium antagonists to modulate mesangial uptake of macromolecules.[75] Additionally, calcium antagonists may slow the progression of renal disease by diminishing the enhanced metabolic activity of remnant kidneys as well as diminishing renal calcium deposition.[58,76] The demonstration that calcium antagonists are protective against acute ischemia[77] and nephrotoxic injuries[8,13,22] suggests that the pathogenetic processes that might be involved in renal damage (e.g., calcium overloading) are inhibited by these agents.[58,78]

In addition, it is interesting to speculate that calcium antagonists may exert their salutary effects by directly inhibiting transcellular calcium movements.[79] We have recently demonstrated that in resistance vessels, increased transmural pressure activates a calcium entry process that is blocked by calcium antagonists.[79] Thus, it is possible that calcium antagonists may attenuate pressure-induced injury by directly inhibiting transcellular calcium movements.

Finally, it has been suggested that elevated free radical formation may mediate renal injury in diverse settings.[79a,79b] Calcium is essential for the activation of proteases and phospholipases involved in the biochemical events leading to free radical generation. Furthermore, elevated cytosolic calcium is implicated in the stimulation of free radical formation upon reperfusion of ischemic tissues.[79c] Thus, calcium antagonists may decrease free radical formation through their effects on cell calcium. Further investigations are required to ascertain the importance of this mechanism in the renal protective actions of calcium antagonists.

Additional studies will be required to determine the mechanisms whereby calcium antagonists do not accelerate renal damage despite putative persistent glomerular capillary hypertension. Nevertheless, it appears either that these agents reduce the deleterious effects of elevated glomerular capillary pressure, or that factors in addition to elevated hydrostatic pressure may mediate progressive glomerular injury.

Clearly, additional studies will be required to assess the attributes of calcium antagonists compared with nonspecific vasodilator therapy and angiotensin-converting enzyme (ACE) inhibitors, as in antihypertensive therapy in patients with chronic renal insufficiency.

Role in Diabetic Nephropathy

Although ACE inhibitors have been advocated as being advantageous in patients with diabetic nephropathy, the role of calcium antagonists in this setting remains to be established. Studies by Brenner and associates have provided a theoretical framework for assessing pharmacologic interventions as a means of retarding the progression of renal failure in chronic renal disease, including diabetic nephropathy.[80,81] These investigators have demonstrated that in experimental animals, a reduction in nephron number leads to an adaptive increase in flow and pressure in the remaining glomeruli. This intraglomerular hypertension in the surviving nephrons appears to be instrumental in further reducing the number of nephrons, with an inexorable progression of renal insufficiency. Brenner et al.[80,81] have demonstrated that, by virtue of their ability to obviate the effects of ANG II at the level of the efferent arteriole, ACE inhibitors can normalize the glomerular capillary hydraulic pressure without reducing the glomerular filtration rate in rats with diabetes mellitus. Consequently, maintenance of normal glomerular capillary hydraulic pressure markedly reduced the development of proteinuria and glomerular structural lesions. These results have been interpreted as indicating that therapy directed at reducing the glomerular capillary pressure effectively retards the progressive loss of renal function in rats with diabetes mellitus. Based on these and similar data, Brenner et al.[80,81,82] and Myers and Meyer[83] have proposed that ACE inhibition may be advantageous in patients with diabetic nephropathy or other forms of progressive renal disease, especially if given early in the course.

In contrast to recent observations with ACE inhibitors, there are relatively few studies on the effects of calcium antagonists in experimental diabetic nephropathy, and the results are inconsistent. Jackson et al.[84] compared the effects of enalapril with verapamil on renal function in the diabetic rat. Renal function was assessed in Sprague-Dawley rats subjected to unilateral nephrectomy and subsequent streptozotocin administration. Unilateral nephrectomy was performed prior to induction of diabetes, since this maneuver had previously been shown to accelerate the development of light and immunohistopathologic glomerular changes in the diabetic rat.[85] One month after induction of diabetes, rats were randomized to a no-treatment group, to an enalapril-treated group, or to a verapamil-treated group. Treatment of diabetic rats with either enalapril (5 mg/kg/day) or verapamil (5 mg/kg/day) reduced blood pressure to a similar degree in each of the two groups, and to levels similar to that of nondiabetic rats. Enalapril treatment reduced the elevated (as compared to nondiabetic rats) creatinine clearance in diabetic rats, but C_{Cr} was unaltered by verapamil administration. Furthermore, enalapril reduced the degree of proteinuria at 3 months, whereas protein excretion in verapamil-treated rats did not differ from the levels of untreated diabetic rats.

Subsequently, Whitty and Jackson[86] extended these observations. They compared the effects of enalapril and verapamil on renal function in the diabetic rat. Using an approach similar to their earlier study,[84] renal function was assessed sequentially in Sprague-Dawley rats subjected to unilateral nephrectomy and subsequent streptozotocin administration. One month after induction of diabetes, rats were allocated to three groups: group 1 receiving enalapril (5 mg/kg/day), group 2 receiving verapamil (5 mg/kg/day), and the third group of diabetic rats receiving neither antihypertensive agent. Following initiation of antihypertensive therapy, rats were studied sequentially over the subsequent 2-month period. Despite similar reductions in systolic blood pressure, the two drugs induced disparate effects on renal function. Enalapril reduced the degree of proteinuria at 3 months, whereas protein excretion in verapamil-treated rats was similar to that of untreated diabetic rats. Determinations of renal hemodynamics in a small number of animals from each of the three groups, 3 months after induction of diabetes, revealed disparate findings. GFR (estimated from ^{51}Cr EDTA clearance) was unchanged by either enalapril or verapamil administration. In contrast, effective renal plasma flow (estimated from ^{125}I-iodohippurate clearance) was elevated during enalapril, but not verapamil, treatment. Consequently, calculated filtration fraction decreased in response to enalapril (from 0.40 to 0.26%), whereas verapamil did not alter filtration fraction as compared to untreated diabetic rats. After perusal of the data of this paper,[86] it is uncertain whether it was an update of their other study.[84]

In contrast, Matsushima et al.[87] observed that captopril and nicardipine were equally effective in inhibiting the increment of renal growth in diabetic rats. Utilizing a similar experimental model of streptozotocin-treated rats previously subjected to unilateral nephrectomy, these investigators compared the ability of captopril or nicardipine to attenuate diabetes-induced renal hypertrophy. Untreated diabetic rats developed marked renal hypertrophy with kidney weight increasing from 0.53 ± 0.02 to 0.90 ± 0.03g/100g body weight, in accord with the observations of Sayer-Hansen.[88] Concomitantly, creatinine clearance increased from 13.3 ± 1.5 to 18.8 ± 1.0 dl/day. Administration of captopril (20 mg/day po) for one week markedly attenuated this hyperfiltration and prevented the increase in kidney weight. Although nicardipine did not attenuate the hyperfiltration, it also prevented the increment in renal mass (0.74 ± 0.03 to 0.77 ± 0.03g/100g body weight). Furthermore, both agents did not alter urinary excretion of protein or N-acetyl-β-D-glucosaminidase (NAG). Thus, in the present study, both an ACE inhibitor and a dihydropyridine antagonist were equally efficacious in preventing renal hypertrophy. The demonstration that nicardipine exerted a protective effect without attenuating the hyperfiltration raises questions regarding the precise role of altered renal hemodynamiocs in mediating diabetic glomerulopathy. Whether glomerular capillary hydraulic pressure, glomerular capillary flow, or vascular wall tension is the critical element in mediating the glomerular injury remains to be established. As noted in Chapter 8, Dworkin has proposed that vascular wall tension depends equally on the transcapillary pressure gradient and the vessel radius. Thus, a reduction in capillary radius may also attenuate injury independent of changes in transcapillary pressure. Finally, Myers has suggested that the beneficial effects of ACE inhibition in ameliorating proteinuria may relate to the effects of these agents in enhancing the size-selectivity barrier rather than altering glomerular hemodynamics (personal communication). Whether calcium antagonists may also enhance the size-selectivity barrier remains to be established.

Calcium Antagonist-induced Renal Dysfunction

Although the preceding pages have considered the beneficial effects of calcium antagonists on renal hemodynamics and renal function, a few isolated reports have raised the possibility that calcium antagonists might have adverse effects on renal function in rare, susceptible patients. That calcium antagonists may cause renal dysfunction in patients experiencing frank hypotensive episodes while receiving such drugs is not surprising. However, Diamond et al.[89] have reported that nifedipine caused acute, reversible deterioration in renal function in four patients with chronic renal insufficiency in the absence of hypotension. The investigators speculated that nifedipine blocked ANG II-mediated efferent tone. As detailed previously, because glomerular filtration rate is a function of the pressure created by afferent dilation and efferent constriction, either constriction of the afferent arteriole or dilation of the efferent arteriole or both could result in a loss of pressure and a decrease in GFR. These observations should be placed in perspective. First, it should be noted that calcium antagonist-induced renal dysfunction appears to be rare. Furthermore, there is recent evidence suggesting that calcium antagonists do not interfere with the action of ANG II on the efferent tone in vitro.[90,91]

Effect of Calcium Antagonists on Renal Function in Patients with Renovascular Hypertension

A clinical setting in which calcium antagonists might theoretically influence renal function is patients with renovascular hypertension. Within the past several years, increasing attention has been devoted to the potential adverse effects of ACE inhibitors on renal function in susceptible patients. Specifically, it has been shown that ACE inhibitors may induce acute reversible renal insufficiency in the presence of bilateral renal artery stenosis, or stenosis of a solitary kidney, or in diabetic patients with class III or IV congestive heart failure.[92] It is believed that ACE inhibitors mediate renal insufficiency by blocking ANG II-mediated efferent tone.

Recently, Ribstein et al.[93] have compared the effects of nifedipine with those of captopril in 6 patients with bilateral renal artery stenosis and 4 patients with renal artery stenosis in a solitary kidney. Patients were challenged with an acute administration of nifedipine, 20 mg, and subsequently with the acute administration of captopril, 50 mg. Nifedipine induced a decline in MAP of $19 \pm 4\%$. The GFR did not decrease but rather increased slightly ($+13 \pm 6\%$). In contrast, acute administration of captopril induced a fall in GFR ($-23 \pm 11\%$) despite a lesser decrement in MAP (Fig. 5). The authors proposed that the relatively beneficial effect of calcium antagonists on GFR was attributable to preferential afferent arteriolar vasodilation. Regardless of mechanism, these preliminary findings suggest that patients with renal artery stenosis are not at risk for developing acute renal insufficiency when treated with calcium antagonists.

Miyamori et al,[94] have recently extended these observations. They compared the effects of captopril vs. nifedipine on split renal function in six patients with renovascular hypertension secondary to unilateral renal artery stenosis. Patients received either captopril (37.5 to 75 mg per day in three divided doses) or nifedipine (20 to 40 mg twice daily). The order of administration of these drugs was randomized and both drugs were given for 4 weeks. Split renal function was determined during the pretreatment period and on the last day of each drug treatment. The GFR of individual kidneys was determined utilizing a single intravenous injection of ^{99m}Tc-diethylenetriamine pentaacetic acid (DTPA). Effective renal plasma flow (ERPF) of individual kidneys was determined utilizing 250 mCi of ^{131}I-iodohippurate sodium. The GFR in the stenotic kidney decreased markedly during captopril administration

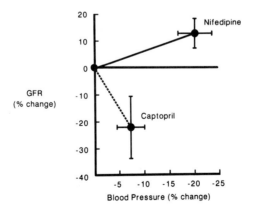

FIGURE 5. Comparison of the acute effects of captopril and nifedipine on GFR in patients with bilateral renal artery stenosis (n = 6) or with arterial stenosis of a solitary kidney (n = 4). In contrast to the reduction of GFR induced by captopril, GFR tended to increase with nifedipine. Redrawn from data of Ribstein et al.[82]

(from 24 ± 6 SE to 11 ± 2 ml/min, $p < 0.01$), whereas it decreased only slightly during nifedipine administration (to 19 ± 5 ml/min). The ERPF increased in the nonstenotic kidneys in response to both drugs. The authors concluded that by virtue of its preferential vasodilatory effect on the preglomerular arterioles, calcium antagonists such as nifedipine may be preferred as antihypertensive agents in patients with renovascular hypertension.

Summary

Several lines of evidence have demonstrated that calcium antagonists preferentially attenuate afferent arteriolar vasoconstriction. Thus, it is possible that calcium antagonists might have a role in ameliorating the course of patients who are at increased risk for developing acute renal failure. A number of recent studies indicate that calcium antagonists protect against the development of acute renal failure in the setting of cadaveric renal transplantation. Additional investigation is required to delineate other settings in which calcium antagonists may have a renal protective effect. Potential examples include administration of radiocontrast and aminoglycoside nephrotoxicity. Finally, the long-range consequences of the renal hemodynamic actions of calcium antagonists must be delineated. Specifically, the consequences of a presumed calcium antagonist-induced increase in glomerular capillary pressure in concert with the off-setting of effects of a reduction in elevated systemic blood pressure and attenuation of renal calcium deposition require elucidation in prospective, long term studies.

Acknowledgments. We thank Audrey Kincaid for her expert secretarial help and Dr. James R. Oster for his critical review.

References

1. Loutzenhiser R, Epstein M: Effects of calcium antagonists on renal hemodynamics. Am J Physiol 249:F619–F629, 1985.

2. Loutzenhiser R, Epstein M: Calcium antagonists and the kidney. Hosp Pract 22:63–76, 1987.

3. Loutzenhiser R, Epstein M: Modification of the renal hemodynamic response to vasoconstrictors by calcium antagonists. Am J Nephrol 7:7–16, 1987.

4. Koch-Weser J: Vasodilator drugs in the treatment of hypertension. Arch Intern Med 133:1017–1027, 1974.

5. Epstein M, Oster JR: Role of calcium channel blockers in the treatment of hypertension. In Epstein M (ed): Hypertension. Practical Management. Miami, Battersea Medical Publications, 1988.

6. Hof RP: Analysis of peripheral vascular actions of the new calcium antagonist isradipine. Am J Med 84(suppl 3B):18–25, 1988.

7. Epstein M, Loutzenhiser R: Interrelationship of calcium antagonists and atrial natriuretic peptides. J Hypertens (in press).

8. Lee SM, Hillman BJ, Clark RL, Michael UF: The effects of diltiazem and captopril on glycerol-induced acute renal failure in the rat: Functional, pathologic, and microangiographic studies. Invest Radiol 20:961–970, 1985.

9. Mergner WJ, Smith MW, Sahaphong S, et al: Studies on the pathogenesis of ischemic cell injury. VI. Accumulation of calcium by isolated mitochondria in ischemic rat kidney cortex. Virchows Arch (Cell Pathol) 26:1–16, 1977.

10. Eliahou H, Iaina A, Serban S: Verapamil's beneficial effect and cyclic nucleotides in gentamicin-induced acute renal failure in rats. Proceedings of the IXth International Congress of Nephrology, 1984, p 323A.

11. Lee SM, Pattison ME, Michael UF: Nitrendipine protects against aminoglycoside nephrotoxicity in the rat. J Cardiovasc Pharmacol 9(suppl 1):S65–S69, 1987.

12. Lee SM, Michael UF: The protective effect of nitrendipine on gentamicin acute renal failure in rats. Exp Mol Pathol 43:107–114, 1985.

13. Watson AJ, Gimenez LF, Klasssen DK, et al: Calcium channel blockade in experimental aminoglycoside nephrotoxicity. J Clin Pharmacol 27:625–627, 1987.

14. Malis CD, Cheung JY, Leaf A, et al: Effects of verapamil in models of ischemic acute renal failure in rats. Am J Physiol 243:S735–S742, 1983.

15. Goldfarb D, Iaina A, Serban I, et al: Beneficial effects of verapamil in ischemic acute renal failure in the rat. Proc Soc Exp Biol Med 172:389–392, 1983.

16. Hertle L, Garthoff B: Calcium channel blocker nisoldipine limits ischemic damage in rat kidney. J Urol 134:1251–1254, 1985.

17. Wagner K, Schultze G, Molzahn M, Neumayer HH: The influence of longterm infusion of the calcium antagonist diltiazem on postischemic acute renal failure in conscious dogs. Klin Wochenschr 64:135–40, 1986.

18. Talner LB, Davidson AJ: Renal hemodynamic effects of contrast media. Invest Radiol 2:310–317, 1968.

19. Bentley MD, VanHoutte V, Schryver SM, et al: Contraction of isolated canine renal arteries induced by the radiocontrast medium sodium diatrizoate and meglumine diatrizoate. J Lab Clin Med 109:595–600, 1987.

20. Byrd L, Sherman RL: Radiocontrast-induced acute renal failure: A clinical and pathophysiologic review. Medicine 58:270–279, 1979.

21. Caldicott WJH, Hollenberg NK, Abrams HS: Characteristics of response of renal vascular bed to contrast media. Invest Radiol 5:539–547, 1970.

22. Bakris GL, Burnett JC: A role for calcium in radiocontrast-induced reductions in renal hemodynamics. Kidney Int 27:465–468, 1985.

23. Oliet A, Lumbreras C, Mateo S, et al: Calcium channel blockade minimizes the renal toxicity of radiocontrast agents. J Cardiovasc Pharmacol 12(suppl 6):S164, 1988.

24. Cacoub P, Deray G, Baumelou A, Jacobs C: No evidence for protective effects of nifedipine against radiocontrast-induced acute renal failure (letter). Clin Nephrol 29:215–216, 1988.

25. Agatstein EH, Farrer JH, Kaplan LM, et al: The effect of verapamil in reducing the severity of acute tubular necrosis in canine renal autotransplants. Transplantation 44:355–357, 1987.

26. Golueke PJ, Kahng KU, Lipkowtiz GS: Effect of verapamil on posttransplant acute renal failure in the canine kidney. Transplantation 45:502–504, 1988.

27. Duggan KA, MacDonald GJ, Charlesworth JA, Pussell BA: Verapamil prevents posttransplant oliguric renal failure. Clin Nephrol 24:289–291, 1988.

28. Wagner K, Albrecht S, Neumayer H: Prevention of post-transplant acute tubular necrosis by the calcium antagonist diltiazem: a prospective randomized study. Am J Nephrol 7:287–291, 1987.

29. Neumayer HH, Wagner K: Prevention of delayed graft function in cadaver kidney transplants by diltiazem: Outcome of two prospective, randomized clinical trials. J Cardiovasc Pharmacol 10:S170–S177, 1987.

30. Frei U, Harms A, Schindler R, et al: Kidney graft pretreatment by diltiazem reduces the rate of acute renal failure after transplantation. Proc Intl Symp on Calcium Antagonists. Basel, Switzerland, February 11-12, 1988, abstract 35.

31. Neumayer HH, Schreiber M, Wagner K: Prevention of delayed graft function by diltiazem and iloprost. Transplant Proc 21:(February), 1989 (in press).

32. Myers BD: Cyclosporine nephrotoxicity. Kidney Int 30:964–974, 1986.

33. Curtis JJ, Luke RG, Dybovsky E, et al: Cyclosporine in therapeutic doses increases renal allograft vascular resistance. Lancet 2:477, 1986.

34. Myers BD, Ross J, Newton L, et al: Cyclosporine-associated chronic nephropathy. N Engl J Med 311:699–705, 1984.

35. Sabbatini M, Esposito C, Uccello F, et al: Effects of cyclosporine on glomerular dynamics: micropuncture study in the rat. International Congress on Cyclosporine, November 1987, abstract, p 117.

36. Rooth P, Dawidson I, Diller K, Taljedal I-B: Beneficial effects of calcium antagonist pretreatment and albumin infusion on cyclosporine A-induced impairment of kidney microcirculation in mice. Transplant Proc 19:3602–3605, 1987.

37. Dieperink H, Leyssac PP, Starklint H, et al: Antagonist capacities of nifedipine, captopril, phenoxybenzamine, prostacyclin and indomethacin on cyclosporine A induced impairment of rat renal function. Eur J Clin Invest 16:540–548, 1986.

38. Duarte R: Cyclosporine: Renal effects and prostacyclin. Ann Intern Med 102:420, 1985.

39. Kawaguchi A, Goldman MH, Shapiro R, et al: Increase in urinary thromboxane B in rats caused by cyclosporine. Transplantation 40:214–216, 1985.

40. Coffman TM, Carr DR, Yarger WE, Klotman PE: Evidence that renal prostaglandin and thromboxane production is stimulated in chronic cyclosporine nephrotoxicity. Transplantation 43:282–285, 1987.

41. Kawaguchi A, Goldman MH, Shapiro R, et al: Urinary thromboxane excretion in cardiac allograft rejection in immunosuppressed rats. Transplantation 43:346, 1987.

42. Loutzenhiser R, Epstein M, Horton C, Sonke P: Reversal of renal and smooth muscle actions of the thromboxane mimetic U-44069 by diltiazem. Am J Physiol 250:F619–F626, 1986.

43. Epstein M, Hayashi K, Loutzenhiser R: Direct evidence that thromboxane mimetic U-44069 preferentially constricts the afferent arteriole. Kidney Int 35:291, 1989.

44. Sumpio B, Baue AE, Chaudry IH: Treatment with verapamil and adenosine triphosphate-MgCl$_2$ reduces cyclosporine nephrotoxicity. Surgery 101:315–322, 1987.

45. Neumayer H, Wagner K: Prevention of delayed graft function in cadaver kidney transplants by diltiazem. Lancet 2:1355–1356, 1985.

46. Brockmoller J, Neumayer HH, Wagner K, et al: Interaction between cyclosporine and diltiazem. Submitted for publication.

47. Poochet JM, Pirson Y: Cyclosporine-diltiazem interaction. Lancet 1:979, 1986.

48. Grino JM, Sabate J, Castelao AM, Alsina J: Influence of diltiazem on cyclosporine clearance. Lancet 1:1387, 1986.

49. Rozencweig M, vonHoff DD, Slavik M, Muggia FM: Cis-diammine-dichloroplatinum (II): A new anticancer drug. Ann Intern Med 86:802–812, 1977.

50. Loehrer PJ, Einhorn LD: Drugs five years later: Cisplatin. Ann Intern Med 100:704–713, 1984.

51. Madias NE, Harrington JT: Platinum nephrotoxicity. Am J Med 65:307–314, 1978.

52. Offerman JJG, Meijer S, Sleijfer DTh, et al: Acute effects of cis-diamminedichloroplatinum (CDDP) on renal function. Cancer Chemother Pharmacol 12:36–38, 1984.

53. Offerman JJG, Mulder NJ, Sleijfer DTh, et al: Influence of captopril on cis-diamminedichloroplatinum-induced renal toxicity. Am J Nephrol 5:433–436, 1985.

54. Offerman JJG, Sleijfer DTh, Mulder NJ, et al: The effect of captopril on renal function in patients during the first cis-diammine-dichloroplatinum II infusion. Cancer Chemother Pharmacol 14:262–264, 1985.

55. Sleijfer DTh, Offerman JJG, Mulder NJ, et al: The protective potential of the combination of verapamil and cimetidine on cisplatin-induced nephrotoxicity in man. Cancer 60:2823–2828, 1987.

56. Cheng JT, Witty RT, Robinson RR, Yarger WE: Amphotericin B nephrotoxicity: Increased renal resistance and tubule permeability. Kidney Int 22:626–633, 1982.

57. Tolins JP, Raij L: Adverse effect of amphotericin B administration on renal hemodynamics in the rat. Neurohumoral mechanisms and influence of calcium channel blockade. J Pharmacol Exp Ther 245:594–599, 1988.

58. Goligorsky MS, Chaimovits C, Raporport J, et al: Calcium metabolism in uremic nephrocalcinosis: preventative effect of verapamil. Kidney Int 27:774–779, 1985.

59. Harris DCH, Hammond WS, Burke TJ, Schrier RW: Verapamil protects against progression of experimental chronic renal failure. Kidney Int 31:41–46, 1987.

60. Klahr S, Schreiner G, Ichikawa I: The progression of renal disease. N Engl J Med 318:1657–1666, 1988.

61. Brenner BM, Meyer TW, Hostetter TH: Dietary protein intake and the progressive nature of kidney disease: the role of hemodynamically mediated injury in the pathogenesis of progressive glomerular sclerosis in aging, renal ablation and intrinsic renal disease. N Engl J Med 307:652–659, 1982.

62. Hostetter TH, Olson JL, Rennke HG, et al: Hyperfiltration in remnant nephrons: a potentially adverse response to renal ablation. Am J Physiol 241:F85–F93, 1981.

63. Pelayo JC, Harris DCH, Shanley PF, et al: Glomerular hemodynamic adaptations in remnant nephrons: Effects of verapamil. Am J Physiol 254:F425-F431, 1988.

64. Sterzel RB: Effects of nitrendipine (N) on the course of chronic renal diseases in rats. J Cardiovasc Pharmacol 12(suppl 6):S163, 1988.

65. Eliahou HE, Cohen D, Herzog D, et al: The control of hypertension and its effect on renal function in rat remnant kidney. Nephrol Dial Transplant 3:38–44, 1988.

66. Yoshioka T, Shiraga H, Yoshida Y, et al: "Intact nephrons" as the primary origin of proteinuria in chronic renal disease. Study in the rat model of subtotal nephrectomy. J Clin Invest 82:1614–1623, 1988.

67. Jackson B, Johnson CI: The contribution of systemic hypertension to progression of chronic renal failure in the rat remnant kidney: effect of treatment with an angiotensin converting enzyme inhibitor or a calcium inhibitor. J Hypertens 6:495–501, 1988.

68. Eliahou HE, Cohen D, Hellberg B, et al: Effect of the calcium channel blocker nisoldipine on the progression of chronic renal failure in man. Am J Nephrol 8:285–290, 1988.

69. Loutzenhiser R, Epstein M, Horton C, Sonke P: Reversal by the calcium antagonist nisoldipine of norepinephrine-induced reduction of GFR: Evidence for preferential antagonism of preglomerular vasoconstriction. J Pharmacol Exp Ther 232:382–387, 1985.

70. Loutzenhiser R, Horton C, Epstein M: Effects of diltiazem and manganese on renal hemodynamics: Studies in the isolated perfused rat kidney. Nephron 39:382–388, 1985.

71. Steele T, Challoner-Hue L: Renal interactions between norepinephrine and calcium antagonists. Kidney Int 26:719–724, 1984.

72. Fleming JT, Parekh N, Steinhausen M: Calcium antagonists preferentially dilate preglomerular vessels of hydronephrotic kidney. Am J Physiol 253:F1157–F1163, 1987.

73. Dworkin LD, Feiner HD: Glomerular injury in uninephrectomized spontaneously hypertensive rats: A consequence of glomerular hypertension. J Clin Invest 77:797–809, 1986.

74. Dworkin LD, Benstein J, Feiner HD, Parker M: Nifedipine prevents glomerular injury without reducing glomerular pressure (P_{GC}) in rats with desoxycorticosterone-salt (DOC-salt) hypertension. Kidney Int 33:374 (abstract), 1988.

75. Raij L, Keane WF: Glomerular mesangium. Its function and relationship to angiotensin II. Am J Med 79: 24–30, 1985.

76. Schrier RW, Arnold PE, Van Putten VJ, Burke TJ: Cellular calcium in ischemic acute renal failure: Role of calcium entry blockers. Kidney Int 32:313–321, 1987.

77. Burke TJ, Arnold PE, Gordon JA, et al: Protective effect of intrarenal calcium membrane blockers before and after renal ischemia. J Clin Invest 74:1830–1841, 1984.

78. Farber JL: The role of calcium in cell death. Life Sci 29:1289–1295, 1981.

79. Hayashi K, Epstein M, Loutzenhiser R: Myogenic vasoconstriction of renal microvessels in normotensive and hypertensive rats: Studies in the isolated perfused hydronephrotic kidney. Circulation Res. 1989, in press.

79*a*. Paller MS: Free radical scavengers in mercuric chloride-induced renal failure in the rat. J Lab Clin Med 105:459-463, 1985.

79*b*. Canavese C, Stratta P. Vercellone L: The case for oxygen free radicals in the pathogenesis of ischemic acute renal failure. Nephron 49:9-15, 1988.

79*c*. McCord JM: Oxygen-derived free radicals in postischemic tissue injury. N Engl J Med 312:159-163, 1985.

80. Anderson S, Brenner BM: Pathogenesis of diabetic glomerulopathy: hemodynamic considerations. Diabetes Metab Rev 4:163–177, 1988.

81. Hostetter TH, Rennke HG, Brenner BM: The case for intrarenal hypertension in the initiation and progression of diabetic glomerulopathies. Am J Med 72:375–380, 1982.

82. Zatz R, Dunn BR, Meyer TW, et al: Prevention of diabetic glomerulopathy by pharmacological amelioration of glomerular capillary hypertension. J Clin Invest 77:1925–1930, 1986.

83. Myers BD, Meyer TW: Angiotensin-converting enzyme inhibitors in the prevention of experimental diabetic glomerulopathy. Am J Kidney Dis 13:20–24, 1989.

84. Jackson B, Cubela R, Debevi L, et al: Disparate effects of angiotensin converting enzyme inhibitor and calcium blocker treatment on the preservation of renal structure and function following subtotal nephrectomy or streptozotocin-induced diabetes in the rat. J Cardiovasc Pharmacol 10:S167–S169, 1987.

85. Steffes MW, Brown DM, Mauer SM: Diabetic glomerulopathy following unilateral nephrectomy in the rat. Diabetes 27:35–41, 1978.

86. Whitty MR, Jackson B: Diabetic nephropathy in the rat: differing renal effects of an angiotensin converting enzyme inhibitor and a calcium inhibitor. Diabetes Research 8:91–96, 1988.

87. Matsushima Y, Kojima S, Kawmura M, et al: Effects of captopril and nicardipine on renal hyperfiltration and hypertrophy in uninephrectomized diabetic rats. Nippon Jinzo Gakkai Shi (Japanese J Nephrol) 30: 279–283, 1988.

88. Sayer-Hansen K: Renal hypertrophy in experimental diabetes mellitus. Kidney Int 23:643–646, 1983.

89. Diamond JR, Cheung JY, Fang LST: Nifedipine-induced renal dysfunction: alterations in renal hemodynamics. Am J Med 77:905–909, 1984.

90. Loutzenhiser RD, Epstein M: Renal hemodynamic effects of calcium antagonists. J Cardiovasc Pharmacol 12(suppl 6):S48–S52, 1988.

91. Loutzenhiser R, Hayashi K, Epstein M: Calcium antagonists augment glomerular filtration rate (GFR) of angiotensin II-vasoconstricted isolated perfused rat kidneys (IPRK) by dilating afferent but not efferent arterioles. J Cardiovasc Pharmacol 12(suppl 6):S149, 1988.

92. Packer M, Lee WH, Medina N, et al: Influence of diabetes mellitus on changes in left ventricular performance and renal function produced by converting enzyme inhibition in patients with severe chronic heart failure. Am J Med 82:1119–1126, 1987.

93. Ribstein J, Mourad G, Mimran A: Contrasting acute effects of captopril and nifedipine on renal function in renovascular hypertension. Am J Hypertens 1:239–244, 1988.

94. Miyamori I, Yasuhara S, Matsubara T, et al: Comparative effects of captopril and nifedipine on split renal function in renovascular hypertension. Am J Hypertens 1:359–363, 1988.

Index

Entries in **boldface type** indicate complete chapters.

CAT = calcium antagonist